Novel Applications of Virtual Communities in Healthcare Settings

Christo El Morr
York University, Canada

A volume in the Advances in Healthcare Information Systems and Administration (AHISA) Book Series

IGI Global
DISSEMINATOR OF KNOWLEDGE

Published in the United States of America by
IGI Global
Medical Information Science Reference (an imprint of IGI Global)
701 E. Chocolate Avenue
Hershey PA, USA 17033
Tel: 717-533-8845
Fax: 717-533-8661
E-mail: cust@igi-global.com
Web site: http://www.igi-global.com

Library of Congress Cataloging-in-Publication Data

Names: El Morr, Christo, 1966- editor.
Title: Novel applications of virtual communities in healthcare settings / Christo El Morr, editor.
Description: Hershey PA : Medical Information Science Reference, [2018] | Includes bibliographical references.
Identifiers: LCCN 2017011898| ISBN 9781522529583 (hardcover) | ISBN 9781522529590 (ebook)
Subjects: | MESH: Mental Health | Internet | Community Networks | Self-Help Groups | Community Mental Health Services | Telemedicine--methods | United Kingdom | Review
Classification: LCC RA971.23 | NLM WM 26.5 | DDC 362.10285--dc23 LC record available at https://lccn.loc.gov/2017011898

This book is published in the IGI Global book series Advances in Healthcare Information Systems and Administration (AHISA) (ISSN: 2328-1243; eISSN: 2328-126X)

British Cataloguing in Publication Data
A Cataloguing in Publication record for this book is available from the British Library.

All work contributed to this book is new, previously-unpublished material.
The views expressed in this book are those of the authors, but not necessarily of the publisher.

For electronic access to this publication, please contact: eresources@igi-global.com.

Advances in Healthcare Information Systems and Administration (AHISA) Book Series

ISSN:2328-1243
EISSN:2328-126X

Editor-in-Chief: Anastasius Moumtzoglou, Hellenic Society for Quality & Safety in Healthcare and P. & A. Kyriakou Children's Hospital, Greece

MISSION

The **Advances in Healthcare Information Systems and Administration (AHISA) Book Series** aims to provide a channel for international researchers to progress the field of study on technology and its implications on healthcare and health information systems. With the growing focus on healthcare and the importance of enhancing this industry to tend to the expanding population, the book series seeks to accelerate the awareness of technological advancements of health information systems and expand awareness and implementation.

Driven by advancing technologies and their clinical applications, the emerging field of health information systems and informatics is still searching for coherent directing frameworks to advance health care and clinical practices and research. Conducting research in these areas is both promising and challenging due to a host of factors, including rapidly evolving technologies and their application complexity. At the same time, organizational issues, including technology adoption, diffusion and acceptance as well as cost benefits and cost effectiveness of advancing health information systems and informatics applications as innovative forms of investment in healthcare are gaining attention as well. **AHISA** addresses these concepts and critical issues.

COVERAGE

- Virtual health technologies
- Clinical Decision Support Design, Development and Implementation
- Decision Support Systems
- IT Applications in Physical Therapeutic Treatments
- IS in Healthcare
- IT security and privacy issues
- Management of Emerging Health Care Technologies
- IT Applications in Health Organizations and Practices
- Medical informatics
- Measurements and Impact of HISA on Public and Social Policy

IGI Global is currently accepting manuscripts for publication within this series. To submit a proposal for a volume in this series, please contact our Acquisition Editors at Acquisitions@igi-global.com or visit: http://www.igi-global.com/publish/.

The Advances in Healthcare Information Systems and Administration (AHISA) Book Series (ISSN 2328-1243) is published by IGI Global, 701 E. Chocolate Avenue, Hershey, PA 17033-1240, USA, www.igi-global.com. This series is composed of titles available for purchase individually; each title is edited to be contextually exclusive from any other title within the series. For pricing and ordering information please visit http://www.igi-global.com/book-series/advances-healthcare-information-systems-administration/37156. Postmaster: Send all address changes to above address.

Titles in this Series

For a list of additional titles in this series, please visit:
https://www.igi-global.com/book-series/advances-healthcare-information-systems-administration/37156

Patent Law and Intellectual Property in the Medical Field
Rashmi Aggarwal (Institute of Management Technology Ghaziabad, India) and Rajinder Kaur (Panjab Universit, India)
Medical Information Science Reference • ©2017 • 257pp • H/C (ISBN: 9781522524144) • US $200.00

Handbook of Research on Data Science for Effective Healthcare Practice and Administration
Elham Akhond Zadeh Noughabi (University of Calgary, Canada) Bijan Raahemi (University of Ottawa, Canada) Amir Albadvi (Tarbiat Modares University, Iran) and Behrouz H. Far (University of Calgary Canada)
Medical Information Science Reference • ©2017 • 400pp • H/C (ISBN: 9781522525158) • US $255.00

Design, Development, and Integration of Reliable Electronic Healthcare Platforms
Anastasius Moumtzoglou (P&A Kyriakou Children's Hospital, Greece)
Medical Information Science Reference • ©2017 • 357pp • H/C (ISBN: 9781522517245) • US $205.00

Cloud Computing Systems and Applications in Healthcare
Chintan M. Bhatt (Charotar University of Science & Technology, India) and S. K. Peddoju (Indian Institute of Technology Roorkee, India)
Medical Information Science Reference • ©2017 • 282pp • H/C (ISBN: 9781522510024) • US $205.00

Handbook of Research on Healthcare Administration and Management
Nilmini Wickramasinghe (Epworth HealthCare, Australia & Deakin University, Australia)
Medical Information Science Reference • ©2017 • 825pp • H/C (ISBN: 9781522509202) • US $345.00

Reshaping Medical Practice and Care with Health Information Systems
Ashish Dwivedi (University of Hull, UK)
Medical Information Science Reference • ©2016 • 399pp • H/C (ISBN: 9781466698703) • US $150.00

For an enitre list of titles in this series, please visit:
https://www.igi-global.com/book-series/advances-healthcare-information-systems-administration/37156

IGI Global
DISSEMINATOR OF KNOWLEDGE

701 East Chocolate Avenue, Hershey, PA 17033, USA
Tel: 717-533-8845 x100 • Fax: 717-533-8661
E-Mail: cust@igi-global.com • www.igi-global.com

Editorial Advisory Board

Table of Contents

Detailed Table of Contents

Section 2
Innovation and Future Directions

This chapter will provide an overview of InfoCentral, a virtual community platform launched for advancing digital health information in Canada. Developed and hosted by Canada Health Infoway, InfoCentral has become a hub and resource for stakeholders in digital health to discuss, consider, and evaluate common challenges among digital health system compatibility across the country (i.e., interoperability). A synopsis of the role Infoway contributes toward advancing Canadian digital health, the background and considerations for InfoCentral, along with a series of three flourishing virtual community case studies will be examined. Critical success factors and lessons learned in establishing, supporting and growing productive virtual communities conclude this chapter.

Virtual social connection has become a way of life for many people. The continued implementation of new technologies in social interaction presents an ever-escalating need for researchers and practitioners to understand the implications of mediated interaction and virtual communities on human health and wellbeing. Accordingly, this chapter presents research on the salience of communication and social bonds in relation to human health and wellbeing, explores ways in which individual as well as relational health and wellbeing are affected by the use of social network sites, and argues a case for research on the health-related functions of expressive narratives in virtual settings such as online social networks. Considerations and future directions for research of these issues conclude this chapter.

Preface

Healthcare systems around the world are facing many challenges at different levels. In developed countries, growing elderly population represents a particular challenge; for example in Canada, 14% of the population was 65 or older in 2010 (Canadian Medical Association [CMA], 2013); however, in July 2015 that number was found to be 16.1% (Canadian Medical Association [CMA], 2016; Statistics Canada, 2015). In 2015, for the first time in its history, Canada had more people having an age of 65 and above, than people having an age under 15 (Institute of Aging-University of British Columbia, 2007). The situation is not different in other countries, in Germany, people aged 65 and over represent 21% of the population, in France it is estimated to 19% in France (CMA, 2016). In France, that number is expected to reach 25% in 2030 and nearly 30% in 2050 (Béland & Viriot Durandal, 2013). In the United States more than 20% of residents was estimated to be 65 years or older by 2013, compared with 13 percent in 2010 and 9.8 percent in 1970 (Ortman, Velkoff, & Hogan, 2014). While elderly population health cost impact on increasing health care costs in Canada is modest (nearly 0.9% per year), the health cost per person increases with age (CMA, 2016). Most babies born since 2000 in many countries including Canada, USA, France, Germany, Italy, UK, and Japan are expected to live till a 100 (Christensen, Doblhammer, Rau, & Vaupel, 2009). The case in other countries such as India the number of elderly has tripled over the last 50 years (Dey, Nambiar, & Lakshmi, 2012). The situation is similar in China, by 2050, it is expected that one in every four chines will be elderly (Feng, Liu, Guan, & Mor, 2012). In fact, Asia leads world regions in speed of aging and size of older population (He, Goodkind, & Kowal, 2016). Ageing of the world's population is increasing the number of people living with sequelae of diseases and injuries ("Global, regional, and national incidence, prevalence, and years lived with disability for 310 diseases and injuries, 1990-2015: a systematic analysis for the Global Burden of Disease Study 2015," 2016). It is usually expected that people will suffer from many chronic diseases with age with considerable health cost (Chi, Lee, & Wu, 2011).

However, not only elderly face chronic diseases challenges; global chronic diseases related deaths was estimated to be 35 million out of 58 million annual global deaths in 2005, and the number of people that die annually from cardiovascular diseases is almost twice the number of people who die from all infectious diseases combined (e.g., AIDS, tuberculosis, malaria) (World Health Organization, 2005). Chronic diseases exert a significant impact on health care cost in developing countries (Yach, Leeder, Bell, & Kistnasamy, 2005).

In 2008, about 1 in 5 American had a doctor-diagnosed arthritis, and 1 in 250 children had some form of arthritis or related condition (Marks, 2008). Besides, diabetes and asthma are dominant chronic diseases; 32.8% of males and 38.5% of females in the United States born in 2000 will develop diabetes in their lifetime (Narayan, Boyle, Thompson, Sorensen, & Williamson, 2003). On the other hand, in 2015, 13.9 percent of high school students in the United States were obese, and 16.0 percent were overweight (Kann et al., 2016); while more than one-third (36.5%) of U.S. adults have obesity (Ogden, Carroll, & Fryar, 2015).

This situation has led developed countries to start planning for changes in the healthcare system to face the challenge of caring for elderly at a reasonable cost (CMA, 2016). Innovation, was expected as a main tool to address these set of challenges. There is a clear drive in many countries to booster Industry-Researchers collaboration to innovate and transform innovation into a solution that delivers value for the population. For instance, the Government of Canada launched many initiatives to support the development of new health technologies to address the rising rates of chronic disease (Government of Canada, 2016); the United states have other internal initiatives and external cooperation in eHealth with the European Union (EU) (Health IT, 2016).

Virtual Communities (VCs) constitute a unique opportunity to address these challenges (El Morr, 2010a, 2010b). Virtual communities have been on the rise since the beginning of the web age (World Wide Web Consortium, 2000); known also as online communities, they attracted the attention of researchers from different disciplines: psychology (Blanchard, 2007, 2008; Maloney-Krichmar & Preece, 2005; Nonnecke, Andrews, & Preece, 2006; Nonnecke & Preece, 2000), sociology (Weissman, 2000), computer science (Maret, Vercouter, & El Morr, 2011; Subercaze et al., 2009), health informatics (Demiris, 2005; El Morr & Maret, 2012), culture and lifestyle (Brown et al., 2005; Carter & Fisher, 2004; Rheingold, 2000), and business (Schubert & Hampe, 2005; Singh & Waddell, 2004). Virtual Communities can be defined as a group of people (community members) whose social interaction is supported by a computer system. The community members perform special roles within the community; they meet and possibly collaborate to achieve a purpose (the community raison d'être) and act within a set of policies that govern their interaction (Preece, 2000).

In healthcare, health virtual communities research provided sufficient evidence that VC settings allow mutual support, enhance the quality of life and reduce health service utilization (Gustafson et al., 2001; Temesgen, Knappe-Langworthy, St Marie, Smith, & Dierkhising, 2006). these findings provided coupled with the advance of the web and internet technologies, the rise of computer processing power and storage space, and the reduction in computer and communication cost, provided a mature environment for research and development in Health Virtual Communities (Health VCs). The Health VC promises were galvanized by the advances in mobile technologies and ultimately smart phones and tablets (El Morr & Maret, 2012), as implementing targeted health intervention was then possible anywhere using location based services (El Morr & Kawash, 2007). New trends are pushing advancement in the same direction; in 2016, the Canadian Radio-television and Telecommunications Commission (CRTC) declared broadband high speed internet a "basic service" like landline telephone, water or electricity. The declaration aims to ensure that Internet Service Providers (ISPs) extend their internet offer across the country, including rural areas, offering download speeds of at least 50 Mbps, and upload speed of 10 Mbps (Pewdwell, 2016).

This book will overview the latest of findings in Health Virtual Communities through the exploration of major experiences in Healthcare settings. Healthcare settings should be understood in the wide sense, encompassing mobile health and population health.

ORGANIZATION OF THE BOOK

The book is divided into two sections; in Section 1 (5 chapters), we will investigate opportunities and experiences and evidence regarding Health VCs effectiveness to Health VCs. In Section 2 (3 chapters), we will explore innovative approaches to Health VCs and innovative perspectives. A brief description of each of the chapters follows:

Section 1: Opportunities and Experiences

Chapter 1: Online Mindfulness Interventions – A Systematic Review (Farah Ahmad, Jamie Wang, Christo El Morr)

Chapter 1 is a systematic review of literature on online mindfulness interventions for mental health. It examines the nature of online mindfulness interventions, design features, and effectiveness in improving symptoms of depression, anxiety and stress. The review uncovers the current advances in online delivery of mindfulness; evidence related to effectiveness of online mindfulness interventions on stress, depression and anxiety is explained in depth. The chapter critically assess the evidence and show the missing point as well as propose an extension of online interventions beyond the individual level to include the community dimension provided by a virtual community dimension and a focus on the social determinants of health.

Chapter 2: Socialisation or Social Isolation? Mental Health Community Support in the Digital Age (Kim Heyes)

Chapter 2 examines the experience of online community mental health support groups and suggests that there is a need for face-to-face intervention despite professional and peer to peer online support services positive impact on its participants. The author recommends that through the identification of positive experiences of online mental health support forums, suitable resources can be developed cheaply and effectively in order to reduce the effects of mental illness, and support those who are unable to find support.

Chapter 3: Cancer Virtual Communities in the Era of Personalized Medicine – Perspectives on Scope, Use. and Impact (Jacqueline [Jackie] Lorene Bender)

Chapter 3 takes a theoretical as well as practical approach to Cancer Virtual Communities. The author presents evidence on the scope and characteristics of virtual communities for cancer patients; prevalence and predictors of use, and reasons for non-use; the nature and function of supportive exchanges in cancer virtual communities, including their limitations; and the potential effects, both positive and negative, of participating in cancer virtual communities on health outcomes. Grounded in social support, technology adoption and health behavior theory, this chapter will offer a multi-theory framework for better understanding how cancer virtual communities work and under what conditions.

Chapter 4: Manage My Pain – A Patient-Driven Mobile Platform to Prevent and Manage Chronic Postsurgical Pain (Aliza Weinrib, Muhammad Abid Azam, Vered Valeria Latman, Tahir Janmohamed, Joel Katz, Hance Clarke)

Chapter 4 reviews the burden of chronic pain on patients and the health system and describes a digital pain management platform "Manage My Pain". The authors describe the integration of the platform into the Transitional Pain Service at Toronto General Hospital as a collaborative patient-provider virtual community with the aim of managing complex pain after surgery so as to prevent the transition from acute post-surgical pain to chronic post-surgical pain. User engagement, motivation, and satisfaction are discussed as well as the challenges in implementation.

Chapter 5: Effective Use of Virtual Communities for Health-Purposes in the Elderly – Health Virtual Communities for the Elderly (Elisabeth Beaunoyer, Matthieu J. Guitton)

This chapter proposes a reflection on the current situation and future directions of aged population-targeted virtual communities. It analyzes some of the different factors which can impact the effectiveness of senior-targeted health-related virtual communities (synchronicity, anonymity, supervision, the interface) and suggests elements to rationalize the development of health-oriented virtual community tools and approaches aimed at the elderly. It finally analyzes some the advantages and disadvantages of different types of virtual communities to uncover the types of virtual communities that are suitable or optimal to reach older populations.

Section 2: Innovation and Future Directions

Chapter 6: Virtual Community Engagement to Advance Interoperability in Digital Health (Gina DeBenedetti, Kelly Kuru, Peter Picton, Linda Monico, Tasha Shaw-Verbic)

The chapter will provide an overview of InfoCentral, a Virtual Community platform Canada Health Infoway and launched for the purpose of advancing digital health information in Canada. It describes the rationale the rational of the platform and the functionalities of InfoCentral and how it became a hub and resource for stakeholders' engagement in digital health, to discuss, consider, and evaluate common challenges among digital health system compatibility across the country. Critical success factors and lessons learned in establishing, supporting and growing productive virtual communities conclude the chapter.

Chapter 7: Exploring Healthy Connection – Communication, Social Networks, and Wellbeing (Jessica L. Moore)

Chapter 7 addresses the issue of the link between communication, social networks, and wellbeing. It presents the latest research findings on the salience of communication and social bonds in relation to human health and wellbeing, and explores ways in which individual as well as relational health and wellbeing are affected by the use of social network sites. The author develops a case for research on the health-related functions of expressive narratives in virtual settings such as online social networks. The chapter concludes with considerations and future directions for research of these issues.

Chapter 8: Enablers and Facilitators for Sustainable Implementation of E-Services in Two-Sided Markets and Ecosystems (Vivian Vimarlund)

Chapter 8 analyses and compares implementation approaches in eHealth and Virtual Communities. It develops a vision for two-sided (i.e. producer-consumer) eHealth markets.

The author reviews the implementation assumptions and experiences in one-sided markets and suggest that the implementation of intermediaries that support two-sided e-health markets, specifically virtual communities' markets, implies the commitment of institutions and management engagement programs, as well as the existence of clear guidelines, at the administrative, managerial, and financial level, for both sides of the market and for the virtual community they interact with. The lack of explicit models or methodological frameworks is identified and suggest an invitation to develop a new framework for the sustainable implementation of intermediary platforms in two-sided e-health and Virtual Communities.

Christo El Morr
York University, Canada

REFERENCES

Béland, D., & Viriot Durandal, J.-P. (2013). Aging in France: Population Trends, Policy Issues, and Research Institutions. *The Gerontologist*, *53*(2), 191–197. doi:10.1093/geront/gns149 PMID:23220395

Blanchard, A. L. (2007). Developing a sense of virtual community measure. *Cyberpsychology & Behavior*, *10*(6), 827–830. doi:10.1089/cpb.2007.9946 PMID:18085972

Blanchard, A. L. (2008). Testing a model of sense of virtual community. *Computers in Human Behavior*, *24*(5), 2107–2123. doi:10.1016/j.chb.2007.10.002

Brown, B., Chalmers, M., Bell, M., Hall, M., MacColl, I., & Rudman, P. (2005). Sharing the square: Collaborative Leisure in the City Streets. In H. Gellersen, K. Schmidt, M. Beaudouin-Lafon, & W. Mackay (Eds.), *ECSCW 2005: Proceedings of the Ninth European Conference on Computer-Supported Cooperative Work* (pp. 427-447). Dordrecht, The Netherlands: Springer Netherlands. doi:10.1007/1-4020-4023-7_22

Canadian Medical Association (CMA). (2013). *Health and Health Care for an Aging Population: Policy Summary of The Canadian Medical Association*. Retrieved from https://www.cma.ca/Assets/assets-library/document/en/advocacy/policy-research/CMA_Policy_Health_and_Health_Care_for_an_Aging-Population_PD14-03-e.pdf

Canadian Medical Association (CMA). (2016). *The State of Seniors Health Care in Canada*. Retrieved from https://www.cma.ca/En/Lists/Medias/the-state-of-seniors-health-care-in-canada-september-2016.pdf

Carter, W., & Fisher, S. S. (2004). Mobile sound communities. *Proceedings of the 2004 ACM SIGCHI International Conference on Advances in Computer Entertainment Technology*. Retrieved from http://dl.acm.org/citation.cfm?doid=1067343.1067399

Chi, M. J., Lee, C. Y., & Wu, S. C. (2011). The prevalence of chronic conditions and medical expenditures of the elderly by chronic condition indicator (CCI). *Archives of Gerontology and Geriatrics*, *52*(3), 284–289. doi:10.1016/j.archger.2010.04.017 PMID:20452688

Christensen, K., Doblhammer, G., Rau, R., & Vaupel, J. W. (2009). Ageing populations: The challenges ahead. *Lancet*, *374*(9696), 1196–1208. doi:10.1016/S0140-6736(09)61460-4 PMID:19801098

Demiris, G. (2005). Virtual Communities in Health Care. *Intelligent Paradigms for Healthcare Enterprises*, *184*, 121-137.

Dey, S., Nambiar, D., & Lakshmi, J. K. (2012). Health of the Elderly in India: Challenges of Access and Affordability. In National Research Council (US) Panel on Policy Research and Data Needs to Meet the Challenge of Aging in Asia. Aging in Asia: Findings From New and Emerging Data Initiatives (Vol. 15). Washington, DC: National Academies Press (US).

El Morr, C. (2010a). Health Care Virtual Communities: Challenges and Opportunities. In C.-C. Maria Manuela, J. T. Antonio, & S. Ricardo (Eds.), *Handbook of Research on Developments in E-Health and Telemedicine: Technological and Social Perspectives* (pp. 278–298). Hershey, PA: IGI Global. doi:10.4018/978-1-61520-670-4.ch013

El Morr, C. (2010b). Mobile Virtual Communities in Healthcare: The Chronic Disease Management Case. In S. Mohammed & J. Fiadi (Eds.), *Ubiquitous Health and Medical Informatics: The Ubiquity 2.0 Trend and Beyond* (pp. 258–258). IGI Global. doi:10.4018/978-1-61520-777-0.ch013

El Morr, C., & Kawash, J. (2007). Mobile virtual communities research: A synthesis of current trends and a look at future perspectives. *International Journal of Web Based Communities*, *3*(4), 386. doi:10.1504/IJWBC.2007.015865

El Morr, C., & Maret, P. (Eds.). (2012). *Virtual Community Building and the Information Society: Current and Future Directions*. Hershey, PA: Information Science Reference. doi:10.4018/978-1-60960-869-9

Feng, Z., Liu, C., Guan, X., & Mor, V. (2012). Chinas Rapidly Aging Population Creates Policy Challenges In Shaping A Viable Long-Term Care System. *Health Affairs (Project Hope)*, *31*(12), 2764–2773. doi:10.1377/hlthaff.2012.0535 PMID:23213161

Global, regional, and national incidence, prevalence, and years lived with disability for 310 diseases and injuries, 1990-2015: A systematic analysis for the Global Burden of Disease Study 2015. (2016). *Lancet*, *388*(10053), 1545-1602. doi:10.1016/s0140-6736(16)31678-6

Government of Canada. (2016). *FedDev Ontario Invests in Health Innovations to Support Canadians Living with Chronic Disease*. Retrieved from http://news.gc.ca/web/article-en.do?nid=1102399

Gustafson, D. H., Hawkins, R. P., Boberg, E. W., McTavish, F., Owens, B., Wise, M., . . . Pingree, S. (2001). *CHESS: 10 years of research and development in consumer health informatics for broad populations, including the underserved*. Paper presented at the 10th World Congress on Medical Informatics (Medinfo 2001).

He, W., Goodkind, D., & Kowal, P. (2016). An Aging World: 2015: International Population Report. Retrieved from http://cdn.cnsnews.com/attachments/census_bureau-an_aging_world-2015.pdf

Health IT. (2016). *Public Stakeholder consultation on EU-US cooperation in eHealth/Health IT*. Author.

Institute of Aging-University of British Columbia. (2007). *The Future is AGING: Institute of Aging Strategic Plan 2007 – 2012*. Retrieved from http://www.cihr-irsc.gc.ca/e/documents/ia_strategic_plan_07-12_e.pdf

Kann, L., McManu, T., Harris, W. A., Shanklin, S. L., Flin, K. H., Hawkins, J., . . . Zaza, S. (2016). Youth Risk Behavior Surveillance - United States, 2015. *Surveillance Summaries.* Retrieved from http://stateofobesity.org/high-school-obesity/

Maloney-Krichmar, D., & Preece, J. (2005). A multilevel analysis of sociability, usability, and community dynamics in an online health community. *ACM Transactions on Computer-Human Interaction*, *12*(2), 201–232. doi:10.1145/1067860.1067864

Maret, P., Vercouter, L., & El Morr, C. (2011). Special Issue on Web Intelligence and Virtual Communities. *International Journal of Networking and Virtual Organisations*, *9*(3), 211–213.

Marks, J. S. (2008). *Targeting Arthritis: Improving Quality of Life for More Than 46 Million Americans*. Academic Press.

Narayan, K. M., Boyle, J. P., Thompson, T. J., Sorensen, S. W., & Williamson, D. F. (2003). Lifetime risk for diabetes mellitus in the United States. *Journal of the American Medical Association*, *290*(14), 1884–1890. doi:10.1001/jama.290.14.1884

Nonnecke, B., Andrews, D., & Preece, J. (2006). Non-public and public online community participation: Needs, attitudes and behavior. *Electronic Commerce Research*, *6*(1), 7–20. doi:10.1007/s10660-006-5985-x

Nonnecke, B., & Preece, J. (2000). Lurker demographics: counting the silent. *Proceedings of the SIGCHI conference on Human Factors in Computing Systems.* Retrieved from http://dl.acm.org/citation.cfm?doid=332040.332409

Ogden, C. L., Carroll, M. D., & Fryar, C. D. (2015). *Prevalence of Obesity Among Adults and Youth: United States, 2011–2014*. Retrieved from https://www.cdc.gov/nchs/data/databriefs/db219.pdf

Ortman, J. M., Velkoff, V. A., & Hogan, H. (2014). An Aging Nation: The Older Population in the United States. Retrieved from https://www.census.gov/prod/2014pubs/p25-1140.pdf

Pewdwell, T. (2016). CRTC declares broadband internet a basic service. *The Toronto Star*.

Preece, J. (2000). *Online Communities: Designing Usability supporting Sociability*. John Wiley & Sons Ltd.

Rheingold, H. (2000). *The Virtual Community: Homesteading on the Electronic Frontier*. Cambridge, MA: MIT Press.

Schubert, P., & Hampe, J. F. (2005). *Business Models for Mobile Communities.* Paper presented at the 38th Annual Hawaii International Conference on System Sciences(HICSS '05). doi:10.1109/HICSS.2005.132

Singh, M., & Waddell, D. (2004). *E-business Innovation and Change Management.* IRM Press. doi:10.4018/978-1-59140-138-4

Statistics Canada. (2015). *Canada's population estimates: Age and sex, July 1, 2015.* Retrieved from http://www.statcan.gc.ca/daily-quotidien/150929/dq150929b-eng.htm

Subercaze, J., El Morr, C., Maret, P., Joly, A., Koivisto, M., Antoniadis, P., & Ihara, M. (2009). Towards Successful Virtual Communities. In J. Filipe & J. Cordeiro (Eds.), *Enterprise Information Systems: 11th International Conference, ICEIS 2009* (*Vol. 24*, pp. 677-688). Milan, Italy: Springer Berlin Heidelberg.

Temesgen, Z., Knappe-Langworthy, J. E., St Marie, M. M., Smith, B. A., & Dierkhising, R. A. (2006). Comprehensive Health Enhancement Support System (CHESS) for people with HIV infection. *AIDS and Behavior, 10*(1), 35–40. doi:10.1007/s10461-005-9026-x PMID:16400508

Weissman, D. (2000). *A social ontology.* Yale University Press.

World Health Organization. (2005). *Preventing Chronic Disease: A Vital Investment.* Geneva, Switzerland: WHO.

World Wide Web Consortium. (2000). *A Little History of the World Wide Web.* Retrieved from https://www.w3.org/History.html

Yach, D., Leeder, S. R., Bell, J., & Kistnasamy, B. (2005). Global Chronic Diseases. *Science, 307*(5708), 317. doi:10.1126/science.307.5708.317 PMID:15661976

Acknowledgment

I would like to express my gratitude to my wife Valentina for the many profound discussions we have in the domain of social justice, healthcare and patient care; they are always a source of inspiration in my academic and personal life. I am grateful to our son Alexi whose penetrating remarks, insights and analyses in the many subject we discuss, and high sense of social justice, keep me alert and sensitive. The patience and support of both were crucial for bringing this book to life.

I would like to thank my School of Health Policy and Management colleagues for their support and the wonderful collegial and critical environment they keep in the workplace. Their presence, intellectual achievements and commitment to social justice is inspirational.

I would like to thank Ms. Maria Rohde, Assistant Development Editor from IGI Global, for guiding me in the process of editing this book.

Section 1

Opportunities and Experiences

Chapter 1
Online Mindfulness Interventions:
A Systematic Review

Farah Ahmad
York University, Canada

Jamie Jianmin Wang
York University, Canada

Christo El Morr
York University, Canada

ABSTRACT

The current chapter systematically reviewed literature on online mindfulness interventions. Electronic databases were searched from 2005 to July 2016. The aim was to examine the nature of online mindfulness interventions, design features, and their effectiveness in improving symptoms of depression, anxiety, and stress. The review of selected studies shows that online delivery of mindfulness psycho-education and practice is an area in its infancy. There is evidence that online mindfulness interventions can have a positive impact on mental health in terms of stress, depression, and anxiety; however, large sample studies are needed in order to have conclusive results. Moreover, the extension of online mindfulness interventions beyond the individual level to include a community dimension, such as virtual community features, and a focus on the social determinants of health, needs to be explored in future. The online mindfulness intervention could be a cost-effective way to scale up the promotion of mental wellbeing.

DOI: 10.4018/978-1-5225-2958-3.ch001

INTRODUCTION

Mood and anxiety disorders are on the rise globally as the world population grows and more people reach an age when these disorders are common (World Health Organization, 2017). Estimates show that over 322 million individuals suffer from depression and 264 million suffer from anxiety, worldwide (World Health Organization, 2017). Although the rates are high in low- and -income countries, the situation is not less drastic for developed countries, such as the United States and Canada. The Behavioural Risk Factor Surveillance System (BRFSS) survey of 2008, conducted in the United States, shows that a lifetime diagnosis of depression was experienced by 16% of the population and anxiety disorders by 12% (Centers for Disease Control and Prevention, 2010). In Canada, self-reported diagnosis of mood and anxiety disorders was estimated by 300 million individuals in 2013 (Pearson, Janz, & Ali, 2013). These conditions lead to a poor quality of life and a loss of productivity for the individuals experiencing them, culminating in multiple social and economic consequences for families and societies.

Despite the availability of effective medications and psychological counselling (Arroll et al., 2009; Butler, Chapman, Forman, & Beck, 2006; Hunot, Churchill, Teixeira, & Silva de Lima, 2007; Kapczinski, dos Santos Souza, Batista Miralha da Cunha, & Schmitt, 2003), people experiencing depression and anxiety remain undertreated (Cheung, O'Donnell, Madi, & Goldner, 2017; Mojtabai & Olfson, 2006). Access to care for depression, anxiety, and other mental illnesses is often hampered by social stigma and traditional brick-and-mortar delivery of care, along with cost and affordability. This is of a particular concern for vulnerable populations, including youth. Students of post-secondary education are known to experience multiple personal, familial, and social stressors during transition years (Beiter et al., 2015; Cairns, Massfeller, & Deeth, 2010; American College Health Association, 2013). In 2008, a national survey of university students in the US found that more than half of the students perceived that, within the previous year, academics had "been traumatic or very difficult to handle." Other issues that were at the top included: finances (36.8%), intimate relationships (31.9%), sleep difficulties (31.9%), and career-related issues (30.9%).

In another Canadian study, the counselling services provided to students at a large university were most frequently related to concerns over relationship, anxiety, stress, depression, grief, academics, and career issues (Cairns et al., 2010). Given the growing use of digital technologies, counselling could be delivered remotely. Such Internet-based delivery of cognitive behaviour therapy has been found effective for treating common mental disorders (Zhou, Li, Pei, Gao, & Kong, 2016), but the cost of individualized, one-on-one treatment is still a deterrent for many. In this context, mindfulness, self-practicing meditation is a low-cost technique that could be delivered online to proactively manage symptoms of depressions, anxiety, and stress.

Originated from "the heart" of Buddhist meditation, mindfulness is defined by Kabat-Zinn (2003) as "The awareness that emerges through paying attention on purpose, in the present moment, and non-judgmentally to the unfolding of experience moment by moment." It could be a standalone practice, but often it is integrated into a multi-component treatment package. Studies report positive effects of mindfulness in reducing loneliness (Creswell et al., 2012), depression, anxiety, pain (Marchand, 2012), acute symptoms of depression (Franca & Milbourn, 2015), somatic symptoms, distress (Würtzen et al., 2015), work stress (Grover, Teo, Pick, & Roche, 2016), and Social Anxiety Disorder (Koszycki et al., 2016). In an effort to scale the mindfulness solution, some interventions have been exploring the online mindfulness intervention effects on symptoms of stress, anxiety, and depression (Christensen et al., 2014; Krusche, Cyhlarova, & Williams, 2013; Lappalainen, Langrial, Oinas-Kukkonen, Tolvanen, & Lappalainen, 2015; Levin, Hayes, Pistorello, & Seeley, 2016). Using online tools to scale up mindfulness delivery to a large population is essential as healthcare systems face financial pressure and long wait times. Besides, delivery face-to-face mindfulness to a large population is impractical and virtually impossible with the available resources.

Given (1) the challenges that the population, and particularly students in higher education, are facing in terms of stress, anxiety, and depression, (2) the evidence demonstrating effectiveness of face-to-face mindfulness, (3) the rise of research on online delivery of mindfulness medication, it becomes important to synthesize the available evidence regarding the online mindfulness programs. To our knowledge, there is limited systematic review of such work. Addressing this knowledge gap, we initiated a systematic review of literature on Internet-based mindfulness interventions for youth. As limited studies focused on youth, the study objectives were broadened to examine the nature of online mindfulness interventions, design features, and the effectiveness of these interventions in improving symptoms of depression, anxiety, and stress.

METHODS

Search Strategy

We searched electronic the databases of MEDLINE-Ovid, CINAHL, and PsycINFO from 2005 to July 2016. Keywords and database specific terms (e.g., MeSH terms for MEDLINE, CINAHL headings for CINAHL, and thesaurus for PsycINFO) were used to capture abstracts published on cognitive behaviour therapy, acceptance and commitment therapy or mindfulness, and online tools using randomized controlled designs. The search included all international English literature. Initially, we used terms that restricted the search to youth (e.g., 18-24 years, higher education, college students), with existing diagnoses of mood disorders and one-on-one interventions, but the number of retrieved abstracts was low. Thus, we removed these restrictions to expand the literature search. Further, there were no restrictions applied for sex and geographic location. After excluding 186 duplicates, a total of 647 abstracts were retrieved (See Figure 1).

Figure 1.

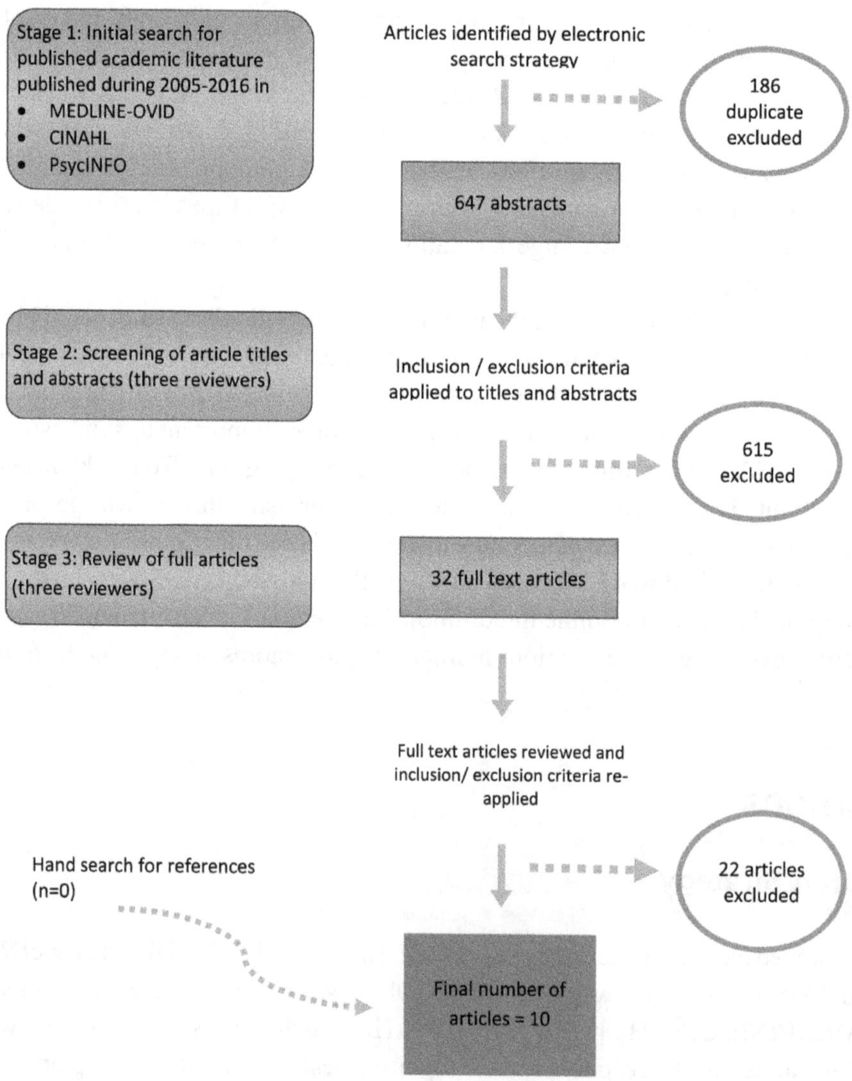

Eligibility Criteria

The inclusion criteria were predetermined and focused on studies that employed randomized controlled trial (RCT) designs, used mindfulness-based intervention(s) via online platforms, recruited adult participants, and assessed effects on depression, anxiety, and/or stress. Exclusion criteria were studies with non-adult populations (children, teens, and seniors), lacking measurement for the aforementioned mental health conditions, and using interventions with no mindfulness elements and web-based delivery.

Selection Process

The inclusion and exclusion criteria were first applied to 647 abstracts (author initial to be added) and 32 were identified as potentially eligible. The full-text versions were retrieved for 32 articles and reviewed by all authors for the final selection. Twenty-two articles were excluded as the interventions focused solely on cognitive behaviour therapy or acceptance and commitment therapy, without any mention of using mindfulness elements. Ambiguities were resolved through team discussions and consensus. Finally, 10 articles were selected for systematic review and synthesis. Bibliographies of these studies were also searched, but no additional articles were identified.

Data Synthesis

The included studies were carefully reviewed and data extracted into Excel spread sheets. The collection of data focused on the characteristics of study population, design features, nature of interventions, and reported outcomes for depression, anxiety, stress, and others. Since there was such heterogeneity in the used interventions, a meta-analysis could not be performed. We employed thematic analysis using the constant comparative technique and identified dominant and unique themes by synthesizing the extracted data. Whether the included studies took the broader framework of social determinants of health into their studies and intervention designs were assessed as well. Risk of potential bias of the included studies was analysed using criteria employed in the Cochrane Collaboration Framework (i.e. use of random sequence, allocation concealment, participants' blinding, and research personnel blinding). Also, criterion for the non-selective reporting (i.e. reporting of all pre-specified outcomes) was used. The attrition was assessed as low or unclear. Low attrition referred to having complete data for the main outcomes along with attrition details and handling of incomplete data.

RESULTS

The search yielded 10 randomized controlled trials, all published after 2011 (Aikens et al., 2014; Boettcher et al., 2014; Cavanagh et al., 2013; Dahlin et al., 2016; Drozd, Raeder, Kraft, & Bjørkli, 2013; Glück & Maercker, 2011; Ly et al., 2014; Morledge et al., 2013; O' Leary & Dockray, 2015; Wolever et al., 2012). Seven of the studies were conducted in European countries and three in the United States (Aikens et al., 2014; Morledge et al., 2013; Wolever et al., 2012). Eight of the studies were conducted on the general population; one study was conducted on patients from primary care (Morledge et al., 2013), and another study was conducted on post-secondary students (Cavanagh et al., 2013). The characteristics of the included studies are listed in Table 1, and the used mental health scales are shown in Table 2.

The study by Dahlin et al. (2016) included mindfulness as an element of the acceptance-based intervention; this study is subsequently referred to as "mindfulness intervention." The term "between-group" refers to the comparison of data between independent groups (e.g. mindfulness-based group versus waitlist group). The term "within-group" refers to the comparison of data within a single group, but at different time points (e.g. pre-to-post or pre-to-follow-up comparisons). The review findings are summarized for the study designs and features, the used interventions, the assessed outcomes, and the identified knowledge gaps related to sample diversity and attention to social determinants of health (See details in Table 3).

Study Designs and Features

Seven of the reviewed studies were two-arm trials and compared the mindfulness (MF)-based intervention with the inactive waitlist control (Aikens et al., 2014; Boettcher et al., 2014; Cavanagh et al., 2013; Dahlin et al., 2016; Drozd et al., 2013; Glück & Maercker, 2011; Ly et al., 2014). Three studies had three-arms wherein the additional arm was a therapeutic intervention (i.e. modified MF by including discussion forum; gratitude centred; or yoga practice) (Morledge et al., 2013; O' Leary & Dockray, 2015; Wolever et al., 2012).

Samples Sizes

Sample sizes varied greatly across the 10 studies. Half of the reviewed studies had a sample larger than 100 participants (Cavanagh et al., 2013; Dahlin et al., 2016; Drozd et al., 2013; Morledge et al., 2013; Wolever et al., 2012). Of the remaining five studies, four (Aikens et al., 2014; Boettcher et al., 2014; Ly et al., 2014; O' Leary & Dockray, 2015) had samples between 50 and 100, and one (Glück & Maercker, 2011) had a sample of less than 50. The per-arm sample sizes were relatively small

Table 1. Characteristics of the included studies

Characteristics	# of studies	Characteristics	# of studies
(N=10)		(N=10)	
Country:		**Sample size:**	
[a]European nations	7	≤ 50	1
United States	3	50 - 100	4
Primary focus:		≥ 100	5
Depression	1	**Age ranges:**	
Anxiety	2	18 – 24 yrs	1
Stress	4	≥25 yrs	8
[b]Other	3	Not specified	1
Recruitment:		**Gender:**	
[c]Active approach	2	Mixed, female dominant sample	9
[d]Passive approach	7	Mixed, male dominant sample	0
Not specified	1	Female only sample	1
Response rate reported:		Male only sample	0
Yes	2	**Education level reported:**	
No	8	Yes	9
Study populations:		No	1
General population	8	**Employment status reported:**	
Patient population	1	Yes	4
University students	1	No	6
Ethnicity reported:		**Household income reported:**	
Yes	2	Yes	2
No	8	No	8

[a]European nations: Austria, Germany, Ireland, Norway, Sweden, UK
[b]Other: multiple foci including mindfulness, depression/anxiety, perceived stress/distress
[c]Active approach: direct invitation by study personnel and health care providers
[d]Passive approach: self-responses to email invitations

in two of the studies (Glück & Maercker, 2011; O' Leary & Dockray, 2015), where the participants allocated to each arm were fewer than 30. Of the three studies (Glück & Maercker, 2011; Ly et al., 2014; Morledge et al., 2013) that detailed the power calculation, sample sizes were determined on the basis of a significance level at .05, two-tailed or one-tailed, and a power of 0.80, with the expectation of obtaining a moderate/unspecified effect size (d = 0.50–0.70) between the MF intervention and the control/other group.

Table 2. Mental health outcomes in the included studies

Study	Depression					Anxiety			Stress			Mindfulness				QoL
	PHQ-9 PHQ-4	BDI-II	CES-D	EDS	MADRS	BAI	GAD-7	PHQ-4	PSS PSQ	DASS	PSWQ	CAMS	FMI	FFMQ	MAAS	QOLI
Aikens, 2014									✓					✓		
Boettcher, 2014		✓				✓										✓
Cavanagh, 2013	✓							✓	✓					✓		
Dahlin, 2016	✓				✓	✓	✓				✓					✓
Drozd, 2013										✓					✓	
Glück, 2011									✓				✓			
Ly, 2014	✓					✓										✓
Morledge, 2013									✓						✓	
O' Leary, 2015				✓					✓							
Wolever, 2012			✓						✓			✓				

Legend: BAI=Beck Anxiety Inventory; BDI-II= Beck Depression Inventory; CAMS= Cognitive & Affective Mindfulness Scale; CES-D= Centre for Epidemiologic Studies – Depression Scale; DASS: Depression, Anxiety & Stress Scale; EDS= Edinburgh Depression Scale; FFMQ= Five Facets Mindfulness Questionnaire; FMI= Freiburg Mindfulness Inventory; GAD-7= Generalized Anxiety Disorder 7-item Scale; LS= Life Satisfaction; MAAS= Mindful Attention Awareness Scale; MADRS= Montgomery Asberg Depression Rating Scale; PHQ= Patient Health Questionnaire; PSS= Perceived Stress Scale; PSQ: Patient Stress Questionnaire; PSWQ= Penn State Worry Questionnaire; QoL= Quality of Life; QOLI= Quality of Life Inventory

Table 3. Summary of the Included RCT Studies

Study	Population	Intervention	Design	Quality[a]
Aikens et al., 2014 USA	Company employees Mean age: unknown Recruited via open email invitation	Web-based, not grp-based Duration: 7 wk Content: virtual class, audio guided exercises, progress tracking survey, customized text messaging, workbook; led by physician trained in mindfulness	2-arms: MF (n=44); WLC (n=45); lost 26 Data: pre, post & 6m F/U (for MF grp) Attrition at F/U: M 30%; WLC 7% Adherence: 28 completed 75%-100% of pgm material & attended on avg. 7.4 classes; practice time on avg 13min/day ITT analysis	1,6,7
Boettcher et al., 2014 Germany	Community sample: some anxiety (BAI > 8), not severely depressed or suicidal; confirmation via SCID Mean age: 38.9yrs Recruited via newspaper/ study website	Web-based, not grp-based Duration: 8wk Content: 20-min intro video, 8 modules (each with 10-min mindfulness exercises); discussion forum on mood disorders	2-arms: MF (n=45), Ctl with general discussion forum (n=46); lost 7 Data: pre, post & 6m f/u (for MF grp) Attrition at F/U: M 57%; Ctl 30% ITT w/ mixed models	1,2,6,7
Cavanagh et al., 2013 UK	College students Mean age: 24yrs Recruited through email invitation & posters	Web-based, not grp-based Duration: 2 wk Content: 10-min audio guided M practice; edu text; 3rd day reminder email; no personal contact	2-arm: MF (n=23); WLC (n=30); lost 46 Data: pre & post Attrition: MF 57%; Ctl 30% ITT analysis	1,6,7
Dahlin et al., 2016 Sweden	Community sample with existing anxiety (PSWQ ≥45); no severe depression, alcohol/ substance and suicidal ideation; SCID confirmed Mean age: 39.5yrs Recruited via Internet ads + poster on university campus/ city centre	Web-based, not grp-based Duration: 9 wk Content: Therapist-guided Internet based acceptance & mindfulness CBT – "the Worry Help" commercial pgm; 7 modules (text, audio, video); therapist contact (15min/wk)	2-arm: MF (n=52); WLC (n=51); lost18 Data: pre, post, 6 month f/u Attrition at F/U: MF 37%; Ctl 16% Adherence: 76% all modules completed; 9.3min/wk M practice avg. ITT analysis	1,2,6,7

Mindfulness (MF); Waitlist Control (WLC); Control (Ctl); Follow-up (F/U); Program (Pgm); Average (Avg); Group (Grp); Minute (Min); Intention to Treat (ITT); Message (Msg); Education (Edu); Week (Wk); Cognitive Behavior Therapy (CBT)

Recruitment Strategies

Recruitment strategies were passive in the majority of the studies. Seven studies (Aikens et al., 2014; Boettcher et al., 2014; Cavanagh et al., 2013; Dahlin et al., 2016; Glück & Maercker, 2011; Ly et al., 2014; Wolever et al., 2012) recruited participants through email invitations, study posters, newsletters or advertisements. Active human contacts for study recruitment were seen in two other studies (Drozd et al., 2013; Morledge et al., 2013). In the study by Drozd el al. (2013), snowball sampling and the so-called "viral recruitment" were employed. First-degree contacts of a master's student's social network were invited directly. These people were further encouraged to relay the study invitation to individuals within their network in order to reach more potential participants. In another study (Morledge et al., 2013) that targeted clinic populations, family physicians and nurses facilitated recruitment by referring

Table 4.

Study	Population	Intervention	RCT Design	Quality[a]
Drozd et al., 2013 Norway	Community sample with access to email Mean age: M grp 32yrs & WLC grp 33yrs Recruited via Facebook network of a master's student	Web-based, not grp-based Duration: 4wk Content: 13 sessions (10min each); 2 components (psychoedu & technique, exercises, homework); email link to session 3 times/wk; no personal contact	2-arm: MF (n=126); Ctl (n=133); lost 133 Data: pre, post & 1,2, 6m f/u Attrition at 1,2,6m F/U: MF 50.8%, 53.9%, 57.9%; Ctl 32%, 38%, 39.8% Multilevel models	1,2,6,7
Gluck et al., 2011 Austria	Community sample with no psychotic or suicidal ideation & no active psychotherapy or substance dependence Mean age: MF grp 33.7yrs & WLC grp 37.2yrs Recruited via open email to a university's student club/ faculty & employees of 3 companies	Web-based, not grp-based Duration: 2 wks Content of Web-based Less Stress: 2 modules (20min/ day for each module for 6 days/wk); contained text, audio, animation; weekly email reminder; no personal contact	2-arm: MF (n=28); WLC (n=21); lost 5 Data: pre, post, & 3m f/u Attrition at F/U: MF 32% & Ctl 14% ITT Analysis	6,7
Ly et al., 2014 Sweden	Community sample with existing depression (PHQ-9 ≥5), confirmed by phone SCID; no other severe psychiatric condition, suicidality or alcohol problems Mean age: 36yrs Recruited via national ads	Web-based & Smartphone, not grp-based Duration: 8 wk both Intv. Content: both Intv. similar except for their theoretical basis; therapist contact (max 20 min/wk); encouraging msg every 2-3 day; wkly general edu msg & self-reflection feedback	2-arm: Behavioral Activation (n=40); MF (n=41); lost 9.. Data: pre, post and 6m f/u Attrition at F/U: MF 13%; Ctl 12% ITT w/ mixed effects model	1,2,6,7

potentially eligible patients to the research personnel. The recruitment strategy was unclear in one of the reviewed study (O' Leary & Dockray, 2015).

Adherence

Adherence to intervention was described in different ways. Only one study (Ly et al., 2014) defined adherence as "the number of weekly reflections the participants sent to their therapist." Five studies (Aikens et al., 2014; Dahlin et al., 2016; Drozd et al., 2013; Ly et al., 2014; Morledge et al., 2013) used the rate for completing all or the majority of the intervention modules. The percentage of participants that completed all, or 50% or more, of the assigned modules ranged from 38.5%–76% (Dahlin et al., 2016; Drozd et al., 2013; Ly et al., 2014) and 35%–100%, respectively (Aikens et al., 2014; Morledge et al., 2013). Four studies (Aikens et al., 2014; Boettcher et al., 2014; Drozd et al., 2013; Morledge et al., 2013) assessed the frequency

Table 5.

Study	Population	Intervention	RCT Design	Quality[a]
Morledge et al., 2013 USA	Primary care patient sample with no psychosis Age: 59.1% were 40-59yrs Recruited via flyers posted in the clinics, direct referrals from healthcare providers or emails/e-newsletters to pgm subscribers	Web-based, not grp-based Duration: 8 wks Content: Internet based Stress Management (ISM) had wkly text/audio lesson & meditation; daily articles/ quotes/ tips; activity logs; no personal contact ISM+: ISM + online msg board	3-arm: MF as ISM (n=183); MF as ISM+ (n=184); Ctl with wkly activity logs (n=184); lost 272. Attrition at F/U: ISM 62%; ISM+ 67%; Ctl 35% Data collected at pre, post, 1m f/u Analytic approaches unclear	1,6,7
O'Leary et al., 2015 Ireland	Primary care patient sample, all women Mean age: 28.4yrs Recruitment approach unclear	Web-based, not grp-based Duration: 3 wk Content: online lessons 4 times/ wk; diaries; MF grp did Body Scan, Gratitude grp did grateful reflection; no personal contact	3-arm: Gratitude (n=29); MF (n=22); WLC (n=10); lost 26 Data: pre, post, 2wk f/u Attrition at F/U: Gratitude 15%; MF 13%; WLC 9% Analytic approaches unclear	6,7
Wolever et al., 2012, USA	Company employees included if PSS>=16; no major/unstable medical/psychological conditions; not a routine yoga practiser Mean age: 42.9yrs Recruited via email invite to all	Web and in-person, not grp-based Duration: 8 wk Content: Intv 1. Mindfulness At Work (MAW) 14hr; instructor led; 2 versions with identical content (one in-person & other virtual class); handouts; real-time teacher-participant communication in both Intv. 2 (Yoga): 12hrs at home (guided by DVD) or at work with meditation instructor	3-arm: MF (n= 96); Yoga (n=90); Ctl (n=53); lost 34. Attrition for 3-arm at post: MF 15%; Yoga 16%; Ctl 11% 2-arm: In-person MF (n=52), online MF (n=44). Attrition for 2-arm at post: in-person MF 4%; MF 27% ITT and other analysis	6,7

[a]Legend: 1= Random sequence used; 2= Allocation concealed; 3= Study participants blinded; 4= Research personnel blinded; 5= Outcome assessment blinded; 6= Attrition low; 7= Non-selective reporting

and time spent on mindfulness practices and exercises. Depending on the design of the intervention, the average time spent on exercises varied from 66 minutes to 90 minutes per week (Aikens et al., 2014; Boettcher et al., 2014; Drozd et al., 2013). One study (Morledge et al., 2013) reported that the frequency of exercising mindfulness meditation averaged 4.07 times per week. Four studies (Cavanagh et al., 2013; Glück & Maercker, 2011; O'Leary & Dockray, 2015; Wolever et al., 2012) did not address the adherence issue.

Attrition

Attrition was high in most of the reviewed studies. Seven of the studies had attrition rates equal to or greater than 30% for the intervention conditions at the endpoint of the studies (Aikens et al., 2014; Cavanagh et al., 2013; Dahlin et al., 2016; Drozd et al., 2013; Glück & Maercker, 2011; Morledge et al., 2013; O'Leary & Dockray, 2015). The extreme case was seen in the study by Morledge et al. (2013) as over 60% of the participants in the two intervention groups dropped out by the end of the follow-up. The lowest attrition, on the other hand, was seen in the study by Ly et al. (2014) where the drop rates for the two intervention groups, behavioural activation and mindfulness-based, were only 13% and 17%.

Interventions

Nine studies used the Internet as the primary venue of intervention administration, and only one used a Smartphone application (Ly et al., 2014). Two studies (Aikens et al., 2014; Wolever et al., 2012) used a hybrid approach to integrating in-person meetings into the web-based interventions The majority of the interventions were module-, session- or class-based (Aikens et al., 2014; Boettcher et al., 2014; Dahlin et al., 2016; Drozd et al., 2013; Glück & Maercker, 2011; Morledge et al., 2013; Wolever et al., 2012), although the rationale for selecting particular sets of modules was largely unclear. The number of modules in seven studies (Aikens et al., 2014; Boettcher et al., 2014; Dahlin et al., 2016; Drozd et al., 2013; Glück & Maercker, 2011; Morledge et al., 2013; Wolever et al., 2012) ranged from 2 to 13 with the average at 8.1 (median = 8). The duration of the interventions across all studies ranged from 2 to 12 weeks, with the average at 6.3 weeks (median = 7.5). The interventions in the reviewed studies unanimously used a multi-component format. Psycho-education and experiential practices (with or without coaches) were the two components most frequently incorporated into the interventions. A focus on participant flexibility also emerged across reviewed interventions.

Psycho-Educational Materials

Psycho-educational materials were either specific to mental health conditions or remedial therapies (or both). In a few cases, it was unclear whether or not participants received knowledge-enhancing materials (Aikens et al., 2014; O' Leary & Dockray, 2015; Wolever et al., 2012), while, in one case, the authors referred to the use of "standardized information" (Glück & Maercker, 2011), but did not elaborate. Education on mental conditions focused on the diagnoses and risk factors of depression, anxiety, and stress, the corresponding treatments, and relapse preventions. The essential ingredients of education on remedial therapies were the introduction of the underlying concepts and the expected benefits and experiences. For example, some interventions included concepts of values and acceptance (Dahlin et al., 2016; Glück & Maercker, 2011; Morledge et al., 2013), procrastination and optimism (Drozd et al., 2013), and compassion and kindness (Morledge et al., 2013). Only one study (Ly et al., 2014) acknowledged that the whole conceptual framework employed was inspired from *The Mindful Way Through Depression* by Williams, Teasdale, Segal, and Kabat-Zinn (2007). In contrast, other reviewed studies were less explicit about theoretical sources of inspiration.

Experiential Practices

Experiential practices focused on mindfulness-based meditation, breathing, and body scanning, which were frequent techniques used in the interventions. Other experiential elements such as relaxation techniques, physical activities, and performance-oriented skills for stress management and problem solving were integrated into some interventions (Aikens et al., 2014; Boettcher et al., 2014; Drozd et al., 2013). Human coaches were employed in a few interventions. In two studies (Dahlin et al., 2016; Ly et al., 2014), master's level psychology students were staffed as coaches or therapists under supervision of licensed psychologists. One study (Aikens et al., 2014) employed an internal medicine physician, with training in mindfulness meditation, as an intervention instructor. The interventions of six studies (Boettcher et al., 2014; Cavanagh et al., 2013; Drozd et al., 2013; Glück & Maercker, 2011; Morledge et al., 2013; O' Leary & Dockray, 2015) reviewed were fully automated. Communication between the participants and the coaches focused primarily on providing supportive feedback, recommendations, problem solving, progress monitoring, and encouragement to continue the care plan. The interaction was largely synchronized and on a weekly, and minimal (15 to 30 minutes per week), basis. Only one study (Wolever et al., 2012) offered live and synchronous communication with an intervention instructor that was an experienced mindfulness meditation teacher.

Participation Flexibility

Participation flexibility was identified to varying levels across the reviewed studies. The delivered modules in three studies (Boettcher et al., 2014; Drozd et al., 2013; Glück & Maercker, 2011) were "chained," meaning the completion of a previous module was a prerequisite to participate in a subsequent one. Participants in two other studies (Aikens et al., 2014; Dahlin et al., 2016) were given the freedom to complete the modules according to their own preferences, although a predetermined order was recommended. The completion order was not specified in the remaining five studies (Cavanagh et al., 2013; Ly et al., 2014; Morledge et al., 2013; O' Leary & Dockray, 2015; Wolever et al., 2012). Two studies (Boettcher et al., 2014; Glück & Maercker, 2011) required their participants to finish the session within a week's time, while another 2 studies (Dahlin et al., 2016; Morledge et al., 2013) allowed 1 to 2 extra weeks to complete the weekly sessions. The remaining six studies (Aikens et al., 2014; Cavanagh et al., 2013; Drozd et al., 2013; Ly et al., 2014; O' Leary & Dockray, 2015; Wolever et al., 2012) did not provide information concerning module completion times.

Another flexibility feature was the use of multimedia in a majority of the studies. In addition to the text-based materials, audio guidance for self-practice and meditation were offered in 5 of the studies (Cavanagh et al., 2013; Drozd et al., 2013; Glück & Maercker, 2011; Ly et al., 2014; Morledge et al., 2013), whereas graphic illustrations and animations were used in one study (Glück & Maercker, 2011). Inclusion of participant reminders was limited to three of the reviewed interventions (Cavanagh et al., 2013; Glück & Maercker, 2011; Morledge et al., 2013); emails or scripted telephone calls were sent to participants aiming at increasing study adherence.

Outcomes

The mental health outcomes of stress, depression, and/or anxiety were assessed in 10 studies, while the levels of mindfulness were measured in 6, and quality of life in 3 studies. The studies used various types of scales (See Table 2). No study evaluated intervention impact on life satisfaction.

Perceived Stress

Perceived stress was measured in eight studies and the results were largely in favour of mindfulness interventions. The superior effects of mindfulness interventions were found in four studies (Aikens et al., 2014; Cavanagh et al., 2013; Dahlin et al., 2016; Drozd et al, 2013) where the comparisons were between mindfulness-based interventions and the inactive waitlist control group. Cavanagh (2013) and Dahlin (2016) reported moderate to large between-group effect sizes (ESs = 0.62–0.87) at post-intervention by comparing MF intervention to the waitlist control group. Aiken et al. (2014) reported within-group effect size at post-intervention and it was high for the MF intervention (ES = 1.03) and low for the waitlist control (ES = 0.18). Drozd et al. (2013) examined MF intervention impact on stress at 1, 2, and 6-month intervals. On conducting growth curve analysis, researchers found that in the MF group, the stress level reduced significantly at 1-month and at six months, although participants showed an increase in stress during the study. In contrast, the stress level in the Drozd's waitlist control group remained largely unchanged after a reduction was seen at the 1-month interval. Likewise, treatment effect was further improved through to the follow-up in Dahlin's study with a large within-group effect size (ES = 1.71). There was, however, a slight, but insignificant, increase in perceived stress at the follow-up according to a study by Aikens (2014).

When comparing the MF-based intervention to 1) its deviated format (supplementing with a message board) and a waitlist control; and 2) a therapeutic yoga and a waitlist control, the treatment effects of all three interventions were superior to the control, but equivalent to each other (Morledge et al., 2013; Wolever et al., 2012); effect sizes were not reported. Negative findings were seen in two studies (Glück & Maercker, 2011; O'Leary & Dockray, 2015). Small and non-superior treatment effects of the MF-based intervention as compared to the waitlist control group were reported in the intention-to-treat (ITT) analysis by Glück et al. (2011). The ESs between the MF-based intervention and the control groups were in a range of 0.08–0.46 at post-intervention and 0.03–0.35 at the follow-up. In the study by O'Leary et al. (2015), no significant differences in terms of treatment effects were found among a MF-based intervention, a gratitude-based one, and a waitlist control group. However, there was a general trend in the study by O'Leary et al. (2015) indicating that both interventions reduced stress over time, as opposed to the negligible change in the control group.

Depressive Symptoms

Depressive symptoms were measured in six studies. Compared to the control conditions, the ability of the MF-based interventions to reduce depressive symptoms was superior. Yet, the effects of MF-based interventions were largely equivalent to other therapeutic interventions in these trials. Ly et al. (2014) compared MF-based and behavioural activation (BA)-based interventions, with no significant differences found between these two interventions for the whole study cohort on reducing depressive symptoms, either at pre-to-post or at post-to-follow-up. The ESs between these two groups was small, ranging from 0.03 to 0.28. Using the Mini-International Neuropsychiatric Interview (MINI), the proportions of participants who clinically recovered between the two groups was comparable both at post-intervention (53% in MF vs. 74% in BA) and at the follow-up (81% in MF and 88% in BA). However, interesting results emerged when Ly et al. (2014) conducted subgroup analyses for participants suffering from mild or severe depression (PHQ-9 > = 10) at baseline. They found that the MF-based intervention, compared to the control group, demonstrated a significant and large impact from pre-to-follow-up for participants with mild depression; between-group ESs ranged from 0.98 to 1.21. A comparison between the BA-based intervention and the control group, by contrast, showed that

BA was more effective for participants with more severe levels of depression; the between-group ESs, however, were small to close to moderate (ESs = 0.39 to 0.47). In three other studies (Boettcher et al., 2014; Cavanagh et al., 2013; Dahlin et al., 2016), comparison was between a MF-based intervention and a waitlist control. The interventions showed significant effects on improving depressive symptoms at post-intervention. The between-group ESs were close to moderate to large (ESs = 0.41 to 0.84). Boettcher (2014) and Dahlin (2016) also followed up participants in the MF-based intervention and found a significant reduction in depression scores from pre-to-follow-up at 6 months with large within-group ESs in a range of 1.00 to 1.04.

In another study by Wolever et al. (2012), MF-based intervention was compared to a therapeutic yoga program and a waitlist control, and both interventions showed greater efficacy in improving depression than the inactive control condition. The differences in terms of the treatment effects between the two interventions, however, were negligible. O'Leary and Dockray (2015) compared MF-based and gratitude interventions with the waitlist control groups; no significant effect on depression was found for the interventions, however, the sample was small. Nevertheless, they noted a trend indicating that both interventions reduced depression over time, despite changes in the control group being negligible.

Anxiety Symptoms

Anxiety symptoms were measured in four of the reviewed studies. The result pattern was similar to that of depressive symptoms: MF-based interventions had a superior effect than control conditions, but a largely equivalent effect compared to other therapeutic interventions in the studies. The MF-based intervention in the study by Boettcher (2014) showed a significantly larger decrease in anxiety symptoms at post-intervention than the waitlist control with between-group ES of 0.99; the treatment effect was sustained at the follow-up (within-group ES = 1.44). Significantly more participants in the MF group reached clinically improved and recovered status, compared to the control group (40.0% in MF vs. 9.1% in the control). The two other studies (Cavanagh et al., 2013; Dahlin et al., 2016) revealed resembling results that, compared to the waitlist control, the intervention groups were more effective in treating anxiety, with the between-group ESs ranging from close to moderate to large (ESs = 0.41 to 0.98). The treatment effect was sustained at the follow-up in the Dahlin et al. 2016 study (within-group ES = 1.69). The differences in terms of the treatment effects on anxiety were insignificant between a MF-based intervention and a BA-based one (Ly et al., 2014); the between-group ESs were negligibly small, both at post-intervention (ES = 0.06) and at follow-up (ES = 0.01).

Mindfulness Levels

Mindfulness levels were measured in six studies. The impact of the interventions on increasing mindfulness was, in general, greater than inactive controls, but largely equivalent to other forms of therapeutic interventions. Significant improvement of mindfulness in the MF-based intervention groups were found in two studies, compared to the control group (Aikens et al., 2014; Cavanagh et al., 2013). The between-group ES at post-intervention was small (ES = 0.42) in one study (Cavanagh et al., 2013), and not available in the other (Aikens et al., 2014). The treatment effects were either maintained or further improved through to the follow-up in the study by Aikens et al (2014); within-group ESs were moderate to large (ESs = 0.52 to 1.08). When the comparison was among a MF-based intervention and, 1) its deviated format (supplementing with a message board) and a waitlist control and, 2) a therapeutic yoga and a waitlist control, the treatment effects of all interventions were superior to the control, but equivalent to each other (Morledge et al., 2013; Wolever et al., 2012); effect sizes were not reported in both studies. In a study by Gluck et al. (2011), a short MF-based intervention was compared to a waitlist control and the ITT analysis found no significant improvement in mindfulness for the intervention group; the between-group ES was small (ES = 0.29). Drozd et al. revealed in their 2013 study that web-based stress intervention increased mindfulness, which in turn, mediated the lower level of stress over time. The effect sizes, however, were not provided.

Quality of Life (QOL)

Quality of life was also assessed in three studies. Boettcher et al. (2014) found a moderate pre-to-post increase in the quality of life for the MF-based intervention (ES = 0.64) while no change occurred for the control group (ES = 0.04); the between-group effect size was small (ES = 0.37). In the study by Dahlin et al. (2016) that compared MF-based intervention to the waitlist control, no significant differences in the change of QOL were found between the two conditions, neither from pre-to-post nor from pre-to-follow-up. In another study by Ly et al. (2014) that compared a MF-based intervention with a BA-based intervention, the treatment effects on QOL were equivalent between the two interventions at pre-to-post and pre-to-follow-up. However, the within-group quality of life scores improved significantly for both MF-based and BA-based interventions at pre-to-post (ES = 0.62 and ES = 0.91, respectively), and at pre-to-follow-up (ES = 0.75 and ES = 0.84, respectively).

Issues, Controversies, and Problems

One of the problems researchers encountered was the occurrence of knowledge gaps due to the types of participant characteristics studied and/or not included in the studies reviewed. Only a few studies reported detailed socio-demographic characteristics of the participants. Participant education level was reported frequently, but employment status was reported by 4 out of the 10 reviewed trials. The least reported characteristics included ethnicity and household income; two studies only. It was also noteworthy that no Canadian study was found. Only one UK-based study focused on post-secondary students. Authors of the included studies were all silent even in the discussion sections on the broader social determinants of health pertaining to mental illnesses, and they did not supply plans and strategies with regard to offering or mobilizing societal resources to support participants who may be at a high risk or in crisis. The interventions were homogenously individual-based. There was no indication that the interventions were developed with an attempt to account for the varying needs of participants, such as age, gender, education, culture, and familial and social relationship background.

Another issue was that the majority of studies used small samples, thus effect sizes varied and did not provide as comprehensive an analysis as studies utilizing larger samples would have, in theory, provided.

DISCUSSION

The systematic review of published studies on mindfulness-based online interventions reveals several insights about the designs of interventions, their impact on depression, anxiety, stress levels, and the broader challenges in this field.

In regard to mental health, the review of included studies showed an overall positive impact of the online delivery of mindfulness awareness and practice. The symptoms of stress, depression, and anxiety improved in the mindfulness groups compared to the control groups across the majority of the reviewed studies, although the effect sizes were moderate.

SOLUTIONS AND RECOMMENDATIONS

Given that most of the studies used small samples, future research with larger samples would help in establishing the effect sizes more precisely. Some of the reviewed studies also measured levels of mindfulness and, overall, reported significant improvement in the mindfulness groups compared to the control groups. Authors of some of the reviewed studies compared online mindfulness interventions with other therapeutic interventions and the effect was largely equivalent amongst these approaches. Indeed, this is an area for further scholarly work. Nonetheless, based on our review, there is sound evidence of the effectiveness of mindfulness online interventions for improving mental health when compared to controlled conditions.

Our review demonstrates that the online delivery of mindfulness psycho-education and practice is an area in its infancy. The reviewed interventions were limited to online delivery of the content to online users. In the reviewed studies, only one-third included interactive features such as discussion forums and electronic messaging. The online mindfulness-based innovations could be further advanced by including user-empowerment features of Web 2.0, such as interaction and collaboration (DiNucci, 1999). This would allow users to interact, collaborate, generate content data, and form a virtual community. A virtual community (VC) is a community of people collaborating to achieve a goal using online (Internet-based) tools (Bender, Jimenez-Marroquin, Ferris, Katz, & Jadad, 2013). Health VCs have received increased attention in the health research community in attempts to educate and support patients while enabling and empowering them to become active participants in managing their own health conditions (El Morr, 2007; El Morr & Kawash, 2007). Likewise, the incorporation of interactive and collaborative features into online mindfulness interventions could form virtual mental health communities, injecting a new community dimension perspective in mental health interventions, which have too often focused narrowly on the individual.

FUTURE RESEARCH DIRECTIONS

Existing evidence reveals that virtual communities (VCs) have a high potential for improving health outcomes. On the client side, health VCs enable individuals with common health-related conditions to provide mutual social support (Johnston, Worrell, Gangi, & Wasko, 2013), and have been found to decrease loneliness and increase emotional well-being, self-esteem, and self-empowerment (Heidelberger, El-Gayar, & Sarnikar, 2011; Loane & D'Alessandro, 2013). On the healthcare provider side, efficient and flexible communication channels are generated through VCs, which offer patient education and advisement continuity on effective chronic disease management, remotely (Chorbev, Sotirovska, & Mihajlov, 2011; Matura, McDonough, Aglietti, Herzog, & Gallant, 2013; Vasconcellos-Silva, Carvalho, & Lucena, 2013). Research has demonstrated the effectiveness and efficiency effects linked to VCs for multiple health conditions, such as chronic kidney disease, pulmonary hypertension, and cancer (Bender et al., 2013; C. El Morr et al., 2014; Matura et al., 2013), and especially for the engagement of patients in the management of their own health (Matura et al., 2013; Vasconcellos-Silva et al., 2013).

Moreover, patient-centred VCs are customizable to individual patient preferences and are responsive to the specific needs and values of patients (Barry & Edgman-Levitan, 2012). Studies suggest that the use of VCs for mindfulness-based interventions offers many benefits, but needs further exploration and research. While mental health conditions have been especially stigmatized in today's society (particularly in visible ethnic minorities) (Hansson, Tuck, Lurie & McKenzie, 2010), VCs present an opportunity to overcome and bypass social stigma by providing e-education and e-support; an opportunity that could be especially availed for university students, as they are frequent users of online technologies and at-risk of experiencing mental stress during their developmental years. VCs could ensure access to personalized, validated information in a private manner, minimizing socially stigmatizing exposures.

Given the anytime and anywhere availability, scaling up of online mindfulness programs holds the potential to facilitate population-based engagement in promoting mental well-being in a cost-effective way. The World Health Organization defines mental well-being as a positive concept "in which every individual realizes his or her own potential, can cope with the normal stresses of life, can work productively and fruitfully, and is able to make a contribution to her or his community" (WHO & Calouste Gulbenkian Foundation, 2014). Mindfulness meditation could be viewed as a mental health promoting approach whereby anyone could meditate and self-manage stress, worries, and other symptoms on an on going basis. Such proactive approaches could help in reducing the occurrences of serious mental health conditions, hence, lowering the need to access specialized care and improving overall quality of life.

Another notable finding in our review was the lack of attention given to the social determinants of mental health. On one side, the reviewed studies reported limited characteristics of the participants; ethnicity and income received the least attention. None of the reviewed studies explained whether social conditions informed the development of mindfulness modules and practice sessions, nor did they provide information on resources related to social conditions, such as housing, employment, child care, places for social interaction, and so forth. This "individualized" focus is a short sightedness on the part of the researchers, as an abundance of evidence demonstrates that social, economic, and physical conditions shape an individual's mental health (WHO & Calouste Gulbenkian Foundation, 2014). Evidence shows that certain groups (e.g., ethnic minorities, communities with low income, and seniors) are at higher disadvantage in experiencing mental stress (Lund et al., 2010; Melzer, Fryers, & Jenkins, 2004), while good social support buffers the effects of weak social conditions on mental health (Kelly, Sacker, Del Bono, Francesconi, &

Marmot, 2011). Therefore, a holistic approach would be important in the development of mindfulness interventions.

This review also revealed that enhanced scholarly reporting is needed around intervention development and implementation processes. For example, the context within which the interventions were developed lacked clarity, as discussed earlier. There was limited information about the theoretical frameworks and/or user-engaged approach in the selection of topics that various modules covered in an intervention. Likewise, the process indicators, including the rate of adherence to the mindfulness-based intervention, and the rate of completion of the various modules within an intervention, were reported by only a limited number of the reviewed studies. The information on the timings of making the modules available to participants (e.g., all open at once or phased approach) was also not always reported. Future research in this area should measure and report such details to enhance the real-life adaptation and adoption of the interventions.

While we conducted a focused literature review, the identification of key strengths and areas to grow is anticipated to inform further scholarly work and the real-life adoption of successful online mindfulness intervention programs on a wider scale.

CONCLUSION

The current chapter systematically reviewed the effectiveness of online mindfulness interventions. Online delivery of mindfulness psycho-education and practice is an area in its infancy. There is evidence that online mindfulness interventions can have a positive impact on mental health in terms of reducing stress, depression, and anxiety; however, large sample studies are needed in order to obtain conclusive results. Moreover, the extension of online mindfulness interventions beyond the individual level to include a community dimension, such as virtual communities, needs to be explored for their potential to augment the positive health impacts of online interventions.

The reviewed studies lacked attention to the social determinants of health. Further research that takes into consideration the social aspects of health is needed, as social conditions have a great impact on physical and mental health. Finally, online mindfulness interventions can be a cost-effective way to scaling up mental health interventions to address stress, anxiety, and depression at the individual and population levels. Although future research is necessary, this study uncovers the potential benefits of online mindfulness interventions in reducing stress, anxiety, and depression.

REFERENCES

Aikens, K. A., Astin, J., Pelletier, K. R., Levanovich, K., Baase, C. M., Park, Y. Y., & Bodnar, C. M. (2014). Mindfulness goes to work. *Journal of Occupational and Environmental Medicine, 56*(7), 721–731. doi:10.1097/JOM.0000000000000209 PMID:24988100

American College Health Association. (2013). *American College Health Association-National College Health Assessment II: Canadian Reference Group Data Report Spring 2013*. Hanover, MD: American College Health Association.

Arroll, B., Elley, C. R., Fishman, T., Goodyear-Smith, F. A., Kenealy, T., Blashki, G., & MacGillivray, S. et al. (2009). Antidepressants versus placebo for depression in primary care. *Cochrane Database of Systematic Reviews*, (3): CD007954. PMID:19588448

Barry, M. J., & Edgman-Levitan, S. (2012). Shared decision making - The pinnacle of patient-centered care. *The New England Journal of Medicine, 366*(9), 780–781. doi:10.1056/NEJMp1109283 PMID:22375967

Beiter, R., Nash, R., McCrady, M., Rhoades, D., Linscomb, M., Clarahan, M., & Sammut, S. (2015). The prevalence and correlates of depression, anxiety, and stress in a sample of college students. *Journal of Affective Disorders, 173*, 90–96. doi:10.1016/j.jad.2014.10.054 PMID:25462401

Bender, J. L., Jimenez-Marroquin, M. C., Ferris, L. E., Katz, J., & Jadad, A. R. (2013). Online communities for breast cancer survivors: A review and analysis of their characteristics and levels of use. *Supportive Care in Cancer, 21*(5), 1253–1263. doi:10.1007/s00520-012-1655-9 PMID:23179491

Boettcher, J., Astrom, V., Pahlsson, D., Schenstrom, O., Andersson, G., & Carlbring, P. (2014). Internet-based mindfulness treatment for anxiety disorders: A randomized controlled trial. *Behavior Therapy, 45*(2), 241–253. doi:10.1016/j.beth.2013.11.003 PMID:24491199

Butler, A. C., Chapman, J. E., Forman, E. M., & Beck, A. T. (2006). The empirical status of cognitive-behavioral therapy: A review of meta-analyses. *Clinical Psychology Review, 26*(1), 17–31. doi:10.1016/j.cpr.2005.07.003 PMID:16199119

Cairns, S. L., Massfeller, H. F., & Deeth, S. C. (2010). Why do postsecondary students seek counselling? *Canadian Journal of Counselling and Psychotherapy, 44*(1), 34–50.

Cavanagh, K., Strauss, C., Cicconi, F., Griffiths, N., Wyper, A., & Jones, F. (2013). A randomised controlled trial of a brief online mindfulness-based intervention. *Behaviour Research and Therapy*, *51*(9), 573–578. doi:10.1016/j.brat.2013.06.003 PMID:23872699

Centres for Disease Control and Prevention. (2010). Current depression among adults --- United States, 2006 and 2008. *Morbidity and Mortality Weekly Report*, *59*(38), 1229–1235. PMID:20881934

Cheung, R., O'Donnell, S., Madi, N., & Goldner, E. (2017). Factors associated with delayed diagnosis of mood and/or anxiety disorders. *Health Promotion and Chronic Disease Prevention in Canada: Research. Policy & Practice*, *37*(5), 137–148.

Chorbev, I., Sotirovska, M., & Mihajlov, D. (2011). Virtual communities for diabetes chronic disease healthcare. *International Journal of Telemedicine and Applications. Art.*, *721654*, e7.

Christensen, H., Batterham, P., Mackinnon, A., Griffiths, K. M., Kalia Hehir, K., Kenardy, J., & Bennett, K. et al. (2014). Prevention of generalized anxiety disorder using a web intervention, iChill: Randomized controlled trial. *Journal of Medical Internet Research*, *16*(9), e199. doi:10.2196/jmir.3507 PMID:25270886

Creswell, J. D., Irwin, M. R., Burklund, L. J., Lieberman, M. D., Arevalo, J. M. G., Ma, J., & Cole, S. W. et al. (2012). Mindfulness-based stress reduction training reduces loneliness and pro-inflammatory gene expression in older adults: A small randomized controlled trial. *Brain, Behavior, and Immunity*, *26*(7), 1095–1101. doi:10.1016/j.bbi.2012.07.006 PMID:22820409

Dahlin, M., Andersson, G., Magnusson, K., Johansson, T., Sjögren, J., Håkansson, A., & Carlbring, P. et al. (2016). Internet-delivered acceptance-based behaviour therapy for generalized anxiety disorder: A randomized controlled trial. *Behaviour Research and Therapy*, *77*, 86–95. doi:10.1016/j.brat.2015.12.007 PMID:26731173

DiNucci, D. (1999, July). Fragmented future. *Print*, *53*(4), 32.

Drozd, F., Raeder, S., Kraft, P., & Bjørkli, C. A. (2013). Multilevel growth curve analyses of treatment effects of a Web-based intervention for stress reduction: Randomized controlled trial. *Journal of Medical Internet Research*, *15*(4), e84. doi:10.2196/jmir.2570 PMID:23607962

El Morr, C. (2007, May). *Mobile virtual communities in healthcare: Managed self care on the move*. Paper presented at the International Association of Science and Technology for Development – Telehealth Conference, Montreal, Canada.

El Morr, C., Cole, C., & Perl, J. (2014). A health virtual community for patients with chronic kidney disease. *Procedia Computer Science*, *37*, 333–339. doi:10.1016/j.procs.2014.08.049

El Morr, C., & Kawash, J. (2007). Mobile virtual communities research: A synthesis of current trends and a look at future perspectives. *International Journal for Web Based Communities*, *3*(4), 386–403. doi:10.1504/IJWBC.2007.015865

Franca, R. D., & Milbourn, B. (2015). A meta-analysis of mindfulness based interventions (MBIs) show that MBIs are effective in reducing acute symptoms of depression but not anxiety. *Australian Occupational Therapy Journal*, *62*(2), 147–148. doi:10.1111/1440-1630.12198 PMID:25865879

Glück, T. M., & Maercker, A. (2011). A randomized controlled pilot study of a brief web-based mindfulness training. *BMC Psychiatry*, *11*(1), 175. doi:10.1186/1471-244X-11-175 PMID:22067058

Grover, S. L., Teo, S. T. T., Pick, D., & Roche, M. (2016). Mindfulness as a personal resource to reduce work stress in the job demands-resources model. *Stress and Health*. doi: 10.1002/smi.2726

Hansson, E., Tuck, A., Lurie, S., & McKenzie, K. (2010). Improving mental health services for immigrant, refugee, ethno-cultural and racialized groups: Issues and options for service improvement. Report for the Task Group of the Services Systems Advisory Committee, Mental Health Commission of Canada.

Heidelberger, C. A., El-Gayar, O., & Sarnikar, S. (2011, January). *Online health social networks and patient health decision behavior: A research agenda.* Paper presented at the Forty-fourth Hawaii International Conference on System Sciences. doi:10.1109/HICSS.2011.328

Hunot, V., Churchill, R., Teixeira, V., & Silva de Lima, M. (2007). Psychological therapies for generalised anxiety disorder. *Cochrane Database of Systematic Reviews*, (1): CD001848. PMID:17253466

Johnston, A. C., Worrell, J. L., Di Gangi, P. M., & Wasko, M. (2013). Online health communities: An assessment of the influence of participation on patient empowerment outcomes. *Information Technology & People*, *26*(2), 213–235. doi:10.1108/ITP-02-2013-0040

Kabat-Zinn, J. (2003). Mindfulness-based interventions in context: Past, present, and future. *Clinical Psychology: Science and Practice*, *10*(2), 144–156. doi:10.1093/clipsy.bpg016

Kapczinski, F., dos Santos Souza, J. J. S. S., Batista Miralha da Cunha, A. A. B. C., & Schmitt, R. R. S. (2003). Antidepressants for generalized anxiety disorder. *Cochrane Database of Systematic Reviews*, (3): CD003592. PMID:12804478

Kelly, Y., Sacker, A., Del Bono, E., Francesconi, M., & Marmot, M. (2011). What role for the home learning environment and parenting in reducing the socioeconomic gradient in child development? Findings from the Millennium Cohort Study. *Archives of Disease in Childhood*, *96*(9), 832–837. doi:10.1136/adc.2010.195917 PMID:21666278

Koszycki, D., Thake, J., Mavounza, C., Daoust, J. P., Taljaard, M., & Bradwejn, J. (2016). Preliminary investigation of a mindfulness-based intervention for social anxiety disorder that integrates compassion meditation and mindful exposure. *Journal of Alternative and Complementary Medicine (New York, N.Y.)*, *22*(5), 363–374. doi:10.1089/acm.2015.0108 PMID:27070853

Krusche, A., Cyhlarova, E., & Williams, J. M. G. (2013). Mindfulness online: An evaluation of the feasibility of a web-based mindfulness course for stress, anxiety and depression. *BMJ Open*, *3*(11), e003498. doi:10.1136/bmjopen-2013-003498 PMID:24293203

Lappalainen, P., Langrial, S., Oinas-Kukkonen, H., Tolvanen, A., & Lappalainen, R. (2015). Web-based acceptance and commitment therapy for depressive symptoms with minimal support: A randomized controlled trial. *Behavior Modification*, *39*(6), 805–834. doi:10.1177/0145445515598142 PMID:26253644

Levin, M. E., Hayes, S. C., Pistorello, J., & Seeley, J. R. (2016). Web-based self-help for preventing mental health problems in universities: Comparing acceptance and commitment training to mental health education. *Journal of Clinical Psychology*, *72*(3), 207–225. doi:10.1002/jclp.22254 PMID:26784010

Loane, S. S., & DAlessandro, S. (2013). Communication that changes lives: Social support within an online health community for ALS. *Communication Quarterly*, *61*(2), 236–251. doi:10.1080/01463373.2012.752397

Lund, C., Breen, A., Flisher, A. J., Kakuma, R., Corrigall, J., Joska, J. A., & Patel, V. et al. (2010). Poverty and common mental disorders in low and middle income countries: A systematic review. *Social Science & Medicine*, *71*(3), 517–528. doi:10.1016/j.socscimed.2010.04.027 PMID:20621748

Ly, K. H., Trüschel, A., Jarl, L., Magnusson, S., Windahl, T., Johansson, R., & Andersson, G. et al. (2014). Behavioural activation versus mindfulness-based guided self-help treatment administered through a smartphone application: A randomised controlled trial. *BMJ Open, 4*(1), e003440. doi:10.1136/bmjopen-2013-003440 PMID:24413342

Marchand, W. R. (2012). Mindfulness-based stress reduction, mindfulness-based cognitive therapy, and Zen meditation for depression, anxiety, pain, and psychological distress. *Journal of Psychiatric Practice, 18*(4), 233–252. doi:10.1097/01.pra.0000416014.53215.86 PMID:22805898

Matura, L. A., McDonough, A., Aglietti, L. M., Herzog, J. L., & Gallant, K. A. (2013). A virtual community: Concerns of patients with pulmonary hypertension. *Clinical Nursing Research, 22*(2), 155–171. doi:10.1177/1054773812462867 PMID:23093554

Melzer, D., Fryers, T., & Jenkins, R. (2004). *Social inequities and the distribution of common mental disorders*. Hove: Psychology Press.

Mojtabai, R., & Olfson, M. (2006). Treatment seeking for depression in Canada and the United States. *Psychiatric Services (Washington, D.C.), 57*(5), 631–639. doi:10.1176/ps.2006.57.5.631 PMID:16675755

Morledge, T. J., Allexandre, D., Fox, E., Fu, A. Z., Higashi, M. K., Kruzikas, D. T., & Reese, P. R. et al. (2013). Feasibility of an online mindfulness program for stress management - A randomized, controlled trial. *Annals of Behavioral Medicine, 46*(2), 137–148. doi:10.1007/s12160-013-9490-x PMID:23632913

O Leary, K., & Dockray, S. (2015). The effects of two novel gratitude and mindfulness interventions on well-being. *Journal of Alternative and Complementary Medicine (New York, N.Y.), 21*(4), 243–245. doi:10.1089/acm.2014.0119 PMID:25826108

Pearson, C., Janz, T., & Ali, J. (2013). *Mental and substance use disorders in Canada: health at a glance*. Statistics Canada catalogue no. 82-624-X.

Vasconcellos-Silva, P. R., Carvalho, D., & Lucena, C. (2013). Word frequency and content analysis approach to identify demand patterns in a virtual community of carriers of Hepatitis C. *Interactive Journal of Medical Research, 2*(2), e12. doi:10.2196/ijmr.2384 PMID:23827772

Williams, J. M. G., Teasdale, J. D., Segal, Z. V., & Kabat-Zinn, J. (2007). *The mindful way through depression: Freeing yourself from chronic unhappiness*. New York: The Guilford Press.

Wolever, R. Q., Bobinet, K. J., McCabe, K., Mackenzie, E. R., Fekete, E., Kusnick, C., & Baime, M. (2012). Effective and viable mind-body stress reductin in the workplace: A randomized controlled trial. *Journal of Occupational Health Psychology*, *17*(2), 246–258. doi:10.1037/a0027278 PMID:22352291

World Health Organization. (2017). *Depression and other common mental disorders: Global health estimates*. Geneva: World Health Organization.

World Health Organization and the Calouste Gulbenkian Foundation. (2014). *Social determinants of mental health*. Geneva: World Health Organization.

Würtzen, H., Dalton, S. O., Christensen, J., Andersen, K. K., Elsass, P., Flyger, H. L., & Johansen, C. et al. (2015). Effect of mindfulness-based stress reduction on somatic symptoms, distress, mindfulness and spiritual wellbeing in women with breast cancer: Results of a randomized controlled trial. *Acta Oncologica*, *54*(5), 712–719. doi:10.3109/0284186X.2014.997371 PMID:25752972

Zhou, T., Li, X., Pei, Y., Gao, J., & Kong, J. (2016). Internet-based cognitive behavioural therapy for subthreshold depression: A systematic review and meta-analysis. *BMC Psychiatry*, *16*(1), 356. doi:10.1186/s12888-016-1061-9 PMID:27769266

KEY TERMS AND DEFINITIONS

Between-Group Measurement: A measurement about the difference in outcome between two groups of participants in a certain experiment.

Effect Size: A quantification of the difference in an outcome between two groups of participants in a certain experiment.

Mindfulness: “The awareness that emerges through paying attention on purpose, in the present moment, and non-judgmentally to the unfolding of experience moment by moment” Zinn (2003).

Online: Internet based or web based.

Virtual: An experience that is not in the same physical area.

Virtual Community: A group of people meeting online to achieve a goal.

Within-Group Measurement: A measurement about the difference in outcome between two different situations (e.g. usually before and after an intervention has been implemented) within the same group of participants in a certain experiment.

World Health Organization (WHO): An international organization that thrive to “build a better, healthier future for people all over the world” (WHO website).

Chapter 2
Socialization or Social Isolation?
Mental Health Community Support in the Digital Age

Kim Heyes
Manchester Metropolitan University, UK

ABSTRACT

This research project specifically examines the experience of online community support groups as reported by users. The project began out of concern that healthcare providers in the Global North are directing people with mental health problems to online services, without seemingly understanding the impact that this may have on the individuals. The research findings will be of particular interest to mental health practitioners and service providers in the UK and elsewhere in the Global North, and aims to influence decisions made for policies around developing new online mental health services.

INTRODUCTION

There are many people living and surviving in the community with mild to severe mental health problems who do not have easy access to professional health and social care services. Globally, we have started to see a demand for more choice in how healthcare provision is provided, however constant cuts to healthcare budgets in the Global North mean that options such as telehealthcare and online services are seen as a cheaper alternative, and are often billed as a more effective solution

DOI: 10.4018/978-1-5225-2958-3.ch002

(Chambers *et al.*, 2016). This is despite much research showing that there is little to no benefit of this method of support, particularly that of peer to peer online support communities (Eysenbach *et al.,* 2004).

This chapter specifically examines the experience of online community support groups as reported by users. Twenty-five participants answered between one and six open questions posted on three different mental health forums. The research began out of concern that healthcare providers in the Global North are directing people with mental health problems to online self-care or peer to peer support services, which may not be suitable for all mental health patients. Despite a paucity of research showing completion rates of professional online therapeutic support interventions are rare (Simco *et al.*, 2014), those that do complete the set programmes have been found to benefit from the support (Learmonth *et al.*, 2008). However, statistics released in January 2017 by NHS Digital (the UK National Health Service) show that more people than ever are turning up at hospital emergency departments in the UK to receive support for mental health issues (NHS Digital, 2017). Since 2011, the numbers of people going to emergency hospital departments because of their mental ill health has increased by over 50%, and this is also the case for those under the age of 18 (NHS Digital, 2017). This shows that despite a growing number of professional and peer to peer online support services, there may still a growing need for face-to-face intervention.

This chapter suggests that through the identification of positive experiences of online mental health support forums, suitable resources can be developed cheaply and effectively in order to reduce the effects of mental illness, and support those who are unable to find support elsewhere.

BACKGROUND

Worldwide the spending is disproportionately low on mental health (between approximately 2 and 50 USDs per capita), and the lack of financial support has resulted in cuts to services, especially public sector services that support people with mental health problems within their local communities (WHO, 2015). Others are unable to access such support, perhaps due to living arrangements, or because of the negative stigma associated with mental health (Corrigan *et al.,* 2005; Link *et al.*, 1999; Star, 1955). Globally, one in ten people are estimated to have a mental health issue, yet up to two thirds of these do not access any type of support services (WHO, 2015). It is of great concern that budget cuts and negative attitudes to mental health issues may lead to an increase in people isolated through lack of professional service support, so it is vital to understand the social factors that shape the way people may seek support in different formats.

The wellbeing of people with mental ill health is highly related to the experience of social isolation and the lack of social support (Corry 2008; Steptoe *et al.* 2013). More recently, there has been a shift in thinking when it comes to treatments with many patients (in general) taking an active role in deciding on the best method of healthcare provision for themselves (Allen *et al.*, 2016). Brown and Calnan (2016) found that the level of trust between providers and service users was of vital importance. If trust is lost, it can exacerbate mental health issues and increase isolation (Heyes, 2017). However if trust is fostered, then the result is likely to be positive and isolation is reduced. Therefore, it is important that service users have a choice regarding their preferred method of care in order to get the best possible outcome for the individual (Allen *et al.*, 2016; Heyes, 2017).

User-led initiatives (which can also be organised around other health and lifestyle issues), such as cancer support groups and bariatric surgery patient support groups, are part of a wider sociological phenomenon of social movements around self-care and peer patient support (Das & Faxvaag, 2014; Tanis, 2008). These groups are usually informally created, such as individuals with mental ill health issues setting up their own peer to peer support groups, or backed by non-governmental organisations. The central aim of these is to bring users together for mutual support and to reduce isolation (Barak *et al.*, 2008; Mind, n.d.). Therefore, there is a need to examine the specific mechanisms that make up social support to understand who is benefitting from the current provisions (Kawachi and Berkman, 2001; Eysenbach *et al.*, 2004). There are also a great deal of online mental health professionally led community support groups, although there has been less analysis of these (Eysenbach *et al.* 2004). It is apparent that there is a paucity of academic knowledge in this area, which demands research attention in order to maximise the effectiveness of such groups in the wider context of social and health care support (Eysenbach *et al.* 2004).

Political Framework

Understanding a particular political framework when discussing mental ill health is important, as it is often the case that the whole discourse around mental health is a result of political decisions (WHO, 2005). UK social policy focuses on enabling people to live and manage symptoms, as far as possible, within the community and providing that they have the mental capacity to cope (Mental Capacity Act, 2005; The Care Act, 2014; The Mental Health Act, 2007). However, the majority of people with mental ill health living 'within the community' do not benefit from the resources available to them (Morris, 2012). Isolation from meaningful community engagement often leads to loneliness and further co-morbidity issues, such as depression or substance misuse, particularly if subjected to discrimination and abuse (Link *et al.*, 1997). Crabtree and Haslam's (2010) study on positive and negative implications of group identification demonstrated that a group support setting could reinforce supportive frameworks, and that this could outweigh the negativity felt by stigmatisation by non-group members. They recommended that a qualitative study should be conducted to explore the causal variables of relationships within the group settings and the effects that these may have on each individual (Crabtree and Haslam, 2010). There is a vast amount of knowledge about how community support groups are perceived by service users, whether they find them useful and in what ways they are helpful (Cruwys *et al.*, 2013; Steffens *et al.*, 2016; Welbourne *et al.*, 2013), yet there is still little understood about how people utilise online support for mental health issues. Welbourne *et al.*, (2013) suggest that this may be because motivations are often different for other online peer to peer patient groups, so research findings in one online health support area may not necessarily translate to others.

The most recent policy in the UK, The Care Act (2014), was launched on 1st April 2015. The Act focuses on the wellbeing of the individual with care needs, and also that of the carer (as long as they are not a paid service). By signposting these individuals to face-to-face community support services, there is a reliance on creating sufficient support systems in the local area. The cost objectives to creating these communities is to save money in the long run through 'fixing' problems that could arise from isolating people with care needs initially. Often carers of people with disabilities (physical or mental) suffer from mental health problems or physical ill health as a result of their caring role, consequently having to seek expensive health provisions for themselves (paid for through public funding) (Whybrow and Heyes, 2016). Therefore, social connections are important in preventing further or future health issues.

A study by the NIHR (Pinfold *et al.*, 2015), focused on the effects of communities on individuals with severe mental health issues (SMI). This exploration found that the family network can be viewed in many different ways, and these are not always positive, despite good intentions. The findings suggest that those with little familial interaction, but regular interaction with stable service providers (social services/ support worker/ priest and so on) were the happiest in their environment, and were likely to have a better health outcome than those with close family ties and/ or inconsistent relationships with service providers (Pinfold *et al.*, 2015). The lack of understanding around mental health has also lead to some people being segregated from family and friend connections, which could lead to further isolation or seeking identity in other ways, such as within online communities (Link et al, 1999; Pescosolido, 2010).

Isolation and Stigma

Isolation continues to be a significant risk factor for morbidity, across the age spectrum (Holt-Lunstad *et al.*, 2015). There are many people for whom isolation is not an option, but something that is forced on them through age or ill-health, and a vast number of those people may not get the help they need (Hawkley and Cacioppo, 2010; Uchino, 2006). Online support may mean that vastly more people get access to the support they need as and when it is required rather than having to wait for a GP or counselling appointment (Learmonth *et al.*, 2008).

The stigma surrounding mental ill health is still concerning, particularly as it has been found to have a detrimental effect on help-seeking (Clement *et al,* 2015). Recent data collected by Schomerus *et al.* (2016) showed that even when members of the general public expressed understanding of mental ill health, attitudes towards acceptance of people with mental health issues are not altered. Although this experiment was a relatively small sample (n=1679), the findings show how important it is for mental health professionals to approach public attitudes in the future. Similarly, a recent study by NSUN (National Survivor User Network) for mental health in the UK (Beresford *et al.*, 2015), found that service users believed that stigma was still evident in social dealings on a daily basis. The general belief held, was that stigma around mental health was formed by an outdated understanding of the medical model (Beresford *et al.*, 2015).

Mental health issues, tend to be predominantly diagnosed using the medical model of the Diagnostic and Statistical Manual of Mental Disorders (DSM), however there are many people living and surviving in the community with mild to severe mental health problems who do not have access to medical or psychological support and/or would not welcome professional labelling or intervention. It is not fully understood what causes mental illness, or indeed if mental illness really exists (see Szasz, 1961, for arguments around this). Frances (2013) argues that the DSM is a way of creating control within society and of the medical profession, maintaining governance over what is normal and abnormal. The DSM is not necessarily an accurate portrayal of mental ill health, but it is generally accepted as the diagnostic criteria for most of the world's mental state (Frances, 2013).

Medical approaches to treating individuals with mild to moderate mental ill health issues in the UK can vary from involuntary incarceration, to providing signposting information about charitable services that can help with grief or suicidal thoughts, medication, and referral to counselling or online support services. However, Evans-Lacko *et al.,* (2013) argue that despite this range of possible medical actions, in general, medication is relied upon in general practice and in hospital care. They go onto note that mental illness should be treated as seriously as physical illness and that this need for dealing earnestly with mental health issues is increasingly important (Evans-Lacko *et al.,* 2013). However, there is a dominant and continuing lack of will in treating and understanding mental ill health, both socially and medically (for example see Maclure, 1988; Cuijpers, 2003; and Frances, 2013). It is therefore important to understand how individuals feel about their own mental health, and their choices and preferences in how they want to receive help and support (Heyes and Whybrow, 2016; The Care Act, 2014).

Health research is also still fixated on the idea of the medical model, with little psychological research into online mental health forums utilising a social constructionist approach (Burr, 2015). However, some health researchers (Link et al, 1999; Pescosolido, 2010), focus on interpersonal dynamics and social networks which highlight the issues of social withdrawal and link to community theories. Yuill et al., (2010) advocate the idea that a true perspective on health can only come from a consideration of both medical and social models for mental health, creating a pathway for multidisciplinary research in mental health.

Online Communities

Online forums have become commonplace amongst internet users worldwide. The number of worldwide users hit 3 billion in 2014, and is now approximately 3.5 billion in 2017, which is approximately 46% of the world's population (internetlivestats.com, 2017: online). Several hundred thousand forums now exist on the internet, with the number growing exponentially on a daily basis (Carroll, 2014). In Japan in 2007, the top discussion forum, 2-channel, was receiving in excess of 2.5 million posts per day (Carroll, 2014). This has since closed down, but currently one of the most popular worldwide sites, Reddit, receives approximately 1.5m users per day, with around 40,000 subscribers to their mental health threads (Reddit.com, 2015: online).

The idea that society has easy access to everything because it is on the internet may be a misnomer. The NHS in the UK (for example) puts information on the internet to make sure that it is easily and readily accessible, most businesses have websites that are 'user friendly', and adverts tell us to look online for further information. However, it is not easily accessible to the 54% of the world's population that do not have internet access. There are also varying reasons as to why the 46% that could in theory access the internet, may not. Illiteracy, learning difficulties, and fear, are just a few reasons that may prevent online activity. Those who are comfortable with using the internet are therefore given options about how to utilise the choice given to all consumers, whether that is which healthcare services to use, or where to buy their groceries. The people in society that may already be able to gain information from multiple sources are choosing whether to consume information online, and this can be for convenience, personal preference, or accessibility. However, those who do not find online information accessible may miss out, as it may be assumed that information has reached everyone because of its online presence.

Patient forums have gained in popularity (Blank and Adams-Blodnieks, 2005; Neal *et al.*, 2007). The idea of the expert patient in the UK means that those with health needs are encouraged to learn about their conditions so that they can be best placed to manage them (Coulthard *et al.*, 2013; Davidson *et al.*, 2012). There are now many thousands of Mental Health community support groups online, and they provide various methods of information and support. The majority of the specialised forums will link (via 'click through' hyperlinks) to easy to read information produced by public health bodies. However, some rely on the information provided by their members, with potential problems such as misinformation being an issue (Neal *et al.,* 2007). Consumer choice means that people can search the various forums and decide which one they wish to participate in. In order to participate, the consumer must feel as though they will learn to trust the forum, trust the other users, but most importantly, they need to feel as though they can participate and get some support (Easterbrook and Vignoles, 2013; Hornsey and Jetten, 2004; Guo and Cheng, 2016). Noelle-Neumann's (1974) Spiral of Silence theory states that people within society needed to gauge public opinion in order to understand how they can interact on a similar level to avoid isolating themselves. Therefore, it is imperative that the forum chosen by the consumer is one that shares similar ideas and opinions as themselves. As with offline support groups, if the user does not feel as though they are part of the ingroup, they may refrain from the group, and isolation may continue (Tajfel and Turner, 1979). The similarity to offline groups can also mean that those who struggle to participate in offline face-to-face interactions may also struggle to participate in online communities.

Definitions of community vary greatly, however they tend to focus on community being a group of people with a common interest or that are geographically linked (Delanty, 2010, McMillan and Chavis, 1986). Using a virtual platform that does not feel as constricted as face to face contact may enable vulnerable people to explore support systems that they may feel unable to access in the 'real' (offline) world (Bell, 2007). For example, those who hide their mental health issues in everyday society may feel as though they can be open and honest with those in a virtual capacity due to the anonymity of the sphere (Suler, 2004). Most beneficial to users is the anonymity of being online (Daine *et al.,* 2013), particularly if the stigma of having a mental health problem is something that they are trying to escape. However, forums that are receiving 1.5 million hits per day tend to have so many threads added every minute, that it can be difficult for all posts to be seen by users. The consequences of this could be that someone who is asking for help for the first time may be missed, and they will think that they are unwelcome, ignored and therefore, become further isolated (Daine *et al*, 2013).

Woong Yun and Park (2011) looked at the relationships of participants of online communities, and found that often people act the same way within forums as they would do in offline ('real') life. This means that if they are open and trusting in the offline environment, they will be the same online. However, Schiel (2005) states that a person who is not really known to us cannot be a friend and therefore must not be trusted. Blanchard *et al.,* (2011) believed that trust was an important aspect of fostering relationships within virtual communities, and generally, people followed normal social practices expected in an offline community. They found that sanctioning behaviours when someone had acted inappropriately were also an important aspect of fulfilling normal social practices, so when members could rely on others to sanction inappropriate behaviour, trust within the community would grow (Blanchard *et al.,* 2011). However, trolling has become an issue in recent years, particularly within social media, and along with this research, has been shown to decrease trust within virtual spheres, and therefore may increase negative online experiences for users (Herring *et al.,* 2002; Heyes, 2017; Phillips, 2015; Rafferty, 2011).

There is, however, a sense of community created by a shared identity (Ren *et al.,* 2012). In the case of mental health forums, people may be seeking information and advice from people who have had similar experiences (Ren *et al.,* 2012; Tate and Zabinski, 2004). This help may boost self-esteem if the individual has found a community that they can identify with (King and Moreggi, 1998; Ren *et al.,* 2012). The 'field' of virtual community support groups may therefore be a platform that can replicate face-to-face community support groups, and the security of the individuals' identity within this (Tate and Zabinski, 2004; Wood, 1989; Yalom and Leczcz, 2005).

Although the study of online community support groups is somewhat different to the offline groups, the comparison between online and offline is necessary in order to fully understand if there are significant differences. Richardson (2015) ascertains that online and offline should not be considered as completely different entities, as both are communities built through complex multi-dimensional relationships. The on and offline segregation should perhaps therefore be reconsidered as different ways of forging relationships, these being within different social spaces (online) and via different modes (through forums, blogging sites or social media). These different fields may then require different research methods, or the adaption of existing methods in order to revolutionize community psychology and social theory research (Kozinets, 2010).

Baym (1995) had been a participant of an online group before deciding to conduct her research. Over three years she asked questions, took surveys and analysed the text, her method being an ethnographic one that progressed over time, alongside her own understanding of the group. The idea of virtual research evolving as it happens is also supported by Chandler (2016). She found that the lack of rich data in some forums meant that her data collection methods needed to evolve alongside the researchers understanding of forum participation. Chandler (2016) found that in order to maximise the participants to her work on self-harm, she utilised the mass forum Reddit. This provided an inordinate amount of participant responses and yielded some interesting and good quality data. This type of ethnographic research has been termed virtual ethnography, and is a growing phenomenon in online research (Rheingold, 2003). In this particular research (Heyes, 2017), virtual ethnography also involves the idea of the researcher being a 'tolerated observer' (Hine, 2010: 10), a presence that is apparent to the participant, but does not hinder the information given. Markham (2004) believes that ethnographic research in general has flaws, however, the lack of physical cues in virtual ethnography could actually add to, rather than inhibit the analysis of the research.

METHOD

A virtual ethnography study was conducted over a three month period between July 2015 and October 2015. Sixty-five participants answered between one and six questions on one of three forums: 1) a forum created for the purpose of the research called communitysupportmh.freeforums.net; 2) threads set up within Reddit's mental health section; and 3) a peer to peer community support forum that wished to remain anonymous (See Figure 1). No further information was taken about the participants, and there was no follow up contact (apart from to remind them that

Figure 1. Method timeline

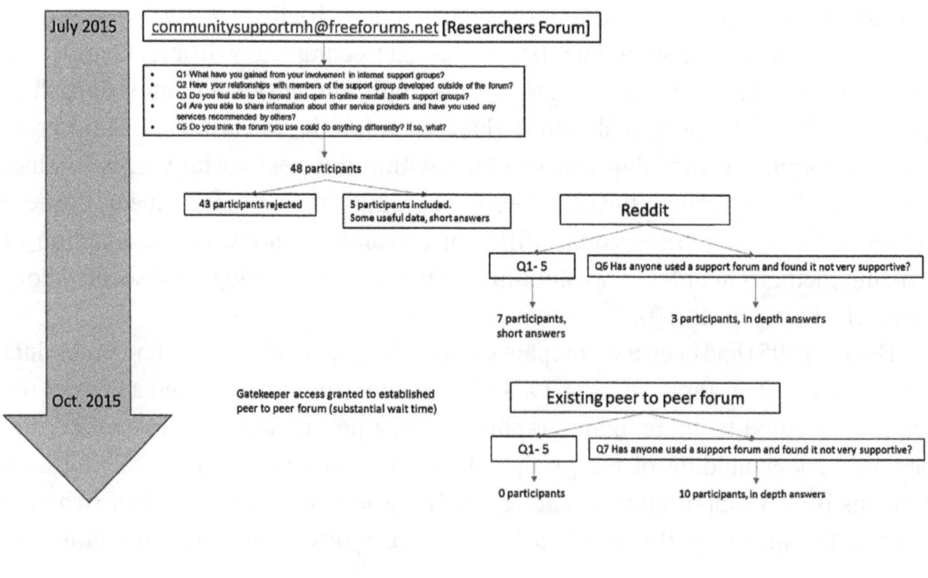

they could withdraw from the study if they wished). Forty-three participants were disqualified from the research due to giving identifying features or not meeting the criteria (i.e. when asked what they gained from being part of a support forum, replied that they had never used one). Gender was not deemed an important factor within this research, and as such, names of the participants were anonymized using an online name generator (http://myusernamegenerator.com/) to avoid gender bias. Open questions were posted as individual threads on each forum in order to create free flowing dialogue. Ethical approval was granted by Manchester Metropolitan University Ethics committee in July 2015.

FINDINGS

The research data was analysed manually using thematic analysis (Boyatzis, 1998; Braun and Clarke, 2006), and second coded using NVivo 11. Through coding, several themes began to emerge. These were reduced to three main issues: safety; support; and network sociality. Minor themes included balance, normality and separate spheres (of offline and online worlds). It emerged that if at least one of the main themes was in place, the participant was likely to have a positive experience of online community support, and therefore, an increased feeling of socialization. If all of the themes were negative, the experience is likely to be negative, and the result would be an increase in social isolation. The minor themes were present in the positive experiences; however, further research needs to be conducted to find the relationship between these themes and the negative experiences (see Figure 2).

Figure 2. A model of online support experiences

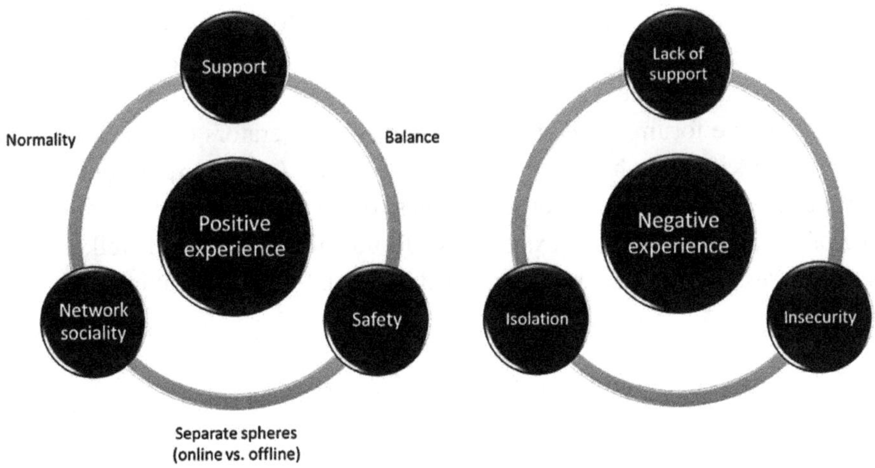

DATA ANALYSIS

The analysis of the themes that emerged can be put into three main categories: Safety, Security and Network Sociality. These encompass a number of other areas that were brought up, including trust, the balance between on and offline life, and how normal the person feels. This section shows how the data were analysed in order for the researcher to defend these three main themes.

Safety

As discussed in the literature review, and confirmed by Brown and Calnan's. (2016) study and Blanchard *et al.*'s (2011) model, trust can be an issue for members of online communities, however, this does not necessarily deter them from online social engagement. Not being able to participate in real life means that alternative methods of group participation are sought, however it may not be identified as 'true' interaction but a 'disembedded subjectivity that is somehow 'lifted out'' (Giddens, 1984, cited in Wittel, 2001: 51), a concept that can help some of the participants feel safer.

Online communities are an unknown entity, and trying to build a sense of a shared social space can be difficult when the participants may have different notions of culture and societal norms (Ostrum, *et al.*, 1993). Safety therefore comes from a sense of 'good' culture within an online mental health community: one that is supportive; offers help and advice; and has participants with similar (perceived) social capital.

However, even when praising one of the forums, many participants still brought up issues and bad experiences they had had previously with other forums. The majority of people still struggled to trust other online participants, being wary of 'exploitative' and 'sneaky people', whilst also expressing defeatist attitudes towards expecting policies to be followed, or for moderators to do anything. The shared culture of the community can then turn into a bad experience and threatens the individual's idea of a safe environment.

Part of online forums is the fact that there are moderators or senior members keeping users safe from harm, which in Urowa's case (names are generated from an online name generator) did not seem to help or keep the participants from harm. Some of the participants gave examples of forums that had started well, but then went on to destroy the trust that people had in them. Unayi, describing it as:

Unayi: *[A forum] was 100% anonymous. The sneaky people trying to squeeze people for personal details happened every few sessions I connected to in the last few weeks it was open. Creepy.*
Trusting anonymous people on the internet is not recommended in any situation. [Reddit, Q6]

The experience of having their safety compromised reminded several participants of experiences of offline interactions. Seven of the participants stated that they do not trust people outside of the internet either, with Unayi admitting that they would not trust their spouse or their friends 'to act in my best interest'. Schiel (2005) agrees, stating that people cannot be treated as friends if they are an unknown entity. The idea that the online community is made up of people that may have no real similar offline capital, means that they could never be trusted as they probably have an ulterior motive (Schiel, 2005).

However, there were many participants who felt as though it was easier to trust people on the internet that those offline, particularly on the basis of their shared identity (Tate and Zabinski, 2004; Suler, 2004):

Udefwl: *(I am) More honest than I can be face to face with people* [Researchers Forum, Q3]
Poufi: *Far more honest than I could be with friends and family* [Researchers Forum, Q3]
Vafez: *I have made some really nice friends on here and they have not judged me for being different.* [MHF, Q7]

Those who feel unable to be open and honest in their offline relationships (perhaps due to the nature of their mental health issues), can find it easier to be open and honest with strangers who share similar health issues, and also easier to offer support. The safety of these interactions comes from the anonymity that may make other people fearful of online interaction (Daine *et al.*, 2013; Guo and Cheng, 2016), and this can cause conflict for the participants when trying to find a safe community in which they feel comfortable enough to become a permanent part of. If they do not feel a sense of safety in online interactions, they are unlikely to feel supported in an online community support forum.

Support

Participants offered their comments as helpful support, even if they had no 'real' (professional) insights to offer. This could be that by providing a support mechanism to others by offering encouragement actually makes them feel better about themselves, rather than directly seeking help for their own issues. They do not feel that they are burdening others with their own stories and have the associated positive feelings of altruism (Brown and Calnan 2016). One of the participants specifically noted that writing their own posts made them feel anxious, but commenting on other people's posts made them feel good.

Other participants did not realise that they were participating to feel better about themselves. An example of this kind of interaction is that of Jaqdudi (Reddit), who had participated and lurked in several forums, was sceptical of the support that they offer. Some of these interactions were trying to show that they were actually part of 'normal' offline interaction, they were just passing by and happened to stop to comment.

Jaqdudi: *I don't honestly have many problems that can't be solved by Googling a specific question or maybe talking to my friends.* [Reddit, Q6]

However, interwoven in between this scepticism of receiving support through forums, they also try and act as though they would still be ok with receiving support – when asked if they have thought about using the forums for more than they already have, the reply was 'Sure, if the need arises'. It is interesting that they have felt the need to be lurking on a mental health forum, and also felt compelled to answer the research question even though they deny the need for support. Jaqdudi was one of the people that posted the most in terms of discussion about the use of forums, but also seemed to be unable to express (perhaps even unaware of) how they use support forums. Through being helpful and answering research questions and supporting others, they may not perceive themselves as needing support at all.

This need for reassurance of being normal was also seen in some of the other participants, expressing how many close friends or family members they have in the offline world, trying to give an air of flippancy to their answers. This guarded behaviour shows that participants such as Jaqdudi, like to be part of a community, but do not feel as though they can ask for support. This may be due to a lack of trust, or that they may be cautious about giving too much information about themselves on a platform that users are often told to be wary of giving too much information to, due to the few that abuse the system. This could drive the participants into becoming part of the out-group in the online communities, resulting in them becoming segregated from the community. However, it could also mean that they are receiving personal gratification through supporting others, and therefore do not need to divulge personal information in order to benefit from being part of the community (Welbourne *et al.,* 2013).

Network Sociality

Being social is something that comes naturally to some people, and as discussed in the literature review, is difficult for those who are seen as being deviant from dominant social norms around their health and wellbeing. Network sociality is not so much wanting to be part of a social community, but is the need for interaction in order to understand one's own identity (Wittel, 2001). Those seeking online health support communities generally want to find or exchange, informational and/ or emotional support (Welbourne *et al.,* 2013). This identity and support seeking is evident throughout the data, and this section will explore isolation, identity and consumerism through the over-arching concept of network sociality.

Through the analysis, it is clear from the number of participants that had been part of multiple forums (at least 8), that the choice afforded by the amount of community support forums subjects users to (at least) as much consumerism as they would be offline. They can decide how many forums they wish to engage in, and whether to lurk, participate or go elsewhere. These choices are helpful to those who may not want to seek advice from a GP or offline services, however the possibility to use orthodox health and wellbeing services is still there for those who may wish to do so, and if necessary they can chose whether to use them concurrently. However, trying to find a supportive community that is right for the individual can prove difficult for people with mental ill health. The stigma of having a mental health problem in offline communities can be the cause of individuals seeking solace in the online world (Goffman, 1963; Link, *et al.*, 1997). Therefore, participating in any community, online or offline, can cause feelings of anxiety and uncertainty about how one's posts will be received and responded to by others.

As one participant states:

Ripem: *Writing about my own issues as a new post gives me anxiety (probably the vulnerability aspect)[sic].* [Reddit, Q1]

The idea of disclosing personal information for someone with mental health problems can be fraught with fear of the consequences. For an individual to decide to disclose this type of information to a new community can be seen as a huge risk. This leads participants to describe a process of 'lurking' on the forums before actually making that crucial first post and connecting to an online community.

One participant mentioned quietly evaluating forums, prior to actively being involved through posting. Although the actual numbers of those who lurk online in forums and never post personal information is not known, the activity is commonly discussed in literature about the use of online forums (Schneider *et al.*, 2013; Rafaeli *et al.*, 2004). The participants want to become part of the community, so lurking can help them to assess if the people already contributing are similar to them, reducing the possibility of alienating themselves from the offset (Blanchard *et al.*, 2010; Bourdieu, 1990; Noelle- Neumann, 1977). Six of the ten participants of the established Mental Health Forum expressed that they were constantly fearful about isolating themselves from the offline world, rather than worrying about not fitting in with the online world.

Three of the participants were unclear on the role of online relationships within the context of broader social experiences, they noted the aim for online forums is to enhance interactions with others. Similarly, Jawodaza notes that interaction with others is important, but s/he struggles with friendships in the 'real world', so utilises the forum as a method of interaction and support without the emotional ties of friendship. S/he also states that having this form of interaction is better than nothing at all:

Jawodaza: *If you feel up for having 'real' company, but are choosing to go online instead, it probably is worth giving yourself a boot up the backside and start getting out a bit more.*
But sometimes it's not that straightforward. I don't have many friends, the friends I do have are older and have their own families/lives.
Though even if I had people to socialise with, sometimes it's really difficult.
So for me it's better to be on here than have nothing. X [sic] [MHF, Q7]

Getting the balance right between online and offline interaction was a common concern amongst the participants on all three forums. Argyle (1969) argues that human interaction is a necessity and Steptoe *et al.* (2013) back up this contention by stating that those who are isolated from physical interaction have a higher risk of mortality. However, Kendall (2002) and Hine (2004; 2008) believe that technology has moved on considerably in recent decades and that limited human face to face interaction may not be as mortifying as it once was. Younger generations have grown up with online social relationships, and therefore, these types of interaction may prove to be more beneficial than having no offline contact at all. Kendall (2002) also states that most people do not use the internet instead of living offline, blending the online and offline worlds provides benefits, without having to worry about one type of interaction dominating one's life.

In line with Kendall's (2002) vision of the benefits of a 'blended world', thirteen of the participants stated that they felt comfortable with a blending of worlds, by utilising online support when they feel as though they are unable to cope with human interaction:

Kabeegi and Exogu both expressed that they found it difficult to talk to people in the real world, particularly if they do not have experience of similar mental health issues. By seeking support online, they feel more comfortable and are able to be honest about their feelings. This could be due to the shared values created through previous interactions on the forums, or a shared illness (and therefore understanding of what each other may be going through).

However, two of the participants saw the interactions between offline and online as separate spheres that provide an alternative place to air feelings and ideas, with no other agenda:

Vafez: *...cant mix with real people outside,.... this forum is great and a life saver for me* [MHF, Q7]

Jaxuq: *i find them helpful as i cant do real interaction with ppl [people] except my parents who work [sic]* [MHF, Q7]

These posts from Vafez and Jaxuq, emphasise interaction online and offline as separate arenas, the online space providing unique opportunities for mental health discussion. There is an interesting theme here, which also emerged elsewhere in the data, of online interaction not being 'real'. However, it clearly is real in the sense that it achieves interactional imperatives in terms of relating to another person and is valued by these respondents. Being online though allows a sense of 'playing at' interaction and experience, the stakes are not so high as face to face. This idea of 'playing' at being online is similar to those who utilise online games to help escape from the real world into a fantasy one (Hine, 2004; Calleja, 2010). Escapism could be therapeutic, allowing some relief from mental health issues, and summoning up support from those who appear to understand you, in a non-threatening way (Calleja, 2010).

However, choosing a forum in which to participate can itself be a difficult task, and one that is not as simple as just lurking until the right one is found because of the emergent and fast-changing nature of these social spaces:

Unayi: *...good ones [forums] can go bad quickly. [A forum] was originally brilliant, then it started to fill up with [..] assholes along with exploitative people...* [Reddit, Q6]

Urowa: *Most of the listeners [through support chat on the forum] did their best to change the subject. Then there was one who first started telling me who I can and can't consider a friend and then gave me a nopology [opposite of apology] when I confronted him.* [Reddit, Q6]

The participants reported that forums could quickly change and 'go bad' with changes in who was using them, arguments and disagreements, breaking out or trolling. Participants were asked if they had had any negative experiences of forums and to expand on why these were not good. Four participants, similar to Unayi and Urowa's experiences in the quotes above, expressed that they had on occasion had disagreements with other forum members and were dissatisfied with the way that it was handled. In these cases, they typically went on to describe how they no longer trusted anyone online or offline, despite the fact that they claimed to have good friends and other social relationships. Urowa however, described their experience as unfortunate rather than confidence destroying, and was disappointed with the way that their particular issue was handled. In this case, the site moderators did not want to get involved, despite having a clear behaviour policy on the site. This is ultimately an illustration spanning all three of the main themes, and showing that they are indeed linked to whether or not a person has a positive or a negative experience of online community support.

Despite these difficulties, eight of the participants argued that identifying with the people in a community support forum can be the key to success and were positive about their experience. Knowing that there were other people having/ or had been through similar experiences seemed to give the participants a sense of relief in having found 'normality':

Imeifl: *I've gained happiness in finally reading about other people like me. I've heard they exist, but until I discovered [a forum], I could never know for certain* [Researchers Forum, Q1]

Thoqwhon: *For me, I can be the 'real me' on here. ... I find it near impossible to let [my friends and family] know that I'm not good and I try to be smiley to deflect concerns.* [MHF, Q7]

These participants seemed to have found a sense of identity authenticity that they could not display elsewhere. Having a sense of being like others and sharing issues is important. They feel accepted within this community and they no longer have to pretend in order to fit into offline society's idea of normal. In the online support forums, the majority of the participants feel that they have become part of an in-group (Tajfel and Turner, 1979; Yalom and Leczcz, 2005; Tate and Zabinski, 2004; Wood, 1989; Bourdieu, 1985) which can boost self-esteem and reduce feelings of anxiety and isolation (King and Moreggi, 1998).

CONCLUSION

This research sought to investigate and clarify what was important about the interactions within virtual mental health support groups and to provide an insight into these communities in order to influence policy and practice. By assessing the impact of online support networks for people with mental ill health, it has become clear that there are gaps in social policies and health care provision. Social constructions that surround mental ill health make it easy for vulnerable people to become invisible in society due to isolation (Corry, 2008; Steptoe *et al.*, 2013), and people can be reluctant to look at alternatives, such as online sources. Face to face mental health support groups, or negative experiences in online community spaces may have detrimental effects on people with mental health issues seeking alternatives.

The research found that there were benefits to most of the participants in terms of creating support networks that would take the place of, or supplement offline communities, and therefore as a result would reduce isolation. There were some negative consequences however, and the reluctance of some participants to fully immerse themselves into online communities meant that they used multiple sites without any affiliation to a particular community. This could make the individual feel further segregated from being supported by a community, and therefore more isolated than before initial online contact.

Users of the community support groups are generally positive about the support that they receive, and find it beneficial to communicate with people with similar experiences. However, the few who have had negative experiences reported that they no longer have any trust in the groups. Those with security issues however, keep using forums but err on the side of caution by not giving away too much personal information.

Good quality online support groups with a high level of peer support seem to be difficult to find, despite the number available. Forums that are successful usually have hundreds or even thousands of users daily, which makes them susceptible to exploitation. In turn, they either close down, or users may leave to find alternatives. They are useful in creating network sociality, providing a community in-group, and helping to boost self-esteem, thus enhancing quality of life for those who are isolated in offline communities. These are however, difficult to set up and can take a long time to attract members, which can be problematic in terms of creating the ideal solution for online community support for mental ill health. The model of online support, in Figure 2, aims to help with building understanding of the impact of this type of social support, although further research needs to be completed in order to recognise how this can be used to influence policy and practice.

One issue that should be addressed around information provided on the internet, is the assumption that everyone accesses it. With around 56% of the world's population still without access to the internet, this assumption can leave vulnerable people without the help they need. However, to those that are able to access it, the amount of information about mental ill health available online can be valuable to people, especially as cuts to funding look set to continue despite numbers of people diagnosed with mental health conditions rising. Lengthy waiting lists for counsellors and specialists may force people to seek alternatives, and those with access to online services may find their consumer prowess is vital in receiving alternative care. However, more research into the effectiveness of this is necessary, and will be a continual process over the coming years as the nature of the consumer changes.

It is also imperative that we do not assume that because the individual has access to the internet, that they will then wish to utilise this as their main method of treatment. Some people will continue to use face-to-face methods as their preference, or they may decide to refuse any treatment at all. Through offering choices in healthcare provision, we must ultimately respect the decision of the individual.

FUTURE RESEARCH DIRECTIONS

The idea of community being similar online to offline is something that has not been explored in great detail within social or community psychology, and it is therefore difficult to ascertain how best to utilise these communities or engage those who are still isolated. The changing nature of online also means that research needs to stay current. The changes in technology and the increase in the use of social media, predict that the interwoven nature of online and offline will become more complex, particularly when vulnerability such as mental ill health is taken into consideration, and where the individual is at in their life stage (Hine, 2008; Third *et al.*, 2014). Bridging to other support mechanisms has not been something that has been found within this research, and it is important that when seeking alternatives to conventional methods of support (i.e. offline), the participants of online support forums need to be careful that they are not self-diagnosing, or hiding a problem that needs medical attention. Therefore, the next stage of this research will be to conduct in depth interviews with users of online mental health community support to understand why they utilise online support, and if they felt it was beneficial.

REFERENCES

Allen, D., Braithwaite, J., Sandall, J., & Waring, J. (2016). Towards a sociology of healthcare safety and quality. *Sociology of Health & Illness*, *38*(2), 181–197. doi:10.1111/1467-9566.12390 PMID:26679563

Argyle, M. (1969). *Social Interaction*. London: Methuen.

Barak, A., Boniel-Nissim, M., & Suler, J. (2008). Fostering empowerment in online support groups. *Computers in Human Behavior*, *24*(5), 1867–1883. doi:10.1016/j.chb.2008.02.004

Baym, N. (1995). The emergence of community in computer-mediated communication. In S. Jones (Ed.), *Cybersociety* (pp. 35–68). Thousand Oaks, CA: SAGE.

Bell, V. (2007). Online information, extreme communities, and Internet therapy: Is the Internet good for our mental health? *Journal of Mental Health (Abingdon, England)*, *16*(4), 445–457. doi:10.1080/09638230701482378

Beresford, P., Perring, R., Nettle, M., & Wallcraft, J. (2015). *From mental illness to a social model of madness and distress*. Retrieved on January 12, 2017 from http://www.shapingourlives.org.uk/wp-content/uploads/2016/05/FROM-MENTAL-ILLNESS-PDF-2.pdf

Blanchard, A. L., Welbourne, J. L., & Boughton, M. D. (2011). A model of online trust: The mediating role of norms and sense of virtual community. *Information Communication and Society*, *14*(1), 76–106. doi:10.1080/13691181003739633

Blank, T. O., & Adams-Blodnieks, M. (2005). The who and the what of usage of two cancer online communities. *Computers in Human Behavior*, *23*(3), 1249–1257. doi:10.1016/j.chb.2004.12.003

Bourdieu, P. (1983). The field of cultural production, or: The economic world reversed. *Poetics*, *12*(4-5), 311–356. doi:10.1016/0304-422X(83)90012-8

Bourdieu, P. (1985). The genesis of the concepts of Habitus and of Field. *Sociocriticism*, *2*, 11–24.

Bourdieu, P. (1990). *The logic of practice*. Cambridge, UK: Polity Press.

Boyatzis, R. E. (1998). *Transforming Qualitative Information*. London: Sage.

Braithwaite, J., Sandall, J., & Waring, J. (2016). Towards a sociology of healthcare safety and quality. *Sociology of Health & Illness*, *38*(2), 181–197. doi:10.1111/1467-9566.12390 PMID:26679563

Braun, V., & Clarke, V. (2006). Using thematic analysis in psychology. *Qualitative Research in Psychology*, *3*(32), 77–101. doi:10.1191/1478088706qp063oa

Brown, P. R., & Calnan, M. W. (2016). Chains of (dis)trust: exploring the underpinnings of knowledge-sharing and quality care across mental health services. In *An Introduction to Social Constructionism*. London: Routledge. doi:10.1002/9781119276371.ch7

Calleja, G. (2010). Digital games and Escapism. *Games and Culture*, *5*(4), 335–353. doi:10.1177/1555412009360412

Carroll, J. M. (2014). *The neighborhood in the Internet: Design research projects in community*. London: Routledge.

Chambers, R., Schmid, M., & Birch-Jones, J. (2016). *Digital Healthcare: the essential guide*. Oxford, UK: Otmoor Publishing.

Chandler, A. (2016). *Self-Injury, Medicine and Society: Authentic Bodies*. London: Palgrave Macmillan. doi:10.1057/978-1-137-40528-9

Clement, S., Schauman, O., Graham, T., Maggioni, F., Evans-Lacko, S., Bezborodovs, N., & Thornicroft, G. et al. (2015). What is the impact of mental health-related stigma on help-seeking? A systematic review of quantitative and qualitative studies. *Psychological Medicine*, *45*(1), 11–27. doi:10.1017/S0033291714000129 PMID:24569086

Corrigan, P. W., Kerr, A., & Knudsen, L. (2005). The stigma of mental illness: Explanatory models and methods for change. *Applied & Preventive Psychology*, *11*(3), 179–190. doi:10.1016/j.appsy.2005.07.001

Corry, P. (2008). *Stigma shout: service user and carer experiences of stigma and discrimination*. London: Time to Change.

Coulthard, K., Patel, D., Brizzolara, C., Morriss, R., & Watson, S. (2013). A feasibility study of expert patient and community mental health team led bipolar psychoeducation groups: Implementing an evidence based practice. *BMC Psychiatry*, *13*(1), 301. doi:10.1186/1471-244X-13-301 PMID:24215655

Crabtree, J. W., Haslam, S. A., Postmes, T., & Haslam, C. (2010). Mental Health Support Groups, Stigma, Self-Esteem: Positive and Negative Implications of Group Identification. *The Journal of Social Issues*, *66*(3), 553–569. doi:10.1111/j.1540-4560.2010.01662.x

Cruwys, T., Dingle, G. A., Haslam, C., Haslam, A. S., Jetten, J., & Morton, T. A. (2013). Social group memberships protect against future depression, alleviate depression symptoms and prevent depression relapse. *Social Science & Medicine*, *98*, 179–186. doi:10.1016/j.socscimed.2013.09.013 PMID:24331897

Cuijpers, P. (2003). Examining the Effects of Prevention Programs on the Incidence of New Cases of Mental Disorders: The Lack of Statistical Power. *The American Journal of Psychiatry*, *160*(8), 1385–1391. doi:10.1176/appi.ajp.160.8.1385 PMID:12900296

Daine, K., Hawton, K., Singaravelu, V., Stewart, A., Simkin, S., & Montgomery, P. (2013). The power of the web: A systematic review of studies of the influence of the Internet on self-harm and suicide in young people. *PLoS ONE*, *8*(10), e77555. doi:10.1371/journal.pone.0077555 PMID:24204868

Das, A., & Faxvaag, A. (2014). What Influences Patient Participation in an Online Forum for Weight Loss Surgery? A Qualitative Case Study. *Interact J Med Res.*, *3*(1), e4. doi:10.2196/ijmr.2847 PMID:24509408

Davidson, L., Bellamy, C., Guy, K., & Miller, R. (2012). Peer support among persons with severe mental illnesses: A review of evidence and experience. *World Psychiatry; Official Journal of the World Psychiatric Association (WPA)*, *11*(2), 123–128. doi:10.1016/j.wpsyc.2012.05.009 PMID:22654945

Delanty, G. (2010). *Community*. London: Routledge.

Department of Health. (2001). *The Expert Patient: A New Approach to Chronic Disease Management*. London: Department of Health.

Digital, N. H. S. (2017). *Hospital accident and emergency activity, 2015-16*. Retrieved on January 11, 2017, from http://www.content.digital.nhs.uk/catalogue/PUB23070

Easterbrook, M., & Vignoles, V. L. (2013). What does it mean to belong? Interpersonal bonds and intragroup similarities as predictors of felt belonging in different types of groups. *European Journal of Social Psychology*, *43*(6), 455–462.

Evans-Lacko, S., Henderson, C., & Thornicroft, G. (2013). Public knowledge, attitudes and behaviour regarding people with mental illness in England 20092012. *The British Journal of Psychiatry*, *202*(s55), 51–57. doi:10.1192/bjp.bp.112.112979

Eysenbach, G., Powell, J., Englesakis, M., Rizo, C., & Stern, A. (2004). Health related virtual communities and electronic support groups: Systematic review of the effects of online peer to peer interactions. *BMJ (Clinical Research Ed.)*, 328. PMID:15142921

Frances, A. (2013). *Saving normal: An insider's revolt against out-of-control psychiatric diagnosis, DSM-5, big pharma and the medicalization of ordinary life*. Retrieved November 15, 2015, from http://search.informit.com.au/documentSummary;dn=464019439257830;res=IELHEA>

Giddens, A. (1984). *The Constitution of Society*. Cambridge, UK: Polity.

Goffman, E. (1963). *Stigma: notes on the management of spoiled identity*. New York: Simon and Schuster Inc.

Guo, T.-C., & Cheng, Z.-C. (2016). Sense of belonging based on novel posting: Individuals processes of social and psychological integration into virtual groups. *Online Information Review*, *40*(2), 204–217. doi:10.1108/OIR-06-2015-0198

Hawkley, L. C., & Cacioppo, J. T. (2010). Loneliness matters: A theoretical and empirical review of consequences and mechanisms. *Annals of Behavioral Medicine, 40*(2), 218–227. doi:10.1007/s12160-010-9210-8 PMID:20652462

Herring, S., Job-Sluder, K., Scheckler, R., & Barab, S. (2011). Searching for Safety Online: Managing "Trolling" in a Feminist Forum. *The Information Society>. International Journal (Toronto, Ont.), 18*(5), 371–384.

Heyes, K. (2017). *Using virtual ethnography to research vulnerable participants online: A case study of mental health online community support forums.* SAGE Research Methods Online; doi:10.4135/9781526403605

Hine, C. (2004). Social research methods and the internet: A thematic review. *Sociological Research Online, 9*(2). doi:10.5153/sro.924

Hine, C. (2008). Virtual Ethnography: Modes, Varieties and Affordances. In N. G. Fielding, R. M. Lee, & G. Blank (Eds.), *The SAGE handbook of online research methods.* London: SAGE. doi:10.4135/9780857020055.n14

Holt-Lunstad, J., Smith, T. B., Baker, M., Harris, T., & Stephenson, D. (2015). Loneliness and social isolation as risk factors for mortality: A Meta-Analytic review. *Perspectives on Psychological Science, 10*(2), 227–237. doi:10.1177/1745691614568352 PMID:25910392

Hornsey, M. J., & Jetten, J. (2004). The individual within the group: Balancing the need to belong with the need to be different. *Personality and Social Psychology Review, 8*(3), 248–264. doi:10.1207/s15327957pspr0803_2 PMID:15454348

InternetLiveStats. (2014). *Internet usage & social media statistics.* Retrieved on January 11, 2017, from http://www.internetlivestats.com

Kawachi, I., & Berkman, L. F. (2001). Social Ties and Mental Health. *Journal of Urban Health: Bulletin of the New York Academy of Medicine, 78*(3), 458–466. doi:10.1093/jurban/78.3.458 PMID:11564849

Kendall, L. (2002). *Hanging Out in the Virtual Pub: Masculinities and Relationships.* Berkeley, CA: University of California Press. doi:10.1525/california/9780520230361.001.0001

King, S. A., & Moreggi, D. (1998). Internet therapy and self-help groups - the pros and cons. In J. Gackenbach (Ed.), *Psychology and the Internet: Intrapersonal, interpersonal, and transpersonal implications* (pp. 77–109). San Diego, CA: Academic Press.

Kozinets, R. (2015). *Netnography: Redefined.* London: SAGE. doi:10.1002/9781118767771.wbiedcs067

Learmonth, D., Trosh, J., Rai, S., Sewell, J., & Cavanagh, K. (2008). The role of computer-aided psychotherapy within an NHS CBT specialist service. *Counselling & Psychotherapy Research*, *8*(2), 117–123. doi:10.1080/14733140801976290

Link, B. G., Phelan, J. C., Bresnahan, M., Stueve, A., & Pescosolido, B. A. (1999). Public Conceptions of Mental Illness: Labels, Causes, Dangerousness, and Social Distance. *American Journal of Public Health*, *89*(9), 1328–1333. doi:10.2105/AJPH.89.9.1328 PMID:10474548

Link, B. G., Struening, E. L., Rahav, M., Phelan, J., & Nuttbrock, L. (1997). On Stigma and Its Consequences: Evidence from a Longitudinal Study of Men with Dual Diagnoses of Mental Illness and Substance Abuse. *Journal of Health and Social Behavior*, *38*(2), 177–190. doi:10.2307/2955424 PMID:9212538

Maclure, M. (1998). Refutation in epidemiology: why else not? In K. J. Rothman (Ed.), *Causal Inference*. Chestnut Hill, PA: Epidemiology Resources.

Markham, A. (2004). Internet as research context. In C. Searle, G. Gobo, J. Gubrium, & D. Silverman (Eds.), *Qualitative Research Practice*. London: Sage. doi:10.4135/9781848608191.d28

McMillan, D. W., & Chavis, D. M. (1986). Sense of community: A definition and theory. *Journal of Community Psychology*, *14*(1), 6–23. doi:10.1002/1520-6629(198601)14:1<6::AID-JCOP2290140103>3.0.CO;2-I

Mind. (n.d.). *Peer support: Helping each other*. Retrieved September 9, 2014 from http://www.mind.org.uk/information-support/guides-to-support-and-services/peer-support/about-peer-support/?o=10153

Morris, J. (2012). *One town for my body, another for my mind*. York, UK: JRF.

Neal, L., Oakley, K., Lindgaard, G., Kaufman, D., Leimeister, J.M., & Selker, T. (2007) Online Health Communities. *Extended Abstracts on Human Factors in Computing Systems,* 2129-2132.

Noelle-Neumann, E. (1974). The Spiral of Silence: A Theory of Public Opinion. *Journal of Communication*, *24*(2), 43–51. doi:10.1111/j.1460-2466.1974.tb00367.x

Ostrum, L., Wilhelmsen, C., & Kaplan, B. (1993). Assessing Safety Culture. *Nuclear Safety*, *34*(2), 163–172.

Pescosolido, B., Martin, J., Long, J., Medina, T., Phelan, J., & Link, B. (2010). A disease like any other? A decade of change in public reactions to schizophrenia, depression, and alcohol dependence. *The American Journal of Psychiatry, 167*(11), 1321–1330. doi:10.1176/appi.ajp.2010.09121743 PMID:20843872

Phillips, W. (2015). *This Is Why We Can't Have Nice Things: Mapping the Relationship Between Online Trolling and Mainstream Culture.* Cambridge, MA: MIT Press.

Pinfold, V., Sweet, D., Porter, I., Quinn, C., Byng, R., Griffiths, C., … Huxley, P. (2015). Improving community health networks for people with severe mental illness: a case study investigation. *Health Serv Deliv Res, 3*(5).

Putnam, R. D. (2000). *Bowling alone: The collapse and revival of American community.* New York: Simon & Schuster. doi:10.1145/358916.361990

Rafaeli, S., Ravid, G., & Soroka, V. (2004). *De-lurking in virtual communities: A social communication network approach to measuring the effects of social and cultural capital.* Paper presented at the 37th annual Hawaii international conference on system sciences. doi:10.1109/HICSS.2004.1265478

Rafferty, R. (2011). *Motivations Behind Cyber Bulling and Online Aggression: Cyber Sanctions, Dominance, and Trolling Online.* Retrieved on May 15, 2017, from https://etd.ohiolink.edu/

Ren, Y., Harper, F. M., Drenner, S., Terveen, L., Kiesler, S., Riedl, J., & Kraut, R. E. (2012). Building member attachment in online communities: Applying theories of group identity and interpersonal bonds. *Management Information Systems Quarterly, 36*(3), 841–864.

Rheingold, H. (1994). *The virtual community: Finding connection in a computerized world.* London: Secker & Warburg.

Richardson, L-J. (2015). Micro-blogging and Online Community. *Internet Archaeology,* 39.

Schiel, T. (2005). Modernity, Ambivalence and the Gardening State. *Thesis Eleven, 83,* 78 -89

Schneider, A., von Krogh, G., & Jager, P. (2013). Whats coming next? Epistemic curiosity and lurking behaviour in online communities. *Computers in Human Behavior, 29*(1), 293–303. doi:10.1016/j.chb.2012.09.008

Schomerus, G., Angemeyer, M. C., Baumeister, S. E., Stolzenberg, S., Link, B. G., & Phelan, J. C. (2016). An online intervention using information on the mental health-mental illness continuum to reduce stigma. *European Psychiatry*, *32*, 21–27. doi:10.1016/j.eurpsy.2015.11.006 PMID:26802980

Seale, C., Anderson, E., & Kinnersley, P. (2006). Treatment advice in primary care: A comparative study of nurse practitioners and general practitioners. *Journal of Advanced Nursing*, *54*(5), 534–541. doi:10.1111/j.1365-2648.2006.03865.x PMID:16722950

Simco, R., McCusker, J., & Sewitch, M. (2014). Adherence to self-care interventions for depression or anxiety: A systematic review. *Health Education Journal*, *73*(6), 714–730. doi:10.1177/0017896913514738

Star, S. (1955, November). *The public's ideas about mental illness.* Paper presented at the Annual Meeting of the National Association for Mental Health, Indianapolis, IN.

Steffens, N. K., Haslam, S. A., Schuh, S. C., Jetten, J., & van Dick, R. (2016). A Meta-Analytic review of social identification and health in organizational contexts. *Personality and Social Psychology Review*. https://doi.org/10.1177/1088868316656701

Steptoe, A., Shankar, A., Demakakos, P., & Wardle, J. (2013). Social isolation, loneliness, and all-cause mortality in older men and women. *Proceedings of the National Academy of Sciences of the United States of America*, *110*(15), 5797–5801. doi:10.1073/pnas.1219686110 PMID:23530191

Suler, J. (2004). The online disinhibition effect. *Cyberpsychology & Behavior*, *7*(3), 321–326. doi:10.1089/1094931041291295 PMID:15257832

Szasz, T. S. (1961). The uses of naming and the origin of the myth of mental illness. *The American Psychologist*, *16*(2), 59–65. doi:10.1037/h0040842

Tajfel, H., & Turner, J. C. (1979). An integrative theory of intergroup conflict. In W. G. Austin & S. Worchel (Eds.), *The Social Psychology of Intergroup Relations* (pp. 33–47). Monterey, CA: Brooks/Cole.

Tanis, M. (2008). Health-related on-line forums: Whats the big attraction? *Journal of Health Communication*, *13*(7), 698–714. doi:10.1080/10810730802415316 PMID:18958781

Tate, D. F., & Zabinski, M. F. (2004). Computer and Internet applications for psychological treatment: Update for clinicians. *Journal of Clinical Psychology*, *60*(2), 209–220. doi:10.1002/jclp.10247 PMID:14724928

Third, A., Forrest-Lawrence, P., & Collier, A. (2014). *Addressing the cyber-safety challenge*. Retrieved September 7, 2015, from https://www.telstra.com.au/content/dam/tcom/about-us/community-environment/pdf/cyber-safety-challenge-risk-resillience.pdf

Uchino, B. N. (2006). Social support and health: A review of physiological processes potentially underlying links to disease outcomes. *Journal of Behavioral Medicine*, *29*(4), 377–387. doi:10.1007/s10865-006-9056-5 PMID:16758315

Welbourne, J. L., Blanchard, A. L., & Wadsworth, M. B. (2013). Motivation in virtual health communities and their relationship to community, connectedness and stress. *Computers in Human Behavior*, *29*(1), 129–139. doi:10.1016/j.chb.2012.07.024

WHO. (2005). *Promoting mental health.* Retrieved August 8, 2016, from http://www.who.int/mental_health/evidence/MH_Promotion_Book.pdf

WHO. (2015). *Global health workforce, finances remain low for mental health.* World Health Organization. Retrieved January 11, 2017, from http://www.who.int/mediacentre/news/notes/2015/finances-mental-health/en/

Whybrow, P., & Heyes, K. (2016). *Caring for Carers.* Research report. Retrieved from Cost of Living Official URL: http://www.cost-ofliving.net/caring-for-carers/

Wittel, A. (2001). Toward a network sociality. *Theory, Culture & Society*, *18*(6), 51–76. doi:10.1177/02632760122052048

Wood, J. V. (1989). Theory and research concerning social comparisons of personal attributes. *Psychological Bulletin*, *106*(2), 231–248. doi:10.1037/0033-2909.106.2.231

Woong Yun, G., & Park, S.-Y. (2011). Selective posting: Willingness to post a message online. *Journal of Computer-Mediated Communication*, *16*(2), 201–227. doi:10.1111/j.1083-6101.2010.01533.x

Yalom, I., & Leszcz, M. (2005). *Theory and Practice of Group Psychotherapy* (5th ed.). New York: Basic Books.

Yeo, A., Legard, R., Keegan, J., Ward, K., McNaughton Nicholls, C., & Lewis, J. (2014). In-Depth Interviews. In J. Ritchie, J. Lewis, C. McNaughton Nicholls, & R. Ormston (Eds.), *A Guide for Social Science Students and Researchers*. London: SAGE.

Yuill, C., Crinson, I., & Duncan, E. (2010). *Key concepts in health studies*. London: SAGE Publications Ltd. doi:10.4135/9781446251676

KEY TERMS AND DEFINITIONS

Ethnography: A method of research that involves non-participatory observation of participants in their normal environment, for example, at a weekly group meeting.

Expert Patient: The empowerment of a user of healthcare services, through the education of their condition and treatment.

Lurking: When users of online spaces watch, read or look at, but do not contribute to the discussion.

NHS: The National Health Service. This is the healthcare service that is provided in the UK. It is paid for with Government funds and is free at the point of access to residents of the UK.

Offline: Anything that happens when not connected to the internet.

Online: Anything that is accessed through, or actions taken, whilst connected to the internet.

Peer to Peer: Discussions or connections that happen with people of the same perceived status, such as users of forums. Medical doctors for example, may be a professional rather than a peer when participating in forum discussions.

Stigma: A negative association with social characteristics, traits or health issues.

Trolling: A means by which individuals attack others online through inflammatory comments.

Virtual Ethnography: A method of research that involves observation of participants in their online environments, for example, an internet chat room.

Chapter 3
Cancer Virtual Communities in the Era of Personalized Medicine:
Perspectives on Scope, Use, and Impact

Jacqueline (Jackie) Lorene Bender
University Health Network, Canada & University of Toronto, Canada

ABSTRACT

Cancer is the most common chronic disease worldwide. Cancer patients report significant unmet supportive care needs. Peer support groups show great promise in meeting cancer patients' supportive care needs, and are considered an important complement to the formal health care system. Virtual communities offer a convenient way for cancer patients to collaborative meet many of their supportive care needs in a timely way. This chapter will present current evidence on: the scope and characteristics of virtual communities for cancer patients; prevalence and predictors of use and reasons for non-use; the nature and function of supportive exchanges in cancer virtual communities, including their limitations; and the potential effects, both positive and negative, of participating in cancer virtual communities on health outcomes. Grounded in social support, technology adoption and health behavior theory, this chapter will offer a multi-theory framework for better understanding for how cancer virtual communities work and under what conditions.

DOI: 10.4018/978-1-5225-2958-3.ch003

INTRODUCTION

Cancer is a leading cause of death, premature death and years of life lost worldwide (World Health Organization [WHO], 2015). In 2012, 14.1 million people were diagnosed with cancer and 8.2 million died from cancer (International Agency for Research on Cancer [IARC], 2014). The number of new cases of cancer is expected to rise by 70% over the next two decades (IARC, 2014). At the same time, cancer survival has improved dramatically as a result of advances in early detection and treatment. It is estimated that there are 32.6 million cancer survivors worldwide (within 5 years of their diagnosis) living with or beyond cancer (IARC, 2014).

Most health systems throughout the world do not yet adequately deal with the confluence of complex, time intensive supportive care issues that people living with cancer and their loved ones have to face daily. These include practical assistance, pain and symptom management support, informational, emotional, psychological, social, spiritual and nutritional support, the need for which can vary over the course of the illness and beyond (Fitch, 2000). Cancer patients are frequently dissatisfied with the quality and amount of information that they receive from health professionals (Jefford & Tattersall, 2002), and rates of psychosocial distress among cancer patients are high, ranging from 30 to 45% across disease subgroups (Zabora, BrintzenhofeSzoc, Curbow, Hooker, & Piantadosi, 2001). Moreover, many cancer patients report significant unmet needs 2 to 10 years post-treatment including physical, financial, informational and psychosocial needs (Burg et al., 2015). Many of these issues are neglected or not adequately addressed because of the fractured nature of care delivery and the lack of mechanisms and incentives to permit their timely management. However, patients whose supportive care needs are met are better able to cope with cancer, have greater quality of life, and rely less on medical services (Kash et al., 2005).

Cancer patients may be able to overcome many of these challenges with support from peers. Support from family, friends and other cancer survivors is recognized as an important complement to the supportive care provided by the formal health care system (Fitch, 2000; Vivar & McQueen, 2005). Family caregivers often serve as the primary source of support (Gass, Weitzen, Clark, & Dizon, 2007). However, support from family caregivers typically drops significantly within the first year of diagnosis (Arora, Finney Rutten, Gustafson, Moser, & Hawkins, 2007). Support from other cancer survivors is highly valued by cancer patients even for those who report high levels of support from family members (Arora et al., 2007). Support form peers can provide a unique sense of community, reassurance and practical information that cannot be gained from other supportive relationships and can improve relations with family and friends by relieving their burden of care (Ussher, Kirsten, Butow, & Sandoval, 2006).

Virtual communities offer a convenient and beneficial way for cancer patients and their loved ones to collaboratively meet many of their support needs (Bender, O'Grady, & Jadad, 2008). Virtual communities overcome many of the practical barriers to face-to-face support while, providing additional advantages such as 24-hour accessibility, anonymity, similarity of experiences and diversity of resources (Wright, 2002). Yet, participation in cancer virtual communities is not a mainstream activity (Bender & Jiang, 2013). Moreover, there are numerous cases of abandonment and closure, as virtual communities struggle to retain members, assess impact and demonstrate return on investment to funders (Bender, Jimenez-Marroquin, Ferris, Katz, & Jadad, 2012; van Uden-Kraan, Drossaert, Taal, Seydel, & van de Laar, 2010; Young, 2013).

This chapter will present current evidence on the: scope and characteristics of virtual communities for cancer patients; prevalence and predictors of use, and reasons for non-use; the nature and function of supportive exchanges in cancer virtual communities, including their limitations; and the potential effects, both positive and negative, of participating in cancer virtual communities on health outcomes. Grounded in social support, technology adoption and health behavior theory, this chapter will offer a multi-theory framework for better understanding how cancer virtual communities work and under what conditions.

In this era of personalized medicine, advances in genetics are paving the way for cancer treatments that are tailored toward specific patient subtypes rather than broad diagnostic groups (Schork, 2015). The European Union describes personalized medicine as a medical model that uses molecular profiling for delivering the right therapeutic strategy for the right person at the right time (European Commission, n.d.). While most descriptions of personalized medicine focus on tailored medicines and medical products for curative purposes, the importance of personalizing the delivery of supportive care must not be forgotten. This chapter will attempt to highlight the importance of paving the way to personalized peer support, and the potential role of virtual communities in achieving this goal.

SCOPE AND CHARACTERISTICS

There are a wide variety of virtual communities available to cancer patients and their loved ones. The abundance and longevity of many cancer virtual communities may be a surrogate indicator of the benefits gained by their members (Jadad, Enkin, Glouberman, Groff, & Stern, 2006). At the same time, the sheer number may be daunting for the lone cancer patient trying to find "someone like me". Furthermore, not all cancer virtual communities are intended or optimally designed for the mutual exchange of cancer related information and support.

Take Facebook, for example. Facebook continues to be the most popular and perhaps successful virtual community, if success is based on sheer number of users. For example, eight in ten (79%) American Internet users use Facebook, more than double the number of Americans who use Instagram (32%), Pinterest (31%), LinkedIn (29%) or Twitter (24%) (Greenwood, Perrin, & Duggan, 2016). Worldwide, there are over 1.79 billion active monthly users on Facebook, 1.18 users log on daily and 4.5 billion 'Likes' are generated daily (Facebook Newsroom, n.d.). Young people between the ages of 25 and 34 remain the most common age demographic on Facebook (Greenwood et al., 2016). However, there is a significant upward trend in Facebook use by older adults, with 62% of online Americans 65+ using Facebook (Greenwood et al., 2016). This is an important trend to keep in mind given the aging demographic and cancer incidence, which increases with age (Canadian Cancer Society [CCS], 2016).

In 2008, we conducted a content analysis of breast cancer groups on Facebook (Bender, Jimenez-Marroquin, & Jadad, 2011). At that time, we found over 620 breast cancer groups on Facebook with a total of 1,090,397 members. The majority of groups were created for fundraising (44.7%) or awareness raising (38.1%) purposes. Only 7% were created for patient or caregiver support and of these, less than 50% of were created by cancer patients themselves. Fundraising and awareness-raising groups were associated with the most members, while support-oriented groups contained the greatest number of posts. Recently, Hale et al conducted a comprehensive examination of the 20 most searched for health conditions on Google represented in Facebook Pages (Hale, Pathipati, Zan, & Jethwani, 2014). Notably cancer was the number one health condition searched for on Google. Consistent with our findings, of the 958 pages produced by their Facebook search, the most common type of page was marketing/promotion (32%) followed by information and awareness (20.7%). Only a small number of pages (9.4%) were devoted to social support, and six conditions were not represented by any support pages. In addition, a large number of page results (29.4%) were not relevant to the health condition searched. Cancer and breast cancer together accounted for 86.9% of the total 'Likes' across all health condition pages.

Taken together these studies suggest that there are a large number of virtual communities available for cancer patients and caregivers on Facebook, but relatively few devoted to social support. This finding might in part be due to the lack of anonymity on Facebook given its popularity and base user profile structure. Social network sites like Facebook are differentiated from other types of virtual communities based on their ability to enable users to display their social networks. Their backbone consists of visible user profiles that display an articulated list of friends who are users on the system (boyde & Ellison, 2008). This unique feature is intended to facilitate connections between individuals that would not otherwise have been made (boyde & Ellison, 2008). In a qualitative study that we conducted examining breast cancer patients' perspectives on the role of virtual communities, nearly all participants explained that they would be uncomfortable discussing breast cancer related issues on Facebook because of its popularity and lack of privacy (Bender, Katz, Ferris, & Jadad, 2013). The visibility of user profiles and personal networks on Facebook reduces the relative anonymity of the encounter and, if open to the public, which all groups in these studies were, they have the potential to attract a much wider audience. The findings from these studies also suggest that it may be difficult for the average cancer patient to find relevant health information and support on Facebook given the large number of irrelevant pages produced by a health search on Facebook.

However, Facebook is not the only place to connect with other cancer patients online. A quick Internet search produces a number of cancer virtual communities to choose from, particularly for breast cancer.

In 2010, we attempted to systematically identify and characterize all known online resources that provide English language virtual communities for breast cancer survivors (Bender, Jimenez-Marroquin, Ferris, Katz & Jadad, 2012). The search yielded 111 websites, some of which contained multiple virtual communities (e.g. Facebook and the Association of Cancer Online Resources). Most (65.8%) had a broad focus (e.g., health, cancer or general purpose). One third (34.2%) were exclusive to breast cancer and 11 catered to a specific disease type (e.g. hereditary) or characteristic of breast cancer patient (e.g. young). The majority of virtual communities identified were non-profit (55%) and moderated (69.5%). Most moderators were lay-persons (85.7%). Greater than one-third of virtual communities (36%) were initiated by breast cancer survivors or affected loved ones. Activity levels varied from very high (e.g. over 1 million posts) to very low (e.g. 15 posts). Ten sites accounted for 93.4% of the total number of posts in the breast cancer specific websites sampled, each of which reported more than 100,000 posts.

The results of this study demonstrated that patients and their loved ones are taking a major role in creating virtual communities (Bender, et al., 2012). In fact, the top ten most active sites were initiated by a breast cancer survivor, affected family member or non-profit organization, as opposed to a commercial company. Research by Van Uden-Kraan and colleagues (2010) suggests that patients create virtual communities out of necessity. In their qualitative study with 23 administrators of patient-initiated breast, fibromyalgia and arthritis virtual communities, the authors reported that patients create such resources because of a desire to help others, promote awareness of the disease, or because existing resources do not meet their needs.

Of note, four of the top ten most active sites identified in this study catered to a less common type of breast cancer (e.g. BRCA1/BRCA2 mutations and Herceptin +), characteristic of patient (e.g. young), or stage of disease (e.g. metastatic) (Bender et al., 2012). As O-Reilly forecasted in his description of the evolution of the web, these niche websites demonstrate the potential of the Internet to "reach out to the entire web, to the edges and not just the centre, to the 'long-tail', and not just the head" (O'Reilly, n.d.). The long-tail in health represents the numerous individuals with less common conditions who are poorly served by traditional support systems because they do not fit the model of the "average" patient (Deshpande & Jadad, 2006). Virtual communities enable these individuals to more easily connect, develop a critical mass, and build a shared knowledge base related to their condition (Bender et al., 2008).

As of 2012, 7% of the virtual communities sampled in this study had closed down (Bender et al., 2012). Reasons for closure included changes in the strategic focus of the organization, resources constraints, inactivity, and spam. Building successful, sustainable and scalable virtual communities is challenging and we know little about the factors that determine their success (Kairam, Wang, & Leskovec, 2012). Moderation is considered essential; it includes promoting the group, facilitating participation, responding to messages, and fostering a positive and welcoming atmosphere (O'Grady, Bender, Urowitz, Wiljer, & Jadad, 2010). But moderation can be onerous consuming on average 10 to 15 hours per week (van Uden-Kraan et al., 2010). Moreover, developing and sustaining a successful health related virtual community requires more than 'reactionary moderation' (Young, 2013). Young (2013) explains that to build a thriving virtual community, organizations need to develop and sustain a community management strategy according to the community's life cycle stage and be prepared to evolve with the community throughout its life cycle. Other important sociotechnical attributes of successful virtual communities include the level of anonymity offered by the site, as well as its presence, activity and interactivity, similarity of user experiences and diversity of social capital offered by its members (Preece, 2001; Walther et al., 2005). In addition, our work suggests that the structural characteristics of the organization or governing body play an important role, along with the ability to demonstrate value to funders.

PREVALENCE OF USE, REASONS FOR NON-USE AND FACTORS THAT INFLUENCE USE

As of 2011, one in four (23%) American Internet users living with a health condition like cancer, diabetes or heart disease have gone online to find others with similar health conditions (Fox, 2011). By contrast 15% of American Internet users without an existing health condition reported going online to seek this type of help. Other groups likely to seek health support from peers in online groups include Internet users caring for a loved one, who experienced a medical crisis, and who have experienced a significant change in their health (e.g. weight loss/gain, pregnancy or quitting smoking).

Cancer is not just one disease (CCS, 2016). There are many different types of cancer and while they are alike in some ways, there are more ways in which they differ. Furthermore, no two cancers are the same. Even people with same type of cancer may have different treatment pathways and disease experiences that are further influenced by their personal characteristics and social circumstances, all of which will influence their support needs and support seeking behavior. Until recently, little has been known about the prevalence of online support seeking within and across sub-groups of cancer patients. In 2009, van Uden-Kraan and colleagues conducted a cross-sectional hospital-based study of 679 Dutch patients with breast cancer, rheumatoid arthritis or fibromyalgia (van Uden-Kraan et al., 2009). At that time, they found that 52% of the patients surveyed reported using the Internet as a health resource, and 15% reported specifically using a virtual patient community. However, sub-group analysis was not performed.

To address this gap in knowledge, we conducted a series of cross-sectional hospital-based studies at a major urban cancer centre in Canada to examine the proportion of cancer patients who use virtual communities as a health resource. These studies, which were conducted between 2011 and 2013, involved a total of 552 testicular, thyroid and breast cancer patients who had completed treatment for cancer and were receiving well follow-up care (Bender & Jiang, 2013; Bender et al., 2016; Bender, Wiljer, et al., 2012; Kwan et al., 2017). Typically, testicular cancer affects men between the ages of 20 and 40, thyroid cancer affects men and women between the ages of 15 to 49, and breast cancer affects women between the ages of 50 to 69 (CCS, 2016). The survey response rates ranged from 71 to 75%. The respondents ranged in average age from 36 (testicular), 50 (thyroid) and 63 (breast) years of age, and were on average 48 years of age (SD 16.3). The majority were born in Canada (66%), spoke English as a first language (64%) were married (72%) and had completed college or university (77%).

On average, 25% cancer patients surveyed reported that they had used a virtual community to seek information and support from other cancer patients (Bender & Jiang, 2013). The average proportion of cancer patients who reported using virtual communities in these samples is higher than population based estimates. As mentioned, in 2011, 23% of American Internet users living with a chronic health condition, which included cancer, reported using a virtual community, which corresponds to about 17% of the general adult population at that time.

Of note, technical barriers do not appear to the main reasons why the majority of cancer patients do not use cancer related virtual communities. In order of frequency, reasons for not using virtual communities included: no perceived need/

interest (48%); lack of awareness (33%); not confident using computers or virtual communities (9%); and lack of trust in information on the Internet (6%) (Bender & Jiang, 2013). These findings reflect the modifiable factors that have been shown to influence health related Internet use more generally and include: a positive outcome expectancy, previous use of health websites and positive Internet self-efficacy (Mead, Varnam, Rogers, & Roland, 2003). They also reflect limited eHealth literacy, which is the ability to find, evaluate, and apply information gained in online environments (Norman & Skinner, 2006). An assumption underlying many eHealth resources is that consumers have the skills needed to use them optimally.

To better understand who seeks peer support from cancer virtual communities, we also examined patient characteristics that may be associated with virtual community use (Bender & Jiang, 2013). We performed multivariate logistic regression to assess the relative importance of variables that correlated significantly with virtual community use. Five variables were found to be correlated with virtual community use: age, first spoken language, education, treatments received and unmet supportive care needs. Specifically, respondents who were younger, spoke English as a first language, had received more cancer treatment, and reported more unmet supportive care needs were more likely to use virtual communities. However, only younger age, greater number of unmet supportive care needs and English as a first language were found to be significant predictors of virtual community use.

Age, education, income, and geographic location are well-known predictors of Internet use more generally (Statistics Canada, 2012). While increasing numbers of seniors are going online, there is still a noticeable generational gap – particularly in the type of online activities (Allen, 2013). This study confirms other reports of an under-representation of minorities in virtual patient communities (Fogel, Ribisl, Morgan, Humphreys, & Lyons, 2008; Im, Chee, Im, & Chee, 2008). Most notably, this study provides correlational evidence that suggests that unmet supportive care needs may drive use, confirming qualitative studies that report that use of cancer virtual communities is contingent on need (Sandaunet, 2008). Further research is needed to confirm the direction of causation. For example, whether unmet needs drives use and whether unmet needs decrease over time with use of virtual communities.

In sum, this research suggests that 1 in 4 cancer patients may use virtual communities as a health resource. Cancer patients who are younger, speak English as a first language and report more unmet needs may be more likely to use virtual cancer communities. Reasons for not using virtual communities as a health resource are largely due to a lack of awareness of their existence and their potential benefits. It is worthy of note that when asked, 44% of testicular (Bender, Wiljer, et al., 2012), 63% of thyroid (Bender et al., 2016) and 44.5% of breast cancer survivors (Kwan et al., 2017) reported that they would use a website that contained a cancer related virtual community if created by their cancer centre. It should be noted that these studies were conducted in a single urban cancer centre, and may not reflect the prevalence of virtual community use in rural or community based settings.

NATURE AND FUNCTION OF PARTICIPATION

Numerous studies have examined cancer patients' postings in an effort to understand what is going on in these virtual patient communities, how social support is communicated and what benefits cancer patients gain from participating in them. Researchers have used a variety of methods to study the content of these exchanges including both qualitative and quantitative content analyses, ethnographic observation, qualitative interviews, quantitative surveys and automated text analysis using computer software programs. These studies are mainly concerned with the types of support exchanged within virtual communities, operationalizing social support as the functional provisions of relationships, such as emotional, instrumental and informational support (Weiss, 1974).

Nature of Postings and Impact of Gender

Klemm, Reppert and Visich (1998) used a combination of qualitative and quantitative content analysis to examine the postings in a colorectal cancer mailing list. A total of 300 postings from 48 men and 46 women were analyzed. Eight content categories were identified: information giving/seeking (25.4%), personal opinion (22%); encouragement/support (17.4%); personal experiences (16.4%); thanks (7.7%), humor (4.5%); prayer (2.9%); and miscellaneous (3.2%). Men and women contributed an equal number of postings – an interesting finding given that women outnumber men, 4 to 1, in face-to-face cancer support groups (Cella & Yellen, 1993) and women are frequently interrupted by men in mixed gender groups (Anderson & Leaper, 1998). The anonymity provided by computer-mediated communication may be a factor affecting this phenomenon.

Klemm, Hurst, Dearholt and Trone (1999) conducted a follow-up study to explore the impact of gender on communication in breast, prostate, and mixed cancer online mailing lists. Content analysis of the 947 postings across the three different online groups (involving 126 breast cancer survivors 117 prostate cancer survivors and 43 men and 49 women from the mixed cancers group) revealed the same eight content categories identified in the previous study with the addition of 'activism'. Chi square analysis of the postings revealed significant differences based on gender. Information giving/seeking was most common among the prostate cancer and mixed cancers group, while personal experience ranked first in the breast cancer group followed closely by encouragement/support. In addition, women offered twice as many messages of support in the mixed cancers group as compared to men.

Sullivan (2003) describes the different types of communication in online ovarian and prostate cancer support groups as "rapport" versus "report" talk. Sullivan's phenomenological study of ovarian and prostate cancer mailing lists involving 134 women and 176 men, suggests that men support each other by sharing treatment information while women support each other by sharing personal experiences and feelings. Men in the prostate cancer mailing list shared their personal experiences in the form of personal digests (a personal case history in digest form), and demonstrated empathy toward each other by ensuring that the information shared was accurate, often citing original sources. Sullivan concluded that both groups were supporting each other through the cancer experience albeit in different ways, in keeping with gender norms.

Further research suggests that the impact of gender upon the supportive practices among male and female cancer patients may not be so clear-cut. Gooden and Winefield (2007) conducted a mixed method study using grounded theory and quantitative content analysis to study the communication among 69 women with breast cancer and 77 men with prostate cancer in online discussion boards. In contrast to previous findings, men and women engaged in informational and emotional support fairly equally, with informational needs predominating in both groups: 64% of men's and 60% of women's communication focused on informational needs while 36% of men's and 40% of women's communication focused on emotional needs.

It is clear from these studies that both male and female cancer patients use online support groups to seek and provide information and emotional support, although they may do so in different ways. It also appears that there is more information-oriented than emotionally supportive talk occurring in virtual cancer communities.

Function of Supportive Exchanges

One of the earliest observational studies to examine the functions and benefits gained from participating in cancer virtual communities was published in 1997. In this study Sharf (1997) used participant observation and discourse analysis to examine the communication occurring in the Breast Cancer List, an un-moderated online discussion group serving mainly Canadian and American women. Three major functions were identified: information exchange, psychological support and personal empowerment. Members explained that participation on the list enabled them to become better informed, validated concerns that were ignored by health professionals, provided reassurance that life continues after treatment, and motivation to mobilize action. In addition, the participants reported benefiting from changing their focus from a preoccupation with their own illness to helping others. Anonymity allowed the participants to communicate in ways they felt they could not in face-to-face support groups.

These findings are supported by an ethnographic case study of the Scandinavian Breast Cancer Mailing List conducted by Hoybye and colleagues (2005). Participant observation and semi-structured interviews with 15 survivors on the list revealed that the participants were empowered by the exchanges of knowledge and personal experiences. Participation on the list provided a better understanding of breast cancer and its implications, and motivated users to formulate questions in preparation for their future consultations with health professionals. The members also indicated that the sense of anonymity provided by the medium allowed them to communicate in ways they felt they could not face-to-face.

The relative anonymity of virtual communities has also been reported to be important for prostate cancer survivors. Broom (2005) explored the attitudes toward online support groups among 33 men with prostate cancer of which 8 were online support group users, 20 were general Internet users and 5 did not use the Internet. Each of the 8 men who were users of online support groups explained that the anonymity of the medium allowed them to talk about sensitive aspects of their disease while still maintaining societal perceptions of masculinity publicly. In addition, the ability to silently 'lurk' was highly valued as it provided a way to benefit from the interactions of the group for those not comfortable actively participating. Interestingly, the anonymity and privacy valued by online support group users were viewed as problematic by non-users because they feared that would lead to deception and misinformation.

Collectively, these studies suggest that participation in cancer virtual communities is empowering for cancer patients. Van Uden-Kraan and colleagues sought to identify the empowering effects of virtual communities in a series of investigations. Beginning with a qualitative study involving 32 participants of breast cancer, fibromyalgia, and arthritis virtual communities, the authors identified both empowering processes and outcomes (van Uden-Kraan et al., 2008). Empowering processes included: exchanging information, encountering emotional support, finding recognition, sharing experiences, helping others, and amusement. Empowering effects included: being better informed; feeling confident in their relationship with their physician, their treatment, and social environment; improved acceptance of the disease; enhanced self-esteem and social well-being; and social action. A subsequent survey involving 214 participants of seven different virtual communities for breast cancer survivors revealed that the most common empowering outcomes, experienced by more than 50% of the sample were: being better informed (74%), knowing what questions to ask their physicians (68%), knowing how to manage their disease (60%), and being better prepared for their consultation with their physicians (60%) (Smit et al., 2007).

Researchers have also investigated whether lurkers and posters benefit equally from participating in virtual communities; lurkers are considered to be people who read but do not contribute content to virtual communities. According to a survey of 528 members of breast cancer, fibromyalgia and arthritis communities by Van Uden-Kraan and colleagues (2008), you do not have to post in a virtual community to benefit from it. Lurkers reported the same degree of empowering outcomes as posters, with the exception of "enhanced well-being" for which they scored lower compared to posters. Lurkers were also significantly less satisfied with the online group than posters (van Uden-Kraan, Drossaert, Taal, Seydel, et al., 2008). Research by Burke and Kraut (2016) suggests that the effects on wellbeing may be dependent on posting. Based on data from opt-in surveys combined with de-identified and aggregated counts of Facebook activity from consenting users, Burke and Kraut found that the more people talked one-on-one on Facebook, such as writing wall posts or comments, especially with close friends, the more their well-being improved.

Limitations of Cancer Virtual Communities

One size does not fit all. Most studies of virtual communities report high drop-out rates (Eysenbach, Powell, Englesakis, Rizo, & Stern, 2004). This may be due in part to the challenge of 'fitting in' (Sandaunet, 2008).

Research suggests that cancer virtual communities may not be a space for suffering. Several researchers (Orgad, 2006; Pitts, 2004; Sandaunet, 2008) have observed a discourse of 'restitution' (Frank, 1995) in virtual cancer communities, which privileges coping with illness, rebuilding the body and self, a positive attitude and outcome. Voices of non-survivors, non-fighters, of despair, hopelessness and death were excluded or marginalized (Orgad, 2006). Catharsis, or open expression of feelings including fears and worries, is an important element of coping with cancer (Yalom, 1995). However, even breast cancer patients with metastatic disease and poor prognosis face barriers discussing death in a virtual community of their peers. A qualitative interview study involving 20 women with metastatic breast cancer revealed that participants benefited from participating in the virtual community and were comfortable expressing many concerns, but had difficulty discussing death and dying (Vilhauer, 2009). Reasons for this discomfort included non-response from other members when these topics were broached, and lack of immediate visual cues. Correlational work suggests that the discussion of negative emotions in cancer virtual communities may negatively affect the poster, as well as the reader of the post. Lieberman and Goldstein (2006) found that women who express fear and anxiety in virtual communities have poorer quality of life and more depression and van Uden-Kraan and colleagues found that being confronted with the negative aspects of the disease can have disempowering effects (van Uden-Kraan, Drossaert, Taal, Shaw, et al., 2008).

Research has also demonstrated that virtual cancer communities are predominately used by white cancer survivors. A review of the literature on virtual cancer communities conducted in 2003 revealed that most studies involve college-educated, high-income whites (Klemm et al., 2003). A survey of virtual communities for cancer survivors also conducted in 2003 identified 546 different groups, only 24 of which were ethnic-specific; eight were for African Americans, eight were for Asian Americans and eight were for combined ethnic minority groups (Im et al., 2005). In another study, an online discussion group was used 68% of the time by white women and only 38% of the time by African-American women (Gustafson et al., 2005). The possible reasons for the under-presentation of ethnic minorities in online cancer communities include differences in how ethnic groups make use of the Internet, differences in preferences for support (Fogel et al., 2008; Im et al., 2008), and a North American bias in online breast cancer spaces (Orgad, 2006).

These challenges of 'fitting in' are explored in detail in a qualitative investigation with cancer patients who withdrew from of a virtual community. Sandaunet (2008) conducted a qualitative study involving 25 participants (8 users and 17 non-users) of a breast cancer virtual community to examine the reasons why people stop participating or drop-out of virtual communities. She identified 5 barriers to use: a need to avoid painful details about cancer, not being 'ill enough' to participate, the challenge of establishing a legitimate position in the group, the organization of everyday life, and illness phases that did not motivate for self-help group participation. Of note, technology related aspects of the software were not mentioned in participants' reflections of their non-participation and withdrawal.

Lastly, there is enduring concern about the potential for harm resulting from deception and misinformation in cancer virtual communities (Broom, 2005), and from the use of the Internet in general (Gagliardi & Jadad, 2002; Jadad & Gagliardi, 1998). However, there is little evidence to support the claim (Crocco, Villasis-Keever, & Jadad, 2002). Research suggests that the self-organizing nature of virtual communities may enable its members to identify and correct potentially harmful information (Jadad et al., 2006). Esquivel, Meric-Berstam and Bernstam (2006) analyzed 4600 postings of the Breast Cancer Mailing List during the first quarter of 2005 and found only 10 containing false or misleading information, seven of which were identified by members of the list and corrected, on average, less than five hours after they appeared.

In sum, these studies suggest that the exchanges of knowledge, personal experiences and psychological support that occur in virtual communities is empowering for many cancer patients. Cancer virtual communities seem to provide users with a safe, relatively anonymous space to communicate about sensitive and potentially stigmatizing topics. Sharing experiences with other cancer patients in these spaces can: reduce feelings of isolation and uncertainty; validate concerns ignored by health professionals; provide reassurance, a sense of community and hope for the future; enhance coping and self-management; and lead to better informed and prepared cancer patients. However, these benefits may be restricted to white, North American, English-speaking cancer patients of a certain socioeconomic status given that virtual communities seem to be dominated by their perspectives. Furthermore, most research to date has focused on the use and effect of cancer virtual communities among breast cancer patients. Future work should examine whether and how other cancer survivors, and people from different races and ethnic backgrounds experience benefits from participating in virtual communities.

IMPACT ON HEALTH OUTCOMES

While considerable descriptive evidence from observational studies suggests that virtual communities can benefit cancer patients, far less is known about the impact of virtual communities on health-related outcomes.

A seminal 2004 systematic review conducted by Eysenbach and colleagues (Eysenbach et al., 2004) concluded that there was insufficient evidence to draw firm conclusions about the effects of peer-led health-related virtual communities on health outcomes. The authors found 45 publications describing 38 distinct studies, but only six evaluated "pure" or standalone virtual communities, and none used a randomized controlled trial design (RCT). The remaining studies evaluated complex interventions where the virtual community was one component of a broader intervention that included many potentially therapeutic components (e.g. structured psychotherapy, education and self-management activities), making it impossible to draw conclusions about the impact of the virtual community alone. Of the six evaluations of pure virtual communities, five reported some degree of facilitation by health professionals, with trained individuals formulating topics of interest, moderating discussions, and posting educational material. Possible explanations offered by the authors for the lack of studies and evidence from measured controlled trials included: little commercial or professional interest in evaluating pure virtual communities as opposed to interventions led by health professional, studies investigating natural self-helping processed are difficult to recreate in controlled research environments, and the low levels of participation in many communities which makes it difficult to show an effect.

Since then, the emergence of social media has led to an explosion in health-related virtual communities. In 2016, we undertook a scoping review to map the primary research on health-related virtual communities to determine the value of undertaking a systematic review of effectiveness (Bender & Miller, 2016). We updated the 2004 search strategy with new terms and searched Medline from October 2003 to December 2015 inclusive. We included evaluations, of any type, of the effects of participating in a health-related virtual community alone or in conjunction with a more complex intervention on health outcomes.

This scoping review yielded an additional 179 individual studies and 21 review articles on virtual communities (Bender & Miller, 2016). The majority of reviews grouped evaluations of standalone virtual communities with multicomponent interventions. Three reviews investigated the effects of standalone virtual communities on depression (Griffiths, Calear, & Banfield, 2009), youth with mental health problems (Ali, Farrer, Gulliver, & Griffiths, 2015) and weight management (Chang, Chopra, Zhang, & Woolford, 2013), and found promising but mixed results. None examined the attributes that might explain their effectiveness. Individual studies evaluated virtual communities as multicomponent (n=80), standalone (n=90), or adjunct interventions (n=9). Adjunct interventions used a 2x2 factorial design that compared an intervention without a virtual community to the same intervention with a virtual community. Standalone or adjunct interventions (n=99), mainly targeted cancer (n=30) or mental, behavioural or neurodevelopment conditions (n=23), and health promoting or risk behaviours (n=20), and were evaluated using cross-sectional surveys (n=38), RCTs (n=22) or pre-post designs (n=21). The most common primary outcomes for these studies were perceived effects (n=30), health promoting and risk behaviours (n=20), depression (n=16), as well as empowerment and self-esteem (n=16).

From this scoping review, we identified two effectiveness reviews of cancer virtual communities (Hong, Peña-Purcell, & Ory, 2012; Klemm et al., 2003). The most recent of which was published in 2012. In this review, Hong et al (2012) identified 37 articles describing 24 distinct studies most of which were focused on breast cancer survivors and had small sample sizes. Four studies used an RCT design, but only two evaluated a standalone virtual community. Hoybye and colleagues (2010) compared an un-moderated virtual community for cancer survivors to an educational control condition. No significant differences were found in overall quality of life and mood disturbance in the intervention (n=361) or control group (n=433). However, psychological well-being improved in both groups. Salzer et al (2010) compared an un-moderated virtual community for newly diagnosed breast cancer survivors to an Internet-based control condition that produced conflicting results. Participants in the intervention group (n=51) experienced increased distress and decreased emotional well-being over time, compared to controls (n=27). However, the difference between the groups was not statistically significant. Paradoxically, 60% of the intervention participants felt supported by the virtual community, reporting high levels of satisfaction, a sub-group of which created a mailing list of their own at the end of the study. The authors hypothesized that the homogenous nature of the group (all newly diagnosed breast cancer patients), lack of opportunity to learn from others who are in remission, and absence of a moderator could have limited the potential benefit of the group.

While moderation is considered key to the effective functioning of a virtual community (O'Grady, Bender, Uroowitz, Wiljer, & Jadad, 2010), little is known about how moderation, be it professional, lay or peer, affects health outcomes experienced by participants of virtual communities. Evidence suggests that professionally moderated virtual communities can provide psychosocial benefit to cancer patients. An RCT of three separate email discussion lists, involving a total of 108 breast cancer survivors (36 in each mailing list) that were moderated by a health professional following Spiegel's supportive-expressive therapy (Spiegel & Classen, 2000) resulted in significant reductions in depression, perceived stress and a nearly significant reduction in post-traumatic growth (Winzelberg et al., 2003).

To evaluate the effects of moderation, Klemm (2012) conducted an RCT comparing a moderated virtual community for breast cancer survivors to an un-moderated peer-led group. The moderated group (n=24) was run by trained social workers for a period of 12 weeks using pre-selected topics of relevance to breast cancer survivors. The un-moderated group was run by the subjects themselves (n=26) and was unstructured. There were no significant differences in depressive symptoms between the moderated and peer-led groups. However, the peer-led group had higher pre-treatment levels of depressive symptoms that improved over time to match their moderated counterparts. In addition, the participants in the moderated group contributed and read significantly more posts than the un-moderated group. However, greater participation levels did not translate into better health outcomes.

These studies leave many unanswered questions. Despite the overwhelming positive observational evidence on the benefits of participating in peer-led cancer virtual communities, the question remains as to what, if any, positive or negative effects cancer virtual communities have on participant health outcomes. Whether these effects translate to cancer survivors other than women with breast cancer, or family caregivers. Whether cancer virtual communities benefit from professional or lay moderation beyond the increase in participation. Whether increase in participation is associated with greater perceived benefits. Or who is most likely to benefit and under what conditions? Our scoping review of the field suggests that the evidence base has grown significantly to warrant an update, particularly on the impact of virtual communities for breast cancer. At the same time, future research could enhance the evidence base by employing more rigorous study designs with larger and diverse samples of cancer patients that examine the conditions under which virtual communities are effective and for whom.

THEORETICAL PERSPECTIVES ON USE AND IMPACT

The first step in understanding the role of virtual communities for cancer care is to draw on existing theory to unpack the evidence underlying the assumptions about how and why virtual communities are supposed to work, and for whom. Use of theory could lead to a better understanding of what motivates cancer patients to join and actively participate in virtual communities, the mechanisms by which they work, and how to predict and explain their effects. Greater use of theory has also been shown to lead to more effective eHealth interventions. In a systematic review and meta-analysis of the effects of Internet-based health behavior change interventions, Webb, Joseph, Yardley and Michie (2010) report that interventions that incorporated more extensive use of theory and theory based behavior change techniques had larger effect sizes.

The stark contrast between the overwhelming positive observational evidence on the benefits of virtual communities for cancer patients, and the lack of evidence from measured controlled trials, suggests that we may not be looking for the right effects or using the appropriate outcome measures to capture them. Theory provides a framework for guiding the selection of intervention components that might work, and helps to guide the choice of study design, samples and appropriate outcomes for measuring the effects (Pingree et al., 2010). Furthermore, intervening mechanisms may be easier to measure and may be a more accurate measure of an important treatment effect than distal outcomes affected by multiple causes (Pingree et al., 2010). Without an understanding of the mechanisms underlying the effects of virtual communities, we will not know if a virtual community intervention is simply not working or whether it is having its intended effects.

A review of the research on virtual cancer communities reveals an absence of theory, which has been reported by others (Hong et al., 2012; Klemm et al., 2003; Wright & Bell, 2003). While it is understandable that patient-initiated virtual communities are likely not based on theory, we would argue that evaluations of those interventions should be. In this last section, we employ theories from the fields of social support, health behaviour and technology adoption, to illuminate the social context of virtual support seeking by cancer patients. Specifically, we revisit a multi-theory framework that we proposed for understanding the reasons behind the use of virtual communities as a source of supportive care by breast cancer survivors (Bender et al., 2013). Although previous studies have used stress and coping theories to explain the effects of virtual communities among breast cancer survivors (Davison, Pennebaker, & Dickerson, 2000; Gustafson et al., 2005; Meier et al., 2007; Winzelberg et al., 2003; Wright, 2002), and technology adoption theories to explain intentions to use non-health related virtual communities (Lin,

2006), no known studies have used these theoretical perspectives in combination for this purpose.

We begin by summarizing the results of a mixed-method study from which we developed this framework, that aimed to understand the individual, social and contextual factors that influence breast cancer patients to seek online support and the role that online support plays in relation to more traditional forms of support (Bender et al., 2013). This study involved a survey with 73 breast cancer survivors who were trained face-to-face support group facilitators (73% response rate), supplemented with in-depth interviews with 12 participants from the survey sample. Our goal was to leverage their expertise in providing peer support to better understand the role of online peer support.

This study revealed that virtual communities have the potential to fill gaps in supportive care by addressing the unmet needs of a sub-group of breast cancer survivors. In brief, participants turned to virtual communities to address a specific unmet need, in many cases because they had a less common condition, received insufficient information from health professionals or support from their social network, and lacked access to others who had the same condition. Participants reported seeking help from virtual communities often under conditions of peak stress related to uncertainty, predominantly during the diagnostic and treatment phases to prepare for or decide on a course of treatment, or to learn how to cope with the disease and to manage symptoms and side effects. They explained that they were seeking help to understand "what to expect", and reassurance that their experiences and worries were normal. Once participants' needs were met, many stopped using the virtual community. Factors that motivated use post-treatment were the experience of a new or worsening symptom, the need for subsequent treatment, and a desire to stay informed or help others. Nearly all participants described reaching a point at which they wanted to move beyond cancer, and this included distancing themselves from the virtual community. Compared to support from face-to-face support groups or a health professional, virtual communities seemed to play a distinct role because of their quality of information, reassurance from similar others, availability and immediacy of a response, relative anonymity, control over interpersonal consequences of their illness, low commitment and expected reciprocity (Table 1).

Based on these findings we proposed that Social Comparison Theory (Festinger, 1954), Transactional Theory of Stress and Coping (Lazarus & Folkman, 1984), and a decomposed version of the combined Technology Acceptance Model (Davis, 1989) and the Theory of Planned Behaviour (Ajzen, 1991) with the addition of perceived trust could help explain, the individual, social and contextual factors that influence breast cancer survivors to use virtual communities. We describe the theoretical and practical relevance of the use of these theories in combination in the following sections.

Table 1. Theoretical and practical interpretations of findings (Adapted from Bender et al., 2013)

Theory	Theory Component	Practical Implications
Social comparison theory	Upward comparisons	-Obtain reassurance and learn from others who share specific characteristics that are doing well -Limit exposure to those doing poorly
Transactional model of stress and coping	Problem-focused coping	-Obtain practical answers to specific questions -Reduce illness related uncertainty and anxiety
Technology acceptance model/ Theory of planned behaviour (TAM/TPB)	Attitude: perceived usefulness	-Address specific unmet need in a timely -Obtain reassurance -Validate concerns -Learn what to expect -Learn new coping or symptom management strategies -Learn something new
TAM/TPB	Attitude: perceived ease of use	-Easy to log-on and set up an account -Easy to navigate and find specific information -Easy to post a comment and view the response
TAM/TPB	Attitude: perceived trust	-Well written, accurate and current messages -Empathetic and supportive messages -Credibility of the site owner -Transparent privacy and security measures
TAM/TPB	Subjective norms	-Opinions of relevant others (e.g., survivors) regarding their usefulness and credibility
TAM/TPB	Behavioural control	-Perceived ability to use site to meet need -Perceived ability to control interactions with others including how information is shared -Perceived ability to identify credible information -Verbal persuasion, guidance and opportunities to observe from other cancer survivors using the site

Social Comparison Theory

The two major explanations for why individuals decide to join support groups involve social comparisons (Buunk, Gibbons, & Reis-Bergan, 1997). The first explanation is that in times of stress and uncertainty, people make social comparisons to reduce their anxiety. The second explanation is that participation in support groups reduces feelings of uniqueness or deviance thereby enhancing self-esteem. Both of these explanations gain import from the Theory of Social Comparison (Festinger, 1954) which asserts that under conditions of threat, people seek similar others in order to compare the appropriateness of their thoughts, feelings or behaviours.

People in stressful situations make upward, downward and lateral comparisons with similar and dissimilar others depending on whether their goals are self-evaluation, validation, self-enhancement, self-improvement or modeling (Helgeson

& Gottlieb, 2000). Downward comparisons with people who are worse off can enhance self-esteem, upward comparisons with people who are better off can lead to self-improvement, and lateral comparisons with similar others can serve to normalize experiences (Helgeson & Gottlieb, 2000). A review of the social comparison literature (Taylor & Lobel, 1989) revealed that while cancer patients frequently make downward comparisons to enhance their self-esteem, they prefer to associate with others who have either overcome threatening circumstances or adjusted well to them, avoiding those who are doing poorly. Affiliating with other cancer patients who were doing 'well' provided useful cues to successful coping, as well as hope for the future.

Virtual communities, similar to face-to-face support groups, offer cancer patients many opportunities for social comparisons. Consistent with the reviewed literature (Broom, 2005; Sharf, 1997) participants in our study reported using virtual communities to obtain reassurance that their experiences and feelings were normal and practical information from people who had survived breast cancer - reflecting lateral and upward comparisons. Compared to face-to-face groups, participants in our study described virtual communities as a more effective means to find others with a similar type and experience of breast cancer. Those with less common types of breast cancer and co-morbidities described virtual communities as their main source of support. These findings explain the higher rates of activity we observed in breast cancer communities dedicated to less common conditions (Bender, Jimenez-Marroquin, et al., 2012; Davison et al., 2000).

However, the effects of social comparisons are not always positive, which might, in part, explain why cancer patients drop out of virtual communities. Learning that there are others who are doing better provides two pieces of information: that you are not doing as well as everyone, and that it is possible for you to be better than you are at present (Buunk et al., 1997). Conversely, learning that there are others who are worse off suggests that you are not as badly off as everyone, and it is possible for you to get worse (Buunk et al., 1997). Negative social comparisons can increase anxiety, and decrease self-esteem and perceptions of control (Bogart & Helgeson, 2000). These findings help to explain the reasons why cancer patients report dropping out of virtual communities described by Sandaunet (2008). They also help to explain the increase in distress that Salzer et al (2010) reported in their RCT of a virtual community composed entirely of newly diagnosed breast cancer at the same disease stage. Members of that virtual community likely had no opportunities to make upward social comparisons with others who had overcome anxiety provoking aspects of the breast cancer experience and adjusted well to them.

Stress and Coping Theory

The second theoretical perspective that helps to explain the use and effects of virtual communities is the Transactional Theory of Stress and Coping (Lazarus & Folkman, 1984), which postulates that the impact of a stressful event is mediated by: 1) an individual's appraisal of the event, and 2) the coping resources at his or her disposal. Support from peers is hypothesized to promote coping efforts and lessen negative appraisals of events, which in turn reduce or buffer anxiety. Joining a virtual community to seek support from peers or make social comparisons reflect coping strategies. Specifically, seeking information and making upward comparisons with others who are doing well, reflect active or problem-focused coping strategies, while seeking emotional support and making downward comparisons with others who are worse off, are emotion-focused coping strategies. The predominance of one coping style over the other depends on the context, the personality characteristics of the individual and how the event is appraised.

Surveys indicate that the main reasons cancer patients report for using virtual communities is to obtain information (Meier et al., 2007), and content analyses of the communication occurring in cancer virtual communities demonstrate a greater frequency of information-oriented versus emotionally-supportive exchanges (Gooden et al., 2007). Participants in our study explained that they used virtual communities to obtain information and to learn how to cope from breast cancer survivors who were doing well. These findings are reflective of problem-focused coping strategies. Seeking information is a considered a form of cognitive control and a means to gain mastery over an event (Lazarus & Folkman, 1984). Coping strategies that enhance perceptions of control are an important element in the process of adjustment to cancer (Taylor, 1983). Furthermore, the availability and anonymity offered by the medium, likely serves to enhance cancer patients sense of control by allowing them to access information and support when they want it as opposed to when it is available, and to control their interactions with others including when the choose to disclose personal information and with whom.

Several researchers have successfully used the Theory of Stress and Coping to explain the effects of virtual communities. Gustafson and colleagues (2001, 2005) demonstrated increases in perceptions of social support among users of a multi-dimensional support community for breast cancer survivors. Lieberman and Goldstein (2005) reported reductions in perceived stress among users of online breast cancer discussion lists. A survey of 103 users of 30 different virtual cancer communities demonstrated a modest positive correlation between perceptions of emotional support and global measures of perceived stress (Wright, 2002). Research involving 148 users of 24 different health-related virtual communities revealed that the amount of time spent in virtual communities was directly related to satisfaction with the support received (Wright, 2000). Satisfaction with online support correlated with reduction in perceived stress, suggesting that the degree to which a virtual community meets users' needs may determine the extent of its effects. These findings support Optimal Matching Theory (Cutrona & Russel, 1990), which suggests that the effects of social support will be greatest if matched to the demands of the stressor.

Technology Acceptance Model

Whether or not an individual chooses to use virtual communities as a method of coping in the first place depends on their attitudes and beliefs about virtual communities. The Technology Acceptance Model (Davis, 1989) is perhaps the most widely used theory to explain the relationship between attitudes and use of information technology (IT). The TAM asserts that attitude toward using IT systems is determined by two types of beliefs: *perceived usefulness*, defined as the extent to which using a system will enhance an individual's job; and *perceived ease of use*, defined as the extent to which an individual believes that using the system will be free of effort. The main reasons why most cancer patients do not use virtual communities are consistent with the TAM. Specifically, significantly more cancer patients reported lack of perceived need (48%) as a barrier to use than lack of confidence in using virtual communities (9%) (Bender & Jiang, 2013), which is consistent with applications of the TAM that have shown that perceived need has more predictive power than perceived ease of use (Taylor & Todd, 1995).

The literature suggests that cancer patients' individual motivations to use virtual communities are driven by their health needs. For example, unmet supportive care needs were shown to be predictive of use of virtual communities by cancer patients (Bender & Jiang, 2013). Furthermore, once those needs are met or if those needs are not met, cancer patients withdraw from virtual communities; if a new need arises cancer patients return to virtual communities for support (Bender et al., 2013; Sandaunet, 2008). With colleagues Massimi, Witteman and Ahmed, we argue that departure from a virtual community is not necessarily a failing of the site's design or purpose, but rather a potentially logical reaction to changing life circumstances (Massimi, Bender, Witteman and Ahmed, 2014). In this study, we explained that part of the success of virtual communities stems from their ability to meet a particular need at a particular point in an individual's life. We called for measures that capture the extent to which a virtual community meets participants needs, and innovations to help individuals find the right community at the right time, and transition to other more suitable virtual communities as their needs and life circumstances change.

Theory of Planned Behaviour

The Theory of Planned Behaviour (TPB) (Ajzen, 1991) is an extension of the Theory of Reasoned Action (Fishbein, 1967), on which the TAM is based. The Theory of Planned Behaviour maintains that intentions to perform a health behaviour are influenced not only by *attitudes* toward performing the behavior, but also by *subjective norms* associated with the behavior and *behavioural control* to perform the behaviour. The more favourable the attitude, perceived social pressure, and perceived ability to perform the behaviour, the stronger should be the individual's intention to perform the behaviour in question.

The TPB has been successfully used to predict a wide range of health and non-health related behaviours. Of particular relevance, the TPB was used to investigate factors associated with the use of face-to-face support groups by cancer patients as a method of coping. Using the TPB, Grande, Myers and Sutton (2006) demonstrated that beliefs about face-to-face support groups, important others' beliefs about face-to-face support groups, less perceived difficulty in joining a face-to-face support group, and lack of support from a special person were associated with cancer support group membership, independent of demographic and clinical characteristics.

Virtual communities are similar to IT systems in that they provide technology-mediated access to information that can support decision-making. However, virtual communities differ in one very important way, the information they contain is created through the collaborative efforts of the community. The success of a virtual community is therefore dependent on its *sociability* – the ability to support social interactions (Preece, 2001). One key aspect of sociability is *credibility*, which is the believability of a source or message (Flanagin & Metzger, 2008). Lin (2006) created a decomposed version of the TAM-TPB model tailored to the virtual community context with the addition of *perceived trust* as determinant of attitude along with perceived usefulness and ease of use. Based on a survey of users of non-health related virtual communities, Lin demonstrated that attitude and perceived behavioural control were significant predictors of intention to use, while subjective norms were not. Our research suggests that each of these factors influenced use, the extent to which requires further investigation (Bender et al., 2013). Specifically, the perceived usefulness of a virtual community was judged in part based on its perceived trustworthiness (judged based on the quality, currency and empathic nature of posts). Recommendations from trusted peers influenced use while the negative views of health care professionals regarding virtual communities did not discourage use. Lastly, lack of confidence in using virtual communities was identified as a barrier to use, while the control afforded by the medium in terms of controlling interactions with others was cited as an advantage.

Multi-Theory Framework

Figure 1 presents an integrated theoretical framework for understanding the conditions that influence the use and effects of virtual communities by cancer patients. This multi- theory framework is intended to illustrate the important role virtual communities serve as a problem-focused coping strategy (Stress and Coping Theory) to obtain authentic practical information and emotional support to address a specific unmet need and in doing so reduce illness related uncertainty and anxiety, and enhance

Figure 1. A multi-theory framework for understanding the use and effects of virtual communities by cancer patients (Adapted from Bender et al., 2013)

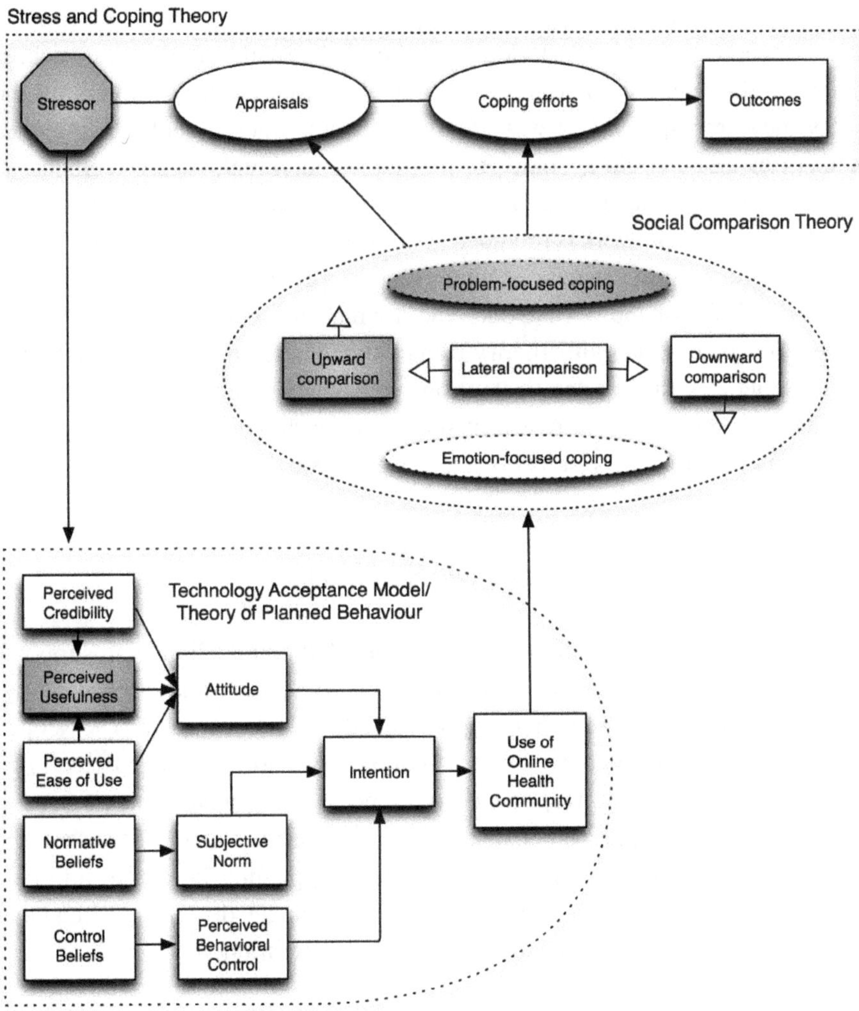

perceptions of control. Although virtual communities offer cancer patients numerous opportunities to make social comparisons with others to judge the appropriateness of their thoughts, feelings and experiences (Social Comparison Theory), they are primarily used to make upward social comparisons with cancer survivors 'who have been through it and are doing well'. Being exposed to cancer patients who are not doing well leads to downward social comparisons, which can cause cancer patients distress and motivate them to leave a virtual community. Lastly, cancer patients are motivated to join and use virtual communities as a coping strategy based on their beliefs about virtual communities, which are largely influenced by their perceptions of their credibility and usefulness, the opinions of other cancer patients, and their self-efficacy to use them effectively (Modified TAM-TPB). A summary of the theoretical constructs and the corresponding practical implications are provided in Table 1

In sum, when used in combination these theories provide a theoretical backbone for understanding what motivates cancer patients to join virtual communities, how and why they are supposed to work, why they sometimes do not work. None of these theories alone could account for the many individual, social, technical and contextual factors that influence the use and effects of cancer virtual communities. This multi-theory framework is intended to help guide the design of effective virtual community interventions for cancer patients, and to predict and explain their effects, including the choice of appropriate outcomes for measuring the effects. Further work is needed to validate this multi-theory framework. There are also other potentially applicable theories that warrant attention, particularly from computer-mediated communication theory. For a review of such theories and how they relate to health related virtual communities, see (Wright & Bell, 2003)].

CONCLUSION AND FUTURE DIRECTIONS

Virtual communities are promising interventions that could fill gaps in supportive cancer care by providing cancer patients with a convenient and effective way to collaboratively meet many of their support needs in a timely way. The scope of virtual communities available to cancer patients is wide reaching extending to individuals with less common types and experiences of cancer who are poorly served by traditional support systems because they do not fit the model of the "average" patient. Virtual communities may be particularly appealing for these individuals because they provide a way for them to more easily connect, develop a critical mass, and build a shared knowledge base related to their condition.

Considerable descriptive evidence suggests that virtual communities help cancer patients by: reducing feelings of isolation; validating concerns; alleviating fears; providing reassurance and hope for the future; enhancing coping and self-management; and lead to better-informed and prepared cancer patients who may use healthcare resources more optimally. Most of this research has focused on breast cancer survivors. More research is needed to understand the role of virtual communities for other cancer survivors and people from different races and ethnic backgrounds.

However, virtual communities are not without their limitations and one size does not fit all. Furthermore, cancer patients' needs and preferences for information and support can change throughout the illness, and their attitudes toward cancer and their coping strategies may constrain their wish for and efforts to obtain support at various stages. Given the abundance of virtual communities that exist for cancer patients, innovations are needed to help patients more easily find an optimal match and transition to new communities as their needs and circumstances change. Moreover, given that cancer patients may have to self-select virtual communities in order to obtain benefit, efforts that seek to use virtual communities to provide care should offer multiple relevant options.

There remain many unanswered questions that should focus future research. Overall, there is a lack of knowledge regarding the effects of virtual communities on cancer patients' health outcomes, along with how and why they work, in what circumstances and for whom. We have proposed a preliminary multi-theory framework to guide future work into the relationships between the context in which virtual communities are applied, the mechanisms by which they work, and the outcomes they produce. Further research is needed to flesh out this multi-theory framework and to evaluate its adequacy as a tool to explain the use and effects of virtual communities for diverse cancer patients.

At the same time, we need to explore and develop new approaches to more accurately capture the effects of virtual communities and to measure their success. Success metrics need to move beyond simply tallying members and posts, to include more nuanced measures that consider the lifecycle of the community and whether and to what extent users' needs are met.

In sum, the provision of support is a very personalized aspect of care. The philosophy of personalized medicine – the right support at the right time - would enhance both the study and delivery of virtual peer support for cancer patients.

REFERENCES

Ajzen, I. (1991). The theory of planned behaviour. *Organizational Behavior and Human Decision Processes*, *50*(2), 179–211. doi:10.1016/0749-5978(91)90020-T

Ali, K., Farrer, L., Gulliver, A., & Griffiths, K. M. (2015). Online Peer-to-Peer Support for Young People With Mental Health Problems: A Systematic Review. *JMIR Mental Health*, *2*(2), e19. doi:10.2196/mental.4418 PMID:26543923

Allen, K. (2013). *Consumption of culture by older Canadians on the Internet.* Statistics Canada.

Arora, N. K., Finney Rutten, L. J., Gustafson, D. H., Moser, R., & Hawkins, R. P. (2007). Perceived helpfulness and impact of social support provided by family, friends, and health care providers to women newly diagnosed with breast cancer. *Psycho-Oncology*, *16*(5), 474–486. doi:10.1002/pon.1084 PMID:16986172

Bender, J., & Jiang, H. (2013). Online communities: Prevalence and predictors of use, and reasons for non-use. In Medicine 2.0. London: Medicine 2.0.

Bender, J., & Miller, A. (2016). Scoping review of virtual health communities as standalone or adjunct interventions. In *Proceedings of the 37th Annual Society of Behavioral Medicine Conference*. Washington, DC: Society of Behavioural Medicine.

Bender, J. L., Jimenez-Marroquin, M. C., Ferris, L. E., Katz, J., & Jadad, A. R. (2012). Online communities for breast cancer survivors: A review and analysis of their characteristics and levels of use. *Supportive Care in Cancer*, *21*(5), 1253–1263. doi:10.1007/s00520-012-1655-9 PMID:23179491

Bender, J. L., Jimenez-Marroquin, M. C., & Jadad, A. R. (2011). Seeking support on Facebook: A content analysis of breast cancer groups. *Journal of Medical Internet Research*, *13*(1), e16. doi:10.2196/jmir.1560 PMID:21371990

Bender, J. L., Katz, J., Ferris, L. E., & Jadad, A. R. (2013). What is the role of online support from the perspective of facilitators of face-to-face support groups? A multi-method study of the use of breast cancer online communities. *Patient Education and Counseling*, *93*(3), 472–479. doi:10.1016/j.pec.2013.07.009 PMID:23928354

Bender, J. L., O'Grady, L., & Jadad, A. R. (2008). Supporting cancer patients through the continuum of care: A view from the age of social networks and computer-mediated communication. *Current Oncology (Toronto, Ont.)*, *15*, S42–S47. PMID:18769582

Bender, J. L., Wiljer, D., Sawka, A. M., Tsang, R., Alkazaz, N., & Brierley, J. D. (2016). Thyroid cancer survivors perceptions of survivorship care follow-up options: A cross-sectional, mixed-methods survey. *Supportive Care in Cancer, 24*(5), 2007–2015. doi:10.1007/s00520-015-2981-5 PMID:26530226

Bender, J. L., Wiljer, D., To, M. J., Bedard, P. L., Chung, P., Jewett, M. A., & Gospodarowicz, M. et al. (2012). Testicular cancer survivors supportive care needs and use of online support: A cross-sectional survey. *Supportive Care in Cancer, 20*(11), 2737–2746. doi:10.1007/s00520-012-1395-x PMID:22382589

Blumer, J. G., & Katz, E. (1974). *The uses of mass communications: Current perspectives on gratifications research*. Beverly Hills, CA: Sage Publications.

Bogart, L., & Helgeson, V. S. (2000). Social comparisons among women with breast cancer: A longitudinal investigation. *Journal of Applied Social Psychology, 30*(3), 547–575. doi:10.1111/j.1559-1816.2000.tb02496.x

Boyde, D., & Ellison, N. (2008). Social network sites: Definition, history and scholarship. *Journal of Computer-Mediated Communication, 13*(1), 210–230. doi:10.1111/j.1083-6101.2007.00393.x

Broom, A. (2005). The eMale: Prostate cancer, masculinity, and online support as a challenge to medical expertise. *Journal of Sociology (Melbourne, Vic.), 41*(1), 87–104. doi:10.1177/1440783305050965

Broom, A. (2005). Virtually he@lthy: The impact of internet use on disease experience and the doctor-patient relationship. *Qualitative Health Research, 15*(3), 325–345. doi:10.1177/1049732304272916 PMID:15761103

Burg, M. A., Adorno, G., Lopez, E. D. S., Loerzel, V., Stein, K., Wallace, C., & Sharma, D. K. B. (2015). Current unmet needs of cancer survivors: Analysis of open-ended responses to the American Cancer Society Study of Cancer Survivors II. *Cancer, 121*(4), 623–630. doi:10.1002/cncr.28951 PMID:25581252

Burke, M., & Kraut, R. E. (2016). The relationship between Facebook use and well-being depends on communication type and tie strength. *Journal of Computer-Mediated Communication, 21*(4), 265–281. doi:10.1111/jcc4.12162

Buunk, B., Gibbons, F., & Reis-Bergan, M. (1997). Social comparison in health and illness - An overview. In B. Buunk, F. Gibbons, & M. Reis-Bergan (Eds.), *Health, coping and well-being*. Lawrence Erlbaum Associates.

Canadian Cancer Society (CCS). (2016). *Canadian Cancer Statistics 2016*. Author.

Chang, T., Chopra, V., Zhang, C., & Woolford, S. J. (2013). The role of social media in online weight management: Systematic review. *Journal of Medical Internet Research, 15*(11), e262. doi:10.2196/jmir.2852 PMID:24287455

Crocco, A. G., Villasis-Keever, M., & Jadad, A. R. (2002). Analysis of cases of harm associated with use of health information on the internet. *Journal of the American Medical Association, 287*(21), 2869–2871. doi:10.1001/jama.287.21.2869 PMID:12038937

Cutrona Russell, D. C. (1990). Type of social support and specific stress: Toward a theory of optimal matching. In S. B. Sarason & G. Pierce (Ed.), Social support: An interactional view. New York: Wiley.

Daher, M. (2012). Cultural beliefs and values in cancer patients. *Annals of Oncology, 23*(suppl 3), 66–69. doi:10.1093/annonc/mds091 PMID:22628419

Davis, F. D. (1989). Perceived usefulness, perceived ease of use, and user acceptance of information technology. *Management Information Science Quarterly, 13*(3), 319–339.

Davison, K. P., Pennebaker, J. W., & Dickerson, S. S. (2000). Who talks? The social psychology of illness support groups. *The American Psychologist, 55*(2), 205–217. doi:10.1037/0003-066X.55.2.205 PMID:10717968

Deshpande, A., & Jadad, A. (2006). Web 2.0: Could it help move the health care system in the 21st century? *Journal of Mens Health & Gender, 3*(4), 332–336. doi:10.1016/j.jmhg.2006.09.004

Esquivel, A., Meric-Bernstam, F., & Bernstam, E. V. (2006). Accuracy and self correction of information received from an internet breast cancer list: Content analysis. *BMJ (Clinical Research Ed.), 332*(7547), 939–942. doi:10.1136/bmj.38753.524201.7C PMID:16513686

European Commission. (n.d.). *Personalised Medicine | Health - Research & Innovation - European Commission.* Retrieved January 27, 2017, from http://ec.europa.eu/research/health/index.cfm?pg=policy&policyname=personalised

Eysenbach, G., Powell, J., Englesakis, M., Rizo, C., & Stern, A. (2004). Health related virtual communities and electronic support groups: Systematic review of the effects of online peer to peer interactions. *BMJ (Clinical Research Ed.), 328*(7449), 1166. doi:10.1136/bmj.328.7449.1166 PMID:15142921

Facebook Newsroom. (n.d.). *Facebook Company Info*. Retrieved January 27, 2017, from http://newsroom.fb.com/company-info/

Festinger, L. (1954). A theory of social comparison processed. *Human Relations*, *7*(2), 117–140. doi:10.1177/001872675400700202

Fishbein, M. (1967). *Readings in attitude theory and measurement*. New York: John Wiley & Sons, Inc.

Fitch, M. I. (2000). Supportive care for cancer patients. *Hospital Quarterly*, *3*(4), 39–46. PMID:11482268

Flanagin, A. J., & Metzger, M. J. (2008). Digital media and youth: Unparalleled opportunity and unprecedented responsibilty. The John D. and Catherine T. MacArthur Foundation Series on Digial Media and Learning. Cambridge, MA: MIT Press.

Fogel, J., Ribisl, K. M., Morgan, P. D., Humphreys, K., & Lyons, E. J. (2008). Underrepresentation of African Americans in online cancer support groups. *Journal of the National Medical Association*, *100*(6), 705–712. doi:10.1016/S0027-9684(15)31346-8 PMID:18595573

Fox, S. (2011). Peer-to-peer Health Care. *Pew Research Center*. Retrieved from http://www.pewinternet.org/2011/02/28/peer-to-peer-health-care-2/

Frank, A. (1995). *The wounded storyteller: Body, illness and ethics*. Chicago: The University of Chicago Press. doi:10.7208/chicago/9780226260037.001.0001

Gagliardi, A., & Jadad, A. R. (2002). Examination of instruments used to rate quality of health information on the Internet: Chronicle of a vouage with unclear destination. *British Medical Journal*, *324*(7337), 569–573. doi:10.1136/bmj.324.7337.569 PMID:11884320

Gass, J. S., Weitzen, S., Clark, M., & Dizon, D. S. (2007). Defining social support systems for women with breast cancer. *American Journal of Surgery*, *194*(4), 501–503. doi:10.1016/j.amjsurg.2007.07.005 PMID:17826065

Gooden, R. J., Winefield, H. R., Gooden, R. J., & Winefield, H. R. (2007). Breast and prostate cancer online discussion boards: A thematic analysis of gender differences and similarities. *Journal of Health Psychology*, *12*(1), 103–114. doi:10.1177/1359105307071744 PMID:17158844

Grande, G. E., Myers, L. B., & Sutton, S. R. (2006). How do patients who participate in cancer support groups differ from those who do not? *Psycho-Oncology*, *15*(4), 321–334. doi:10.1002/pon.956 PMID:16106472

Greenwood, S., Perrin, A., & Duggan, M. (2016). Social Media Update 2016. *Pew Research Centre*. Retrieved from http://www.pewinternet.org/2016/11/11/social-media-update-2016/#fn-17239-1

Griffiths, K. M., Calear, A. L., & Banfield, M. (2009). Systematic review on Internet Support Groups (ISGs) and depression (1): Do ISGs reduce depressive symptoms? *Journal of Medical Internet Research*, *11*(3), e40. doi:10.2196/jmir.1270 PMID:19793719

Gustafson, D. H., McTavish, F. M., Stengle, W., Ballard, D., Hawkins, R., Shaw, B. R., & Landucci, G. et al. (2005). Use and Impact of eHealth System by Low-income Women With Breast Cancer. *Journal of Health Communication*, *10*(sup1), 195–218. doi:10.1080/10810730500263257 PMID:16377608

Hale, T. M., Pathipati, A. S., Zan, S., & Jethwani, K. (2014). Representation of health conditions on Facebook: Content analysis and evaluation of user engagement. *Journal of Medical Internet Research*, *16*(8), e182. doi:10.2196/jmir.3275 PMID:25092386

Helgeson, V. S., & Gottlieb, B. (2000). Support Groups. In S. Cohen, L. Underwood, & B. Gottlieb (Eds.), *Social support measurement and intervention*. Oxford University Press. doi:10.1093/med:psych/9780195126709.003.0007

Hong, Y., Peña-Purcell, N. C., & Ory, M. G. (2012). Outcomes of online support and resources for cancer survivors: A systematic literature review. *Patient Education and Counseling*, *86*(3), 288–296. doi:10.1016/j.pec.2011.06.014 PMID:21798685

Hoybye, M. T., Dalton, S. O., Deltour, I., Bidstrup, P. E., Frederiksen, K., & Johansen, C. (n.d.). Effect of Internet peer-support groups on psychosocial adjustment to cancer: A randomised study. *Br J Cancer, 102*(9), 1348–1354.

Hoybye, M. T., Johansen, C., Tjornhoj-Thomsen, T., Hoybye, M. T., Johansen, C., & Tjornhoj-Thomsen, T. (2005). Online interaction. Effects of storytelling in an internet breast cancer support group. *Psycho-Oncology*, *14*(3), 211–220. doi:10.1002/pon.837 PMID:15386774

Im, E. O., Chee, W., Im, E.-O., & Chee, W. (2008). The use of Internet cancer support groups by ethnic minorities. *Journal of Transcultural Nursing*, *19*(1), 74–82. doi:10.1177/1043659607309140 PMID:18217235

Im, E. O., Chee, W., Tsai, H. M., Lin, L. C., Cheng, C. Y., Im, E.-O., & Cheng, C.-Y. et al. (2005). Internet cancer support groups: A feminist analysis. *Cancer Nursing*, *28*(1), 1–7. doi:10.1097/00002820-200501000-00001 PMID:15681976

Internal Agnecy for Researh on Cancer (IARC). (2014). *GLOBOCAN2012: Estimated Cancer Incidence, Mortality and Prevalence Worldwide in 2012*. Retrieved from http://globocan.iarc.fr/Pages/fact_sheets_cancer.aspx

Jadad, A. R., Enkin, M. W., Glouberman, S., Groff, P., & Stern, A. (2006). Are virtual communities good for our health? *British Medical Journal, 332*(7547), 925–926. doi:10.1136/bmj.332.7547.925 PMID:16627491

Jadad, A. R., & Gagliardi, A. (1998). Rating health information on the Internet: Navigating to knowledge or to Babel? *Journal of the American Medical Association, 279*(8), 611–614. doi:10.1001/jama.279.8.611 PMID:9486757

Jefford, M. H. N., & Tattersall, M. H. N. (2002). Informing and involving cancer patients in their own care. *The Lancet Oncology, 3*(10), 629–637. doi:10.1016/S1470-2045(02)00877-X PMID:12372725

Kairam, S., Wang, D. J., & Leskovec, J. (2012). The life and death of online groups: predicting growth and longevity. *Proceedings of the Web Search and Data Mining (WSDM) Conference*. doi:10.1145/2124295.2124374

Kash, K. M., Mago, R., Kunkel, E. J., Kash, K. M., Mago, R., & Kunkel, E. J. S. (2005). Psychosocial oncology: Supportive care for the cancer patient. *Seminars in Oncology, 32*(2), 211–218. doi:10.1053/j.seminoncol.2004.11.011 PMID:15815967

Klemm, P. (2012). Effects of Online Support Group Format (Moderated vs Peer-Led) on Depressive Symptoms and Extent of Participation in Women With Breast Cancer. *CIN: Computers, Informatics, Nursing, 30*(1), 9–18.

Klemm, P., Bunnell, D., Cullen, M., Soneji, R., Gibbons, P., & Holecek, A. (2003). Online cancer support groups: a review of the research literature. *CIN: Computers, Informatics, Nursing, 21*(3), 136–142.

Klemm, P., Hurst, M., Dearholt, S. L., & Trone, S. R. (1999). Gender differences on Internet cancer support groups. *Computers in Nursing, 17*(2), 65–72. PMID:10194883

Klemm, P., Reppert, K., & Visich, L. (1998). A nontraditional cancer support group. The Internet. *Computers in Nursing, 16*(1), 31–36. PMID:9454992

Kwan, J., Croke, J., Panzarella, T., Ubhi, K., Lui, F., Fyles, A., … Bender, J. (2017). *Well breast cancer surivivors perceptions of alternate follow-up care options: A cross-sectional survey.* In Preparation.

Lazarus, S., & Folkman, R. (1984). *Stress, appriasial and coping*. New York: Springer.

Lieberman, M. A., Goldstein, B. A., Lieberman, M. A., & Goldstein, B. A. (2006). Not all negative emotions are equal: The role of emotional expression in online support groups for women with breast cancer. *Psycho-Oncology*, *15*(2), 160–168. doi:10.1002/pon.932 PMID:15880627

Lin, H. F. (2006). Understanding behavioral intention to participate in virtual communities. *Cyberpsychology & Behavior*, *9*(5), 540–547. doi:10.1089/cpb.2006.9.540 PMID:17034320

Massimi, M., Bender, J. L., Witteman, H. O., & Ahmed, O. H. (2014). Life transitions and online health communities. In *Proceedings of the 17th ACM conference on Computer supported cooperative work & social computing - CSCW '14* (pp. 1491–1501). New York: ACM Press.

Mead, N., Varnam, R., Rogers, A., & Roland, M. (2003). What predicts patients interest in the Internet as a health resource in primary care in England? *Journal of Health Services Research & Policy*, *8*(1), 33–39. doi:10.1177/135581960300800108 PMID:12683432

Meier, A., Lyons, E. J., Frydman, G., Forlenza, M., Rimer, B. K., Meier, A., & Rimer, B. K. et al. (2007). How cancer survivors provide support on cancer-related Internet mailing lists. *Journal of Medical Internet Research*, *9*(2), e12. doi:10.2196/jmir.9.2.e12 PMID:17513283

Norman, C. D., & Skinner, H. A. (2006). eHealth Literacy: Essential Skills for Consumer Health in a Networked World. *Journal of Medical Internet Research*, *8*(2), e9. doi:10.2196/jmir.8.2.e9 PMID:16867972

O'Grady, L., Bender, J., Urowitz, S., Wiljer, D., & Jadad, A. R. (2010). Promoting and participating in online health forums : A guide to facilitation and evaluation for health professionals. *Journal of Communication*, *3*(3), 246–258.

O'Reilly, T. (n.d.). *What Is Web 2.0? 7. Rich User Experiences*. Retrieved January 29, 2017, from http://www.oreilly.com/pub/a/web2/archive/what-is-web-20.html?page=5

OGrady, L. A., Bender, J. L., Uroowitz, S., Wiljer, D., & Jadad, A. R. (2010). Promoting and participating in online health forums: A guide to facilitation and evaluation for health professionals. *Journal of Community Health*, *3*(4), 246–257. doi:10.1179/175380710X12870623776478

Orgad, S. (2006). The cultural dimensions of online communities: A study of breast cancer internet spaces. *New Media & Society*, *8*(6), 877–899. doi:10.1177/1461444806069643

Pingree, S., Hawkins, R., Baker, T., duBenske, L., Roberts, L. J., & Gustafson, D. H. (2010). The value of theory for enhancing and understanding e-health interventions. *American Journal of Preventive Medicine*, *38*(1), 103–109. doi:10.1016/j.amepre.2009.09.035 PMID:20117565

Pitts, V. (2004). Illness and internet empowerment: Writing and reading breast cancer in cyberspace. *Health*, *8*(1), 33–59. doi:10.1177/1363459304038794 PMID:15018717

Preece, J. (2001). Sociability and usability in online communities: Determining and measurign success. *Behaviour & Information Technology*, *20*(5), 347–356. doi:10.1080/01449290110084683

Salzer, M. S., Palmer, S. C., Kaplan, K., Brusilovskiy, E., Ten Have, T., Hampshire, M., & Coyne, J. C. et al. (2010). A randomized, controlled study of Internet peer-to-peer interactions among women newly diagnosed with breast cancer. *Psycho-Oncology*, *19*(4), 441–446. doi:10.1002/pon.1586 PMID:19484712

Sandaunet, A.-G. (2008). A space for suffering? Communicating breast cancer in an online self-help context. *Qualitative Health Research*, *18*(12), 1631–1641. doi:10.1177/1049732308327076 PMID:18955462

Sandaunet, A. G., & Sandaunet, A.-G. (2008). The challenge of fitting in: Non-participation and withdrawal from an online self-help group for breast cancer patients. *Sociology of Health & Illness*, *30*(1), 131–144. doi:10.1111/j.1467-9566.2007.01041.x PMID:18254837

Schork, N. J. (2015). Personalized medicine: Time for one-person trials. *Nature*, *520*(7549), 609–611. doi:10.1038/520609a PMID:25925459

Sharf, B. F. (1997). Communicating breast cancer on-line: Support and empowerment on the Internet. *Women & Health*, *26*(1), 65–84. doi:10.1300/J013v26n01_05 PMID:9311100

Smit, W., van Uden-Kraan, C. F., Drossaert, C. H. C., Seydel, E. R., Taal, E., & Van der Laar, M. (2007). Patients with breast cancer feel empowered by their participation in online support groups. In *Proceedings of the American Society for Clinical Oncology (ASCO) Conference*. Chicago: ASCO Press.

Spiegel, D., & Classen, C. (2000). *Group therapy for cancer patients*. New York: Basic Books.

Statistics Canada. (2012). *Canadian Internet Use Survey, 2012*. Author.

Sullivan, C. F. (2003). Gendered cybersupport: A thematic analysis of two online cancer support groups. *Journal of Health Psychology*, *8*(1), 83–103. doi:10.1177/1359105303008001446 PMID:22113903

Taylor, S., & Todd, P. A. (1995). Assessing IT usage: A test of competing models. *Information Systems Research*, *6*, 144–176. doi:10.1287/isre.6.2.144

Taylor, S. E. (1983). Adjustment to threatening events: A theory of cognitive adaptation. *The American Psychologist*, *38*(11), 1161–1173. doi:10.1037/0003-066X.38.11.1161

Taylor, S. E., & Lobel, M. (1989). Social comparison activity under threat: Downward evaluation and upward contacts. *Psychological Review*, *96*(4), 569–575. doi:10.1037/0033-295X.96.4.569 PMID:2678204

Ussher, J., Kirsten, L., Butow, P., & Sandoval, M. (2006). What do cancer support groups provide which other supportive relationships do not? The experience of peer support groups for people with cancer. *Social Science & Medicine*, *62*(10), 2565–2576. doi:10.1016/j.socscimed.2005.10.034 PMID:16303220

van Uden-Kraan, C. F., Drossaert, C. H., Taal, E., Seydel, E. R., van de Laar, M. A., van Uden-Kraan, C. F., & van de Laar, M. A. F. J. et al. (2008). Self-reported differences in empowerment between lurkers and posters in online patient support groups. *Journal of Medical Internet Research*, *10*(2), e18. doi:10.2196/jmir.992 PMID:18653442

van Uden-Kraan, C. F., Drossaert, C. H., Taal, E., Shaw, B. R., Seydel, E. R., van de Laar, M. A., & van de Laar, M. A. F. J. (2008). Empowering processes and outcomes of participation in online support groups for patients with breast cancer, arthritis, or fibromyalgia. *Qualitative Health Research*, *18*(3), 405–417. doi:10.1177/1049732307313429 PMID:18235163

van Uden-Kraan, C. F., Drossaert, C. H. C., Taal, E., Seydel, E. R., & van de Laar, M. A. F. (2010). Patient-intitated online support groups: Motives for initation, extent of success and success factors. *Journal of Telemedicine and Telecare*, *16*(1), 30–34. doi:10.1258/jtt.2009.001009 PMID:20086265 van Uden-Kraan, C. F., Drossaert, C. H. C., Taal, E., Smit, W. M., Moens, H. J. B., Siesling, S., & van de Laar, M. A. F. J. et al. (2009). Health-related Internet use by patients with somatic diseases: Frequency of use and characteristics of users. *Informatics for Health & Social Care*, *34*(1), 18–29. doi:10.1080/17538150902773272 PMID:19306196

Vilhauer, R. P., & Vilhauer, R. P. (2009). Perceived benefits of online support groups for women with metastatic breast cancer. *Women & Health*, *49*(5), 381–404. doi:10.1080/03630240903238719 PMID:19851944

Vivar, C. G., & McQueen, A. (2005). Informational and emotional needs of long-term survivors of breast cancer. *Journal of Advanced Nursing*, *51*(5), 520–528. doi:10.1111/j.1365-2648.2005.03524.x PMID:16098169

Walther, J. B., Pingree, S., Hawkins, R. P., Buller, D. B., Walther, J. B., Pingree, S., & Buller, D. B. et al. (2005). Attributes of interactive online health information systems. *Journal of Medical Internet Research*, *7*(3), e33. doi:10.2196/jmir.7.3.e33 PMID:15998624

Webb, T. L., Joseph, J., Yardley, L., Michie, S., Webb, T. L., Joseph, J., … Michie, S. (n.d.). Using the internet to promote health behavior change: A systematic review and meta-analysis of the impact of theoretical basis, use of behavior change techniques, and mode of delivery on efficacy. *Journal of Medical Internet Research, 12*(1), e4.

Weiss, R. (1974). The provisions of social relationships. In *Doing unto others*. Prentice Hall.

Winzelberg, A. J., Classen, C., Alpers, G. W., Roberts, H., Koopman, C., Adams, R. E., & Taylor, C. B. et al. (2003). Evaluation of an internet support group for women with primary breast cancer. *Cancer*, *97*(5), 1164–1173. doi:10.1002/cncr.11174 PMID:12599221

World Health Organization. (2015). *WHO | Cancer Fact Sheet Number 297*. WHO.

Wright, K. (2002). Social support within an online cancer community: An assessment of emotional support, perceptions of advantages and disadvantage, and motives for using the community from a communication perspective. *Journal of Applied Communication Research*, *30*(3), 195–209. doi:10.1080/00909880216586

Wright, K. B., Bell, S. B., Wright, K. B., & Bell, S. B. (2003). Health-related Support Groups on the Internet: Linking Empirical Findings to Social Support and Computer-mediated Communication Theory. *Journal of Health Psychology*, *8*(1), 39–54. doi:10.1177/1359105303008001429 PMID:22113899

Yalom, I. (1995). *Theory and practice of group pscyhotherapy*. New York: Basic Books.

Young, C. (2013). Community management that works: How to build and sustain a thriving online health community. *Journal of Medical Internet Research, 15*(6), e119. doi:10.2196/jmir.2501 PMID:23759312

Zabora, J., BrintzenhofeSzoc, K., Curbow, B., Hooker, C., & Piantadosi, S. (2001). The prevalence of psychological distress by cancer site. *Psycho-Oncology, 10*(1), 19–28. doi:10.1002/1099-1611(200101/02)10:1<19::AID-PON501>3.0.CO;2-6 PMID:11180574

KEY TERMS AND DEFINITIONS

Cancer Survivor: "An individual is considered a cancer survivor from the point of diagnosis through the balance of his or her life" (Mullan, 1985).

Long-Tail: The long-tail in health represents the numerous individuals with less common conditions who are poorly served by traditional support systems because they do not fit the model of the "average" patient (Deshpande & Jadad, 2006).

Peer Support: Social support provided by and for individuals who share something in common (Hegleson & Gottlieb, 2000).

Personalized Medicine: A medical model that uses molecular profiling for delivering the right therapeutic strategy for the right person at the right time (European Commission, n.d.).

Social Support: The functional provisions of relationships, such as emotional, instrumental and informational assistance, or the health benefits accrued from simply belonging to a group (Cohen, Gottlieb, & Underwood, 2000).

Supportive Care: "The provision of the necessary services *as defined by* those living with or affected by cancer to meet their physical, social, emotional, informational, psychological, spiritual, and practical needs during the pre-diagnostic, diagnostic, treatment, and follow-up phases of cancer care, encompassing issues of survivorship, palliation and bereavement" (Fitch, 2000).

Virtual Community: "A virtual social space where people come together to get and give information or support, to learn, or to find company" (Preece, 2001).

Chapter 4
Manage My Pain:
A Patient-Driven Mobile Platform to Prevent and Manage Chronic Postsurgical Pain

Aliza Weinrib
Toronto General Hospital, University Health Network, Canada

Muhammad Abid Azam
York University, Canada & Toronto General Hospital, University Health Network, Canada

Vered Valeria Latman
York University, Canada

Tahir Janmohamed
ManagingLife, Canada

Hance Clarke
Toronto General Hospital, University Health Network, Canada

Joel Katz
York University, Canada & Toronto General Hospital, University Health Network, Canada

ABSTRACT

This chapter describes the Manage My Pain digital pain management platform and its integration into the Transitional Pain Service at Toronto General Hospital. A collaboration between ManagingLife, the developer of Manage My Pain, and the Transitional Pain Service led to the creation of a patient-provider virtual community with the aim of managing complex pain after surgery so as to prevent the transition

DOI: 10.4018/978-1-5225-2958-3.ch004

from acute post-surgical pain to chronic post-surgical pain. User engagement, motivation, and satisfaction are discussed with respect to the needs of (1) people living with pain and (2) health care providers. Challenges in implementation are described, along with new features developed for the digital platform as a result of the partnership between ManagingLife and the Transitional Pain Service.

INTRODUCTION

Cindy was diagnosed with severe fibromyalgia in 1996 after a shoulder injury -- in addition, she was suffering from pain due to severe whiplash, spinal stenosis, arthritis, bone spurs, degenerative disc disease, and multiple sclerosis. An orthopedic surgeon informed her she would require surgery on her back and neck; however, she was unable to afford health insurance, and surgery was not an option. The prospect of living with severe pain for the rest of her life, and not being able to work to support herself financially, left her feeling depressed and made it difficult to hope for recovery and a life without pain (ManagingLife, 2012).

In 2011, a doctor suggested that Cindy keep a "health journal" to track her symptoms and manage her painful conditions. The health journal was useful but time-consuming and paperwork-heavy. She looked for a smartphone application that would be more effective and convenient and discovered the app, Manage My Pain. The app enabled her to track important information to manage her pain on a daily basis such as symptoms, pain triggers, and treatments for her pain – all with little hassle and in just a few minutes. Tracking and visualizing her pain through the app helped her learn more about her chronic pain. Moreover, she was able to share her data with her doctors. Manage My Pain helped Cindy create a patient-provider virtual community, which ultimately enhanced her ability to effectively manage her chronic pain (ManagingLife, 2012).

Cindy's struggle with chronic pain resembles that of hundreds of millions of chronic pain sufferers around the world. Unable to afford or access pain management services, many people are left to suffer alone, desperate, and impaired. The implementation of a virtual community within the pain management domain presents the dual opportunities of reducing barriers to chronic pain management for people living in pain, and optimizing the delivery of effective treatment by pain clinicians. This chapter chronicles the integration of the award-winning digital pain management platform, Manage My Pain, into an innovative hospital-based pain service to create a patient-provider virtual community with the aim of preventing and managing chronic pain after surgery.

BACKGROUND

The Burden of Chronic Pain

The *silent epidemic* (Wall & Jones, 1991) of pain is a source of tremendous personal suffering, disability, and healthcare expense. Globally, 20% of the population lives with chronic pain, with one-third reporting that their pain is severe (Breivik, Eisenberg, & O'Brien, 2013; Goldberg & McGee, 2011; Schopflocher, Taenzer, & Jovey, 2011).

Chronic pain is generally defined as pain that persists beyond three to six months (Katz, Pagé, Fashler, Rosenbloom, & Asmundson, 2014; Treede et al., 2015), exceeding the expected timeframe for tissues to heal after injury, surgery, or illness (e.g., cancer). When pain becomes chronic, it can become a primary disorder in its own right: due to changes in pain processing in the central nervous system, *pain itself* is now the problem, rather than signaling the presence of other underlying physical or medical conditions (Siddall & Cousins, 2004; Tracey & Bushnell, 2009). Once pain becomes chronic, its course is expected to be long-term and possibly even life-long. Treatments are focused on pain reduction and self-management, rather than cure.

The burden of chronic pain is best illustrated by a recent study of more than 24,000 community-dwelling individuals comparing those with chronic pain to those with other chronic diseases (Hogan, Taddio, Katz, Shah, & Krahn, 2016a). The decrement in quality of life associated with chronic pain was lower than for most other chronic diseases including heart disease, diabetes, and chronic obstructive pulmonary disease (Hogan et al., 2016a). Moreover, chronic pain is associated with high rates of mood (Arnow et al., 2006) and anxiety disorders (Katz, Pagé, Fashler, Rosenbloom, & Asmundson, 2014).

The financial costs of chronic pain are a substantial burden to individuals as well as to the health care system. In the US, direct and indirect costs associated with medical care and lost work productivity are estimated at between \$560 - \$635 billion annually, exceeding costs associated with heart disease, cancer, and diabetes ("The National Academies Press", 2011). In Canada, the annual, incremental direct healthcare cost to manage chronic pain was reported to be \$1,742 per patient or a total of ~\$11.5 billion each year, and this does not include the indirect costs associated with lost productivity (Hogan, Taddio, Katz, Shah, & Krahn, 2016b).

The gold standard treatment for chronic pain is comprehensive care (Gatchel & Okifuji, 2006; Scascighini, Toma, & Sprott, 2008) involving multidisciplinary pain specialists, most often pain physicians, pain psychologists, and physiotherapists. Unfortunately, comprehensive pain treatment clinics are scarce and overburdened with high caseloads and long wait times (Fashler et al., 2016). With 1 in 5 Canadian adults living with pain (Schopflocher et al., 2011), the ratio of chronic pain patients to Canadian pain treatment facilities is estimated at 52,000:1 (Fashler et al., 2016). These data illustrate that access to appropriate, specialized pain treatment facilities is unacceptably low; as a consequence, many individuals are struggling to manage their chronic pain and communicate about their pain to non-specialist physicians.

Manage My Pain: A Mobile Platform for Chronic Pain Sufferers

Manage My Pain (MMP), developed by ManagingLife, is a digital platform that allows people living with pain to quickly and easily track their pain on a daily basis using a natively designed and responsive app on their Android smartphones, or a responsively-designed web-app through their mobile or desktop browser. Data is instantly summarized in graphs that show trends and trajectories. This summarized data can be shared with health care providers in person or remotely, creating a virtual community between the individual living with pain and their health care provider. A key design principle of this digital platform is, first and foremost, to meet the needs of people living with pain, so that they find the app intuitive and beneficial. Since MMP was launched in 2012, over 24,000 people have created an account and recorded their pain. In total, over 544,000 pain episodes have been documented by users (Figure 1).

Until 2016, MMP was downloaded solely by individuals who were self-motivated to track their pain, and digital pain diaries were shared with providers at the user's

Figure 1. The Manage My Pain digital platform for patients and health professionals. ©ManagingLife, 2017

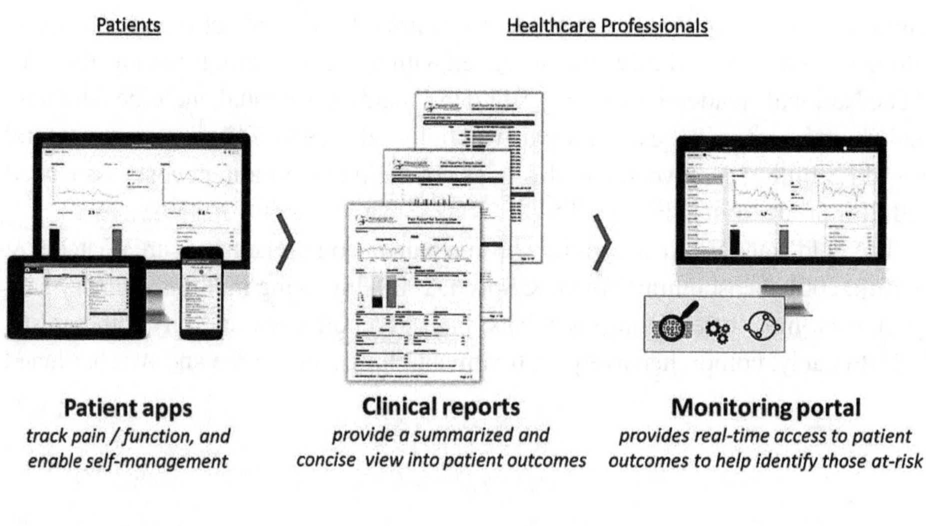

initiative. In 2016, ManagingLife began a partnership with an innovative pain service, the Transitional Pain Service (TPS) at Toronto General Hospital, and this marked a new stage in the application of MMP. As part of this partnership, each patient treated by the pain service would be asked to use the digital platform to record their pain on an ongoing basis, and to communicate their pain and other ratings to their specialized pain team. The goal of this ongoing project is to improve the quality of care provided as well as patient outcomes. As the partnership between ManagingLife and this clinical service evolved, new features, which will be described later, were added to MMP in consultation with the multidisciplinary pain team.

The virtual community formed as a result of this partnership between Managing Life and the Transitional Pain Service, using the MMP application, is a community that links the individual patient to their pain care team, which includes patient coordinators, acute-care nurses, physicians specializing in persistent pain, pain psychologists, and physiotherapists targeting recovery after surgery. Preece (2000) defines a virtual community as one that is composed of individuals satisfying their needs (as our patients are doing post-surgery) or performing their special roles (as our pain team health providers are doing). These individuals must have a reason to form a community – in our case, enhancing post-surgical pain management and patient support after hospital discharge, to allow for open communication regardless of distance, continuity of care, and pro-active and preventative management. In a virtual community, there must be policies to govern interaction (e.g., patients are asked to complete their electronic pain diary once per day). Finally, a computer system is needed which supports social interaction within the community, in this case the MMP application, available as a mobile e-health application or a web-based platform that can be accessed from any web-enabled device. This virtual community has both 'virtual' and 'physical' aspects (El Morr & Kawash, 2007), as patients and providers encounter each other both in the virtual space provided by the digital platform and in the physical space of the pain clinic, at visits that occur bi-weekly or monthly during the six months after surgery. In terms of degree of cooperation (El Morr, 2010), within this virtual community patients provide information and are aware of the engagement of their health providers in the virtual community. Responses to key information come in the form of phone calls between clinic visits in response to actionable health changes, as well as medication changes and so on at clinical visits based on patient self-report using the digital platform. Unlike many virtual communities that are either patient centered (in which patients largely communicate with one another, perhaps guided by a health professional) or professional centered (in which health professionals communicate with one another to build a knowledge network; El Morr, 2010), this virtual community links the patient and his or her specialist pain team, so that continuity of care after surgery can be enhanced, and key information can be shared instantly and with minimal effort among all health care providers in the multidisciplinary pain clinic. This VC has advantages that are consistent with those of health VCs at large: continuity of care, empowering patients and supporting self-managed care, and managing knowledge (in terms of patient's pain information over time, for example; El Morr, 2010).

A Clinical Partner: The Transitional Pain Service at Toronto General Hospital

The TPS (Katz et al., 2015) was founded in 2014 within one of the largest surgical centers in Canada, Toronto General Hospital. The mission of TPS is to offer timely and effective intervention to patients who are at risk of developing chronic pain after undergoing necessary, life-saving procedures, including surgeries for cancer (e.g. thoracic, breast, gastrointestinal, head and neck), cardiac disease (e.g. coronary artery bypass graft, heart valve repair), or organ transplants (e.g. kidney, lung, liver, heart, pancreas). While acute pain after surgery is to be expected, between 10-50% of patients who undergo major surgery go on to develop chronic post-surgical pain – that is, post-surgical pain that continues for more than six months after surgery and possibly for years (CPSP; Katz & Seltzer, 2009; Kehlet, Jensen, & Woolf, 2006). The surgeries that pose the greatest risks for CPSP are usually associated with nerve damage leading to neuropathic pain (Katz & Seltzer, 2009). The one-year incidence of moderate-to-severe postsurgical pain has been estimated at 5 – 10%.

The Transitional Pain Service aims to identify patients at high risk for chronic post-surgical pain, intervene before pain becomes chronic, and support these patients from the earliest days after surgery with state-of-the-art multidisciplinary pain care involving multimodal, opioid sparing medication prescribed by pain physicians and managed with the support of advanced practice nurses, behavioral interventions by pain psychologists, and physiotherapy and acupuncture provided by the physiotherapists specializing in post-surgical care.

Prior to the development of this first-of-its-kind service, multidisciplinary, specialized pain management was not available to post-surgical patients. In fact, multidisciplinary pain care was only available once post-surgical pain had persisted for more than 6 months after surgery. Even then, the patient would need to be properly diagnosed with a chronic pain condition, and referred to a pain management clinic, with an average wait time of 18 months to be seen (Canadian Pain Coalition, 2014). Thus, a patient who developed persistent post-surgical pain could wait more than two years before seeing a pain specialist to optimize their pain treatments, at which point it is likely that pain would be entrenched, opioid medication dose may have escalated, and the patient could be suffering from disability, as well as mental health problems such as depression and anxiety.

The Partnership Between ManagingLife and the Transitional Pain Service

The mission of the Transitional Pain Service is to provide state-of-the-art pain management for complex post-surgical pain from the earliest days after surgery. In order to bring this mission to full fruition, MMP serves an important function in facilitating communication between the patient and the health care team in the early, critical months after surgery. This collaborative project is being implemented to test the feasibility and acceptability of this virtual community to patients recovering from major surgery, with the hope that the mobilization of the virtual community will lead to improved long-term pain outcomes for patients. In addition to this being a clinical implementation project, the TPS has initiated several research projects, with the goal of assessing patient satisfaction and outcomes as a result of incorporating this virtual community into the clinical service.

The goals of the partnership between ManagingLife and TPS are to (a) improve patient care and (b) develop and refine the virtual community with feedback from health care providers and patients. In working toward these goals, the digital platform itself has undergone a process of growth and change. The physicians, nurses, psychologists, physiotherapists, and patient coordinators of the pain service have participated, with the MMP development team, in a series of focus groups and consultations designed to optimize MMP. As part of this process, fruitful cross-pollination has occurred between the clinical service and the MMP development team, leading to the introduction of new features for this virtual community, which will be described below. In addition, the implementation of this virtual community within a large health care institution has presented challenges that will be discussed. Finally, an overview of future directions in the development of the virtual community will be provided.

USER CENTERED DESIGN: MEETING THE NEEDS OF PATIENTS AND HEALTH CARE PROVIDERS

User centered design aims to create products that have a high degree of usability, defined as the "extent to which a product can be used by specified users to achieve specified goals with effectiveness, efficiency and satisfaction in a specified context of use" ("The International Organization of Standardization," 1998). A usable product should be useful, efficient, effective, satisfying, learnable, and accessible (Rubin & Chisnell, 2008). This section will take a closer look at how the virtual community of MMP meets the needs of two key user groups, people with pain and health care providers, first by examining the patient user, and then by looking closely at the clinician user.

The User Living with Chronic Pain

Apps designed for health care institutions risk low user engagement due to misalignment of patient needs with the apps' functionality and user experience (Accenture, 2013). MMP was designed with the needs of the person in pain as a priority, and was first developed and launched as a mobile app for people living with chronic pain after intensive testing for functionality and user experience. It is essential that MMP meet the needs of the patient user, so that the user is engaged, motivated, and satisfied when recording their pain ratings. To meet the needs of the average person living with pain, it is important to understand who they are, what motivates them, and what they are looking for in a virtual community of this nature.

User Characteristics

In Canada, the typical person with chronic pain is likely female, suffering from arthritis or low back pain, and with an average pain duration of 10 years (Moulin, Clark, Speechley, & Morley-Forster, 2002; Schopflocher et al., 2011). The average MMP user has similar characteristics: she is female, between 35 and 50 years of age, and reports one (or more) of five conditions: fibromyalgia, back pain, headaches (including migraines), arthritis, or neck pain. Users live around the world, as MMP has been translated into French, Spanish, German, Simplified Chinese, Korean, and Russian. The person with pain can enter pain records in one language (e.g., French), and their health professional can access the information shared in another language (e.g., German) – this has proved very useful in Switzerland (Ruppen, personal communication, 2012), for example, which has three official languages.

A recent cluster analysis investigated and elucidated key characteristics of users of MMP (Rahman et al, 2017). This data mining analysis employed the k-means clustering algorithm and was based on a sample of more than 24,000 users (comprising more than 544,000 data points). Five clusters of users were found, with each cluster representing a different level of user engagement. The authors found that although MMP has more female users than male users overall, once males register to use the app, they are more likely to use the app over a longer period of time and with greater frequency than female users. This gender difference is consistent with gender differences reported in the utilization of mobile health technology (Zhang et al,

2013; Guo et al, 2015). Furthermore, the investigators found that highly engaged MMP users (1) were older than less engaged users, (2) had more diagnosed pain conditions, (3) were taking a higher number of pain medications, including (4) more opioid-based pain medication.

While the cluster analysis was based on MMP users in the community, patients using MMP as part of care provided by the Transitional Pain Service have their own distinct profile. The average patient seen by the TPS is older, at 52 years of age on average. The gender balance of the TPS patients is 52.7% male and 47.3% female patients. These are complex patients with 65% having more than 3 major medical morbidities. Many patients report indicators of neuropathic pain, including burning, tingling, "electric-shock"-like pain, and sensitivity to touch from bedsheets or clothing, due to damage to nerves sustained during surgery (Cousins, Power, & Smith, 2000).

In order to facilitate ease of use, especially for users who may not be highly "tech savvy", MMP was designed with the naïve user in mind and relies on visual cues, simple language, and customizable user-centric features to promote quick learnability and a frustration-free user experience. The app has been improved repeatedly based in part on user feedback. User feedback has been forthcoming through reviews on the Google Play store, as well as through direct messages to the developers through the "contact us" option within the app. The developers review all feedback and provide comments in response to users in order to ensure that users know that their feedback is valued and acted upon in improving the virtual community. User feedback has been utilized to improve the app's flow and function whenever possible in the next update, and the application has undergone more than 60 iterations (based on the number of updates published on Google Play). The goal of each update is to improve the adoption rate and allow for a smooth, uncomplicated user experience. In addition, a brief, 5-question survey of 100 users who had used the app for at least 12 weeks was undertaken in March 2015 by ManagingLife to solicit feedback from MMP users. Users were asked to rate the utility of the app on a 5-point Likert scale in terms of meeting user needs, such as better characterizing their pain - in addition, users were invited to provide open ended feedback. As a result of ongoing feedback and consultation with users, user satisfaction is excellent, with the "pro" version of the mobile app earning 309 (59%) five star user ratings. Furthermore, MMP was designed to meet accessibility limitations that are present among many persons with chronic pain. Individuals with mobility issues can manage their records from the comfort of home, and can interact with the platform as much or as little as needed, depending on their pain level, mood, schedule, and other relevant factors.

User Motivations

According to a user survey, people with pain reported four main reasons for using MMP.

To Better Understand Their Pain

People with pain often find their pain difficult to understand and predict. When pain is unpredictable, it is more aversive (Chapman, 2009), and therefore one of the key benefits that MMP users report is that the app helps them to better understand their own pain. The central feature of MMP is the "pain record" that enables users to efficiently and regularly enter details about their pain episodes, without overburdening them. Users are asked to complete only one item, a rating of pain intensity using a slider on a visual analogue scale (Figure 2). They have the option of completing seven more items regarding their present pain (see Figure 2) that together take less

Figure 2. Manage My Pain page for adding a new pain record. ©ManagingLife, 2017

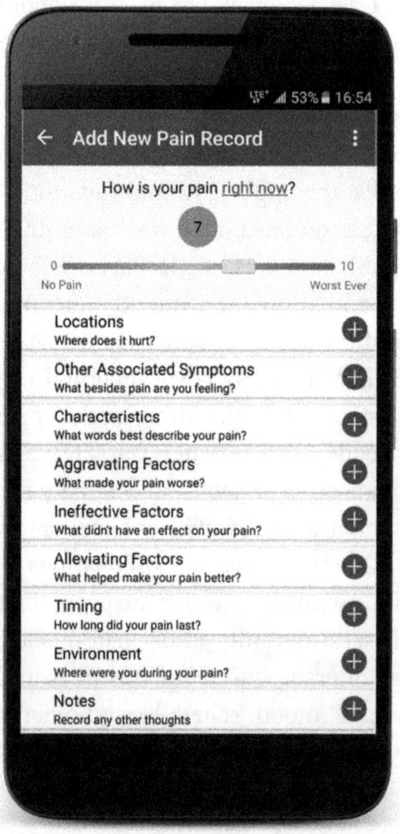

than one minute to complete. In addition, users are prompted daily to record their pain intensity and daily functioning. Over time, users can see the big picture – pain intensity over time, pain triggers presented by frequency, and daily functioning – as this information is presented visually using graphs and charts (Figure 3).

To Provide Information to the Health Care Provider

Since the causes of chronic pain have historically been poorly understood, patients with chronic pain report feeling dismissed, disbelieved and rejected by healthcare professionals (Newton, Southall, Raphael, Ashford, & LeMarchand, 2013). They may be concerned with insensitivity and negative judgment from health care professionals some of whom claim that the pain is all "in their head" (Dewar, White, Posade, & Dillon, 2003; Katz, Rosenbloom, & Fashler, 2015). MMP provides a safe space for users to record their pain and related symptoms without fearing stigma and judgment. The patient's private pain is made visible and more concrete by summary charts

Figure 3. Manage My Pain pain severity tracking chart. ©ManagingLife, 2017

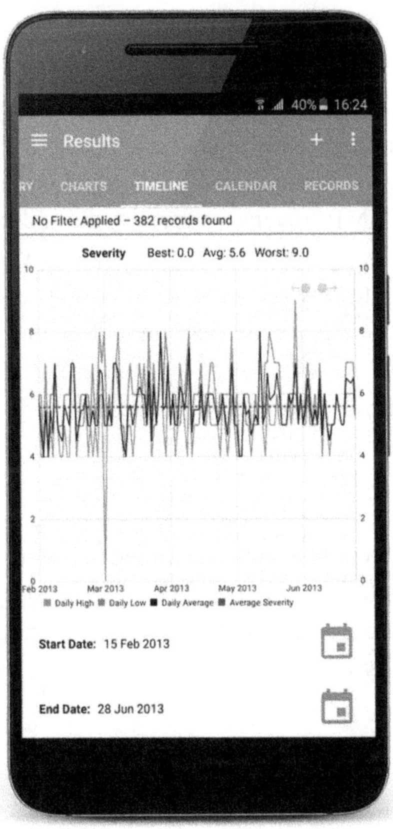

and graphs, leading to improved communication about pain with their health care provider. One user stated: "Not only can I track my pain, but I can keep track of what triggers it, what makes it better, and even input my history. I recently had my initial appointment with a new doctor and all I had to do was pull out this magic app and my entire (complicated) history was readily available and sped the entire process along" (ManagingLife, 2016).

To Have a Space Where They Can Discuss and Share Their Struggles

For many people living with pain, pain interferes with daily life, including social activities with family and friends. Many chronic pain patients report feeling socially isolated and stigmatized (Dewar, Gregg, White, & Lander, 2009). When socially isolated, people with a variety of medical problems turn to virtual communities for support (Marco Leimeister, Schweizer, Leimeister, & Krcmar, 2008). One MMP user reflected on his use of the mobile app, and articulated the way in which it reduced his sense of isolation: "The psychological impact of being asked [by the app] how my day was at 8 pm every evening is ironically very comforting. It feels like I have a friend out there who wants to know how I am doing" (ManagingLife, 2016).

To Support Insurance and Disability Claims

Many people with chronic pain find themselves disabled by pain and without their previous means of employment and financial support. Therefore, one of their key benefits of using MMP is documentation of their pain to support claims for disability benefits. One user called MMP "my insurance sword!" and explained: "I can't always remember everything since my accident. This program gives me the tool to schedule alarms to remind me to enter my pain and meds. Great reports to show doctor and insurance company the severity of my pain on a daily basis. Insurance companies can't see your pain, but they can see a report. Your pain is real. This program allows you to be your own advocate" (ManagingLife, 2016).

The Clinician User

People with pain may wish to share their pain records with a variety of health care practitioners or other stakeholders, including insurance companies. This section will focus on the clinicians who manage pain, describe their needs as users, and outline how the virtual community meets their needs.

Health Care Providers in Pain Management

Effective pain management is best accomplished with a multidisciplinary team; therefore, a variety of health care professionals participate in this virtual community. These health care providers may include:

- Generalist physicians in primary care, known as general practitioners, family doctors, or primary care physicians.
- Pain-specialist physicians – such as anesthesiologists, physiatrists, and psychiatrists – who have advanced training in pain medicine and often work out of specialized pain clinics or rehabilitation facilities.
- Nurses who treat pain patients in community clinics and hospitals, including advanced practice nurses who may manage medications.
- Practitioners focused on coping with pain and psychosocial functioning, including psychologists and social workers.
- Other health care providers focused on physical functioning, such as physiotherapists, occupational therapists, kinesiologists, and exercise physiologists.
- Complementary and alternative medicine practitioners such as registered massage therapists, chiropractors, and yoga instructors.

The introduction of a virtual community into the TPS required an evaluation of the health care providers' needs. To accomplish this, the developers conducted focus groups to assess the needs of the clinician stakeholders, including pain physicians, nurses, psychologists, physiotherapists and patient coordinators. They found that the various health care professionals have similar basic needs in terms of functionality from the virtual community (the needs of the patient coordinators will be discussed in more detail below). For example, pain physicians assess trends in pain intensity and daily activities to evaluate the impact of pain medications. The psychology team also tracks pain intensity and functioning, but uses these metrics differently: they look to pain intensity to assess in part how the patient is perceiving and evaluating their pain, and they look to functioning to track the impact of behavioral interventions aimed at helping the patient do more meaningful and important activities each day. The physiotherapist uses these same metrics with an eye to the impact of acupuncture and daily exercise on pain intensity and functioning. Some information is uniquely useful to certain health care practitioners. For example, advanced practice nurses and physicians are specifically focused on medication side effects, which patients can track on their phones using the mobile app. However, by and large, the information communicated from patients to clinicians within the virtual community is not segmented according to the profession of the clinician, and all clinicians are able to make use of the same interface.

Shared Needs Among Clinician Users

The common ground among health care providers extends to their needs in using the platform. This section will review key needs of the clinician users and how they are addressed within the virtual community.

Accurate Clinical Information

Pain clinicians of all professions need accurate information regarding the patients' pain. Traditionally, this information has been collected using paper-and-pencil questionnaires in clinic. For example, the average post-surgical pain patient comes to TPS once per month for pain assessment and medication consultation. At the monthly visit, the patient is asked to recall their pain over the past month and record their average pain using a standardized and validated questionnaire, e.g., Brief Pain Inventory (Cleeland & Ryan, 1994). This method is simple, low cost, and well-established; however, there are limitations to the accuracy of patient recall.

The memory of pain is influenced by many factors (Redelmeier, Katz, & Kahneman, 2003). In one study (Ariely, 1998) patients were exposed to painful heat and pressure in the lab. If the pain ended on a high note, they remembered more pain than if the pain ended on a low note, even if they experienced the same amount of pain on average. In other words, the intensity of their most recent pain influenced their pain memory (Ariely, 1998). In another study (Eich, Reeves, Jaeger, & Graff-Radford, 1985), patients were asked how much pain they experienced over the previous week. Some of these patients were asked immediately after physiotherapy, which gave them pain relief, whereas others did not receive physiotherapy. The patients who had just competed physiotherapy remembered less pain over the previous week than the patients who did not have physiotherapy, even though their daily electronic pain diaries said that was not the case. In other words, their current pain relief influenced their pain memory (Eich et al., 1985).

It is more accurate to have patients measure their pain in real time between clinic visits. Implementation of this approach is challenging, however, because daily paper-and-pencil diaries generate a lot of data on paper that is then time-consuming to analyze. One key advantage of MMP for the clinician user is that pain ratings can be collected in real-time in the patient's own daily living environment (known as ecological momentary assessment), yielding pain data that is more accurate and precise. Furthermore, it has been shown that patients using digital pain diaries prefer them to paper-and-pencil diaries, with higher rates of patient satisfaction and compliance (Jamison et al., 2001).

Analysis of Patient Trajectories

The ability to assess the trajectory of a patient's pain and functioning in an instant is invaluable for clinicians. Paper-and-pencil assessments collected at clinic visits provide valuable information; however, before meaningful analysis of trends in patient pain and functioning can be understood, the data must be entered into a digital database, total scores for questionnaires must be generated and interpreted, and trends over time must be analyzed (e.g., What is the patient's functioning score today? Is it in the clinical range? Is it an improvement over their score last month?). This requires additional human resources, which are difficult to spare, given the pace and staffing of medical clinics. A key benefit of MMP is that digital data is readily analyzed. No additional labor is required for data entry, analysis or for graphing a patient's pain intensity since the last appointment. Pain trajectories are at the doctor's fingertips and clinicians can assess the impact of previous interventions (e.g., if a new drug was prescribed at the last visit, did pain intensity decrease?), identify at risk-patients (e.g., a patient whose pain is not decreasing adequately and as expected in the weeks after surgery), and – for clinicians involved in clinical research - export and utilize data for research purposes as appropriate.

Time Efficiency

Clinicians treat many patients in one day. Each patient requires high quality, personalized care in a time-efficient manner. Therefore, it is critical that the data collected through the digital platform be delivered to the clinician in a way that does not add to clinician burden, but rather supports the clinician in making efficient and effective decisions regarding the next steps in the overall pain management plan.

The need of clinicians for time-efficient information delivery is met in this virtual community with one-screen (or one-page) summary reports that highlight the most clinically relevant variables using visual representation of data (e.g., color coded graphs) that can be read and understood in 30 seconds (Figure 4). In order to determine what information was most critical and actionable for clinicians from a variety of disciplines, a series of focus groups was conducted with participants from the pain service staff in the Department of Anesthesia and Pain Management and the Pain Research Unit at Toronto General Hospital. A total of approximately 20 health care providers and pain research scientists from a variety of disciplines (i.e., medicine, nursing, psychology, physiotherapy and patient coordinators) provided qualitative feedback on the contents of the one-page report. The health care

Figure 4. Manage My Pain clinician report summary page. ©ManagingLife, 2017

ManagingLife
Helping patients and doctors better manage pain

Pain Report for Sample Patient

Date Range: 01-Aug-2016 to 30-Aug-2016

Generated on 21-Nov-2016 at 10:33 AM by Tahir Janmohamed (ManagingLife Admin)

Summary

Trends

Average Severity: 6.2 ▲0.4
(54 Pain Records) ▲3

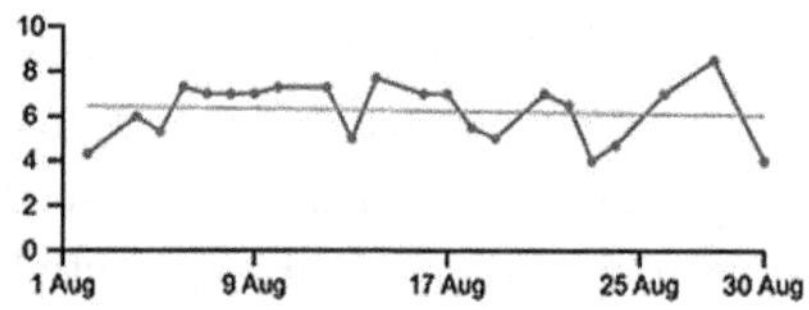

Average Function: 5.6 ▲1.1
(19 Daily Reflections) ▲3

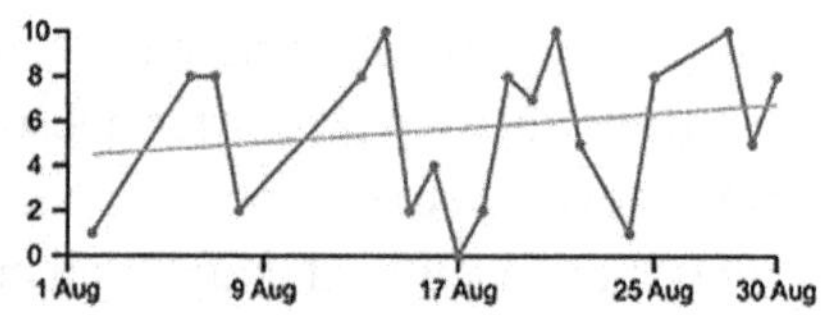

Description

Duration / **Type of Pain**

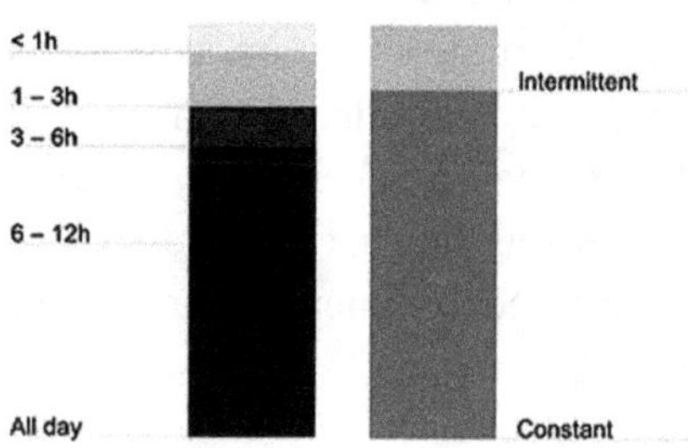

Meaningful Activities

Connected with supportive people online or through text	▲ 3%	67%
Bathed / Showered	▼ 18%	61%
Spent time with friends or family	▼ 7%	50%

Location

Neck	▲ 12%	50%
Genitals	▼ 5%	41%
Abdomen (lower)	▲ 6%	24%

Other Associated Symptoms

No Appetite	▲ 15%	70%
Lethargy	▲ 17%	56%
Mental Fogginess	▲ 10%	47%

Characteristics

Aching	▼ 1%	79%
Sore	▼ 18%	58%
Burning	▲ 1%	54%

Triggers

Aggravating Factors

Sitting	▼ 13%	49%
Bending	▲ 19%	45%
Getting Up Or Sitting Down	NEW	43%

Environment

Home	▲ 17%	74%
Activities Outside Home	▲ 18%	32%
Bed	▼ 21%	30%

Interventions

Alleviating Factors

Rest	▼ 26%	24%
Celecoxib (Celebrex)	NEW	16%
Inactivity	▲ 3%	16%

Ineffective Factors

None Reported

* Indicates how representative values are of patient's pain profile – all frequencies are calculated using only records that contain information from that section.

Page 1 / 1

providers and pain experts highlighted the most useful and important information, what information was missing and should be added, and gave qualitative feedback on the visual presentation of information. After each focus group, a new iteration of the report was created, which was once again available for comment at the next focus group. Three focus groups were conducted in total.

Remote Communication

Most pain clinicians use paper-and-pencil assessments that can only be completed when the patient is in the same physical environment as the clinician. Between visits, there is generally little-to-no communication, unless a patient calls the clinic requesting urgent care. In contrast, within the virtual community, pain information can flow freely from patients to physicians at any time, including between visits. This is highly advantageous during the critical period after surgery, once patients are discharged from hospital. Patients who are seen by the TPS after surgery come from all over the province of Ontario. Returning to the hospital for follow up after surgery is particularly onerous when one has to travel far distances. Therefore, the value of this remote communication is even greater, as patients can keep their pain team apprised of their pain intensity and function at a distance, and make the most of appointments, which require great effort to attend.

CHALLENGES IN IMPLEMENTATION

Integrating an externally-developed mobile health app into a clinical service based in a large healthcare institution comes with a multitude of challenges. In order to facilitate this integration, a close collaboration was needed to refine the features of the digital platform to support the creation of a virtual community that would meet the needs of clinical team members. As part of the implementation process, a series of consultations led to the development of new features for the digital platform, including (1) an assessment of patients' daily functioning, (2) a secure web-based monitoring portal for the clinical team with features added specifically for patient coordinators tracking large numbers of patients, and (3) improved summaries of patient tracking and progress for clinicians. This section will describe these innovations in greater detail, followed by a discussion of our approaches to health data security, ownership, and safeguards for clinician's data access and sharing. Finally, strategies for measuring the impact of deploying MMP on clinical outcomes will be described.

A Close Collaboration Leads to New Features for the Virtual Community

Measuring Functioning With a Daily Reflection

Prior to the collaboration between ManagingLife and TPS, the digital platform did an excellent job of measuring pain and related factors, but did not assess functioning. Functioning refers to the ability of people living with pain to perform daily self-care activities (e.g., bathe or shower, shop for groceries, prepare meals), participate in social activities (e.g., have coffee with a friend, attend community festivals), and perform occupational tasks (e.g., get to work, complete a project, participate in weekly volunteer work), as well as other activities that they find rewarding (e.g., play with grandchildren, learn Sudoku) (Turk et al., 2003).

When assessing treatment progress in individuals with persistent pain, the measurement of functioning is critically important (Dworkin et al., 2008). Focusing solely on pain intensity as the main outcome of treatment can lead to reduced pain at the expense of escalating doses of opioid pain medication (Ballantyne & Sullivan, 2015). While pain intensity may be reduced, due to the serious side effects of opioid medication, the ability to participate in meaningful life activities may not improve, leading to little change in overall quality of life. Thus, without tracking both pain and functioning, the impact of treatment is difficult to determine. Importantly, in patients living with chronic pain, the intensity of pain does not map on to the severity of tissue damage. Once pain has become chronic, the intensity of chronic pain is more strongly associated with emotional and psychosocial factors, such as the perceived meaning of the pain (Ballantyne & Sullivan, 2015). Furthermore, when these psychosocial factors are targeted by behavioral interventions – a standard component of multidisciplinary pain care – then functioning can improve, even when pain intensity does not change (Vowles, Fink, & Cohen, 2014). For all these reasons, functioning is a very important outcome to measure.

The TPS clinical team requested that functioning be measured via the digital platform. However, existing paper-and-pencil questionnaires that assess functioning didn't mesh with the format of the mobile app and its design principles. For example, the World Health Organization Disability Assessment Schedule (World Health Organization, 2000) would take too long to complete daily on a mobile application. In order to minimize patient burden when assessing functioning, two key design principles were implemented: (1) completion of the measure within 60 seconds, (2) use of sliders and checkboxes for ease of use. The MMP team ran a focus group with each discipline represented on the clinical team (e.g., physicians, nurses, psychologists, and physiotherapists) to discuss what facets of functioning they wanted to assess. A study of validated measures of functioning was also undertaken. Finally, four two-hour workshops were conducted. Each workshop started with a mock-up of the new assessment of functioning, followed by reflection and discussion. At the end of this process, the functioning measure had been designed and was ready to be turned over to the developers to code and launch.

The MMP development team and the multidisciplinary TPS clinical and research staff arrived at one question, which users are prompted to complete as a "Daily Reflection" at 8 pm daily: "What did you do that mattered to you today?" Below the question is a slider that users move to rate their day from 0 (i.e., "I did nothing that mattered to me today") to 10 (i.e., "I did everything that mattered to me today") (Figure 5). This formatting mimics the 0 to 10 rating of pain intensity that is familiar to MMP users. Below the slider, a series of checkboxes allow the user to quickly identify the specific meaningful activities they engaged in that day, such as spending time with people they care about or doing an activity that they enjoyed (Figure 5). Users can personalize their list of meaningful activities to reflect the activities that

Figure 5. Manage My Pain data entry page for daily reflections. ©ManagingLife, 2017

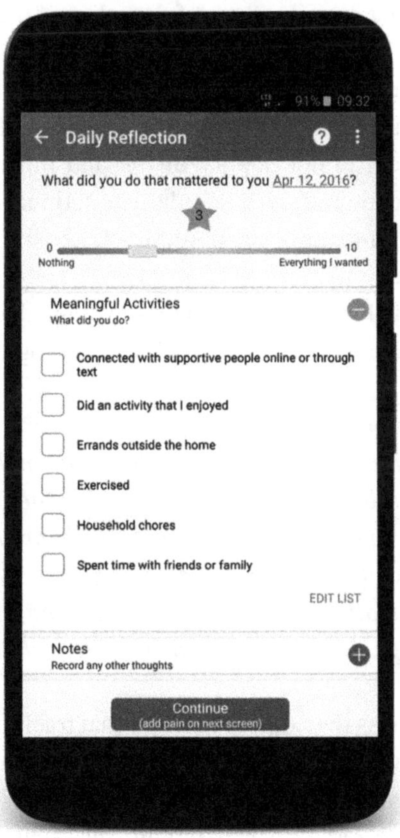

are most important to them (for one patient it could be gardening, whereas for another it might be volunteering). This feature is sensitive to improvements over the course of treatment. For example, one patient at Toronto General Hospital said that her life had changed as a result of the treatment that she received. Prior to treatment, she was so distressed due to her pain that she had suicidal thoughts. During the course of treatment, the patient's engagement in meaningful daily activities increased by ~10% and she reported an increase of ~40% in terms of spending time with friends and family, getting support online or through texting, and exercising.

This kind of engagement in personally meaningful activities is a key component of the behavioral treatment for pain. Acceptance and Commitment Therapy (Hayes, Strosahl, & Wilson, 2011), which is an empirically supported treatment for individuals living with chronic pain ("APA division 12", 2013), emphasizes engagement in personally meaningful activities as a cornerstone of treatment (Polk, Schoendorff, Webster, & Olaz, 2016). Based on this model of behavioural treatment, which is used in the TPS clinic (Azam et al, 2017; Weinrib et al, 2017), the TPS team wanted to capture more than the activities of daily living (bathing, dressing, walking, etc.). The team wanted to capture activities that were based on personal values – a type of meaningful activity that is so important for quality of life, yet often not captured by existing measures of functioning. For example, one patient-user reported that she very much wanted to sing, but hadn't been able to do so due to her pain. After treatment, she was singing again, which was deeply meaningful to her and constituted a substantial improvement to her quality of life and functioning, but it is not an activity that would be captured by a standard functioning measure. In contrast, using the Daily Reflection feature, she could track her singing by including it as a personally meaningful activity.

The new feature of the Daily Reflection was explained to users in a blog post by Dr. Aliza Weinrib, clinical psychologist at TPS. The blog explained:

Sometimes, we can't eliminate pain entirely. I know many of you are all too familiar with this very difficult situation! This is like when I am making soup and I add too much salt. The salt is in there and I can't get it out! The only thing that I can do is add more of the other ingredients – more veggies, more beans, more broth. And then the soup tastes much better. In a similar way, even when you can't get rid of the pain, you can add small, manageable, and meaningful activities to your day. Bit by bit, this can change the flavor of your life (Weinrib, 2016).

It has yet to be shown, as the authors believe, that tracking meaningful activities using the Daily Reflections is, in itself, a helpful intervention for pain. It is well established that tracking behavior has an impact on behavior: "Just the process of tracking itself—often referred to as self-monitoring—can provide many benefits, including increased frequency of desired behaviors and decreased frequency of undesired behaviors, better understanding and awareness of one's behavior and health patterns, and opportunistic engagement in desired behaviors" (Klasnja & Pratt, 2012, p. 186). When people with pain engage in personally meaningful and positive activities, they subsequently report less pain intensity (Hausmann, Parks, Youk, & Kwoh, 2014). In future, the TPS team will assess whether this feature is simply a method of tracking behavior, or has therapeutic impact itself by increasing engagement in meaningful activities and, consequently, improving quality of life.

Improved Summary Reports

Since its inception, patients have been empowered by the MMP application to provide summary reports on their pain to their health care team. Once MMP was introduced to the clinical team at TPS, their feedback was incorporated to make the summary reports as user-friendly as possible for health care professionals from a variety of disciplines. Through a series of iterations and feedback sessions, the report was edited down to a single screen or page of highly visual information.

One of the key pieces of feedback from the clinical team was that the *absolute value* of the patient's pain intensity rating (e.g., 5/10) was not typically as important for the evaluation of the efficacy of clinical interventions as the *change* in the pain intensity rating (e.g., pain intensity has decreased one point on the 0-10 scale). For example, if a physician wanted to know if the patient had less pain since gabapentin was added to the medication regimen at the previous visit one month prior, he needed to see the change in pain values (e.g., pain intensity has gone down two points since the last clinic visit one month ago, in comparison to no change over the previous month). This did not involve any change in how information was collected from patients, but rather required a change in how pain information was analyzed and summarized for clinicians, making it much more useful in treatment planning.

Clinical Monitoring Portal

In addition to the reports (discussed above) that can be generated at the time of the clinic visit for each patient, a substantial advantage of electronic data collection is that it can be viewed remotely and that patients can be monitored as a group. While the physicians, nurses, psychologists and physiotherapists are engaged in one-on-one patient care, the patient coordinators keep an eye on the needs of the patients as a whole – particularly tracking who may need urgent care. Monitoring patients through the web-based MMP clinician portal is therefore an extension of the role of the patient coordinators. Typically, tasks of the patient coordinators in a pain clinic include: (1) taking patient phone calls, (2) triaging concerns about pain and medication with the help of medical staff, (3) scheduling patients' regular appointments and urgent care, (4) coordinating prescription renewals, (5) checking-in patients for medical appointments in the outpatient clinic, and (6) administering standardized paper-and-pencil questionnaires for program evaluation. Patient care coordinators are essential members of the team, particularly as they often are the first line of contact for patients expressing concerns about their pain and medications.

The patient care coordinators from TPS met with the MMP team regarding the clinical monitoring portal. Under the supervision of a responsible physician, the portal allows them to track the post-surgical progress of the patients on the TPS active patient list, viewing pain trajectories in the critical weeks and months after surgery, and taking note of patients whose pain is not resolving and/or who are reporting concerning symptoms, such significant medication side effects. The patient coordinators requested an additional feature. They wanted to have the ability to create a list of patients to follow up as they reviewed patient progress, so that they would have a quick and efficient way to flag patients who require further pro-active follow up or intervention. They also requested the ability to easily search for patients by their hospital number. Both of these features were quickly implemented by the development team to allow for greater functionality and ease of use in monitoring the progress of the patients as a group.

Safeguarding Private Data: Our Approach to Health Data Access and Security

One of the biggest hurdles in the implementation of the MMP platform at Toronto General Hospital was safe stewardship of patient health information. Both organizations take security and privacy very seriously and a lengthy consultation process was initiated with many stakeholders, including research ethics, the legal teams for the hospital and the digital platform, the hospital privacy office, the clinical and research staff of TPS, and the development team for MMP (notably, the hospital information technology department was not involved, as the possibility of integrating MMP data into the electronic medical record was not under consideration). Based on this consultation process, multiple safeguards were put in place to ensure patient data remains protected. These safeguards were formally documented in a legal contract between the two parties after approval by the Research Ethics Board (REB) at University Hospital Network (UHN), which oversees research activity at Toronto General Hospital. A written set of privacy procedures was put in place at UHN, and a UHN privacy officer was designated to be responsible for developing and implementing required policies and procedures. Key protections on electronic protected health information (EPHI) implemented as part of this project are reviewed below.

Data Security

ManagingLife has implemented safeguards to ensure the security and privacy of patient data, which include but are not limited to:

- Transmission of data through a Secure Socket Layer and user authentication using a token-based system and encrypted credentials;
- Encryption of all data in transit and at rest;
- Regular cadence of security and compliance audits against all servers;
- Backing up all data daily off-site through an encrypted channel;
- Storage of all data in electronic format on Amazon Web Services (AWS) secure servers, protected by a firewall and multiple layers of operational and physical security to ensure the integrity and safety of data.

Sharing Patient Data with the Care Team

The care team needed to connect a particular MMP user ID to a specific hospital ID number so that the TPS team would know which MMP user was which specific patient. After a patient undergoes surgery and is recovering in hospital, they are approached by a member of the TPS research team and asked if they would consent to participate in a study of the effectiveness of adding MMP to clinical care. If the patient is interested and gives consent, research staff then generate a unique random ID which they then give to the patient. The patient then goes online to register to use the virtual community and is asked to provide consent for MMP to share their data with TPS. At that point, their user ID is cross-referenced with the TPS patient list, so that the clinical service is aware that one of their patients has engaged with the mobile or web-based application and is voluntarily sharing data.

Authenticating the Clinical User

It was important to define standard operating procedures to ensure that patient data was accessed only by authenticated clinical team members. Clinical users must create their own user name and password using their official UHN email address. A research coordinator must then confirm that this particular health professional is covered by the REB approval for TPS before assigning access, ensuring that only approved staff can access data collected via the virtual community. This ensures access to electronic protected health information is restricted only to employees who require access as part of their job function.

Access to Patient Data After TPS Treatment has Ended

Above and beyond its role in the collaboration with TPS, MMP as a mobile application can be downloaded by anyone, and the patient-user owns their data and controls data sharing. Ordinarily, this would mean that when a TPS patient who is using the platform is discharged from the TPS, his TPS care team would no longer have access to his data. However, given that one goal of this project is for the TPS team to evaluate the impact of deploying a virtual community, an arrangement was made that allowed for patient-user data to be retained and used by the institution for the duration of the study. The patient-user also has continued access to his or her data, and can continue to use the application as he or she wishes.

In these ways, TPS and MMP have addressed concerns regarding the safeguarding of patients' electronic private health information. Addressing these concerns to the satisfaction of all the key stakeholders was one of the major hurdles to overcome in order to implement this project. Figure 6 captures the end result of how the MMP app is used within TPS.

Figure 6. Use of Manage My Pain within the Transitional Pain Service. ©ManagingLife, 2017

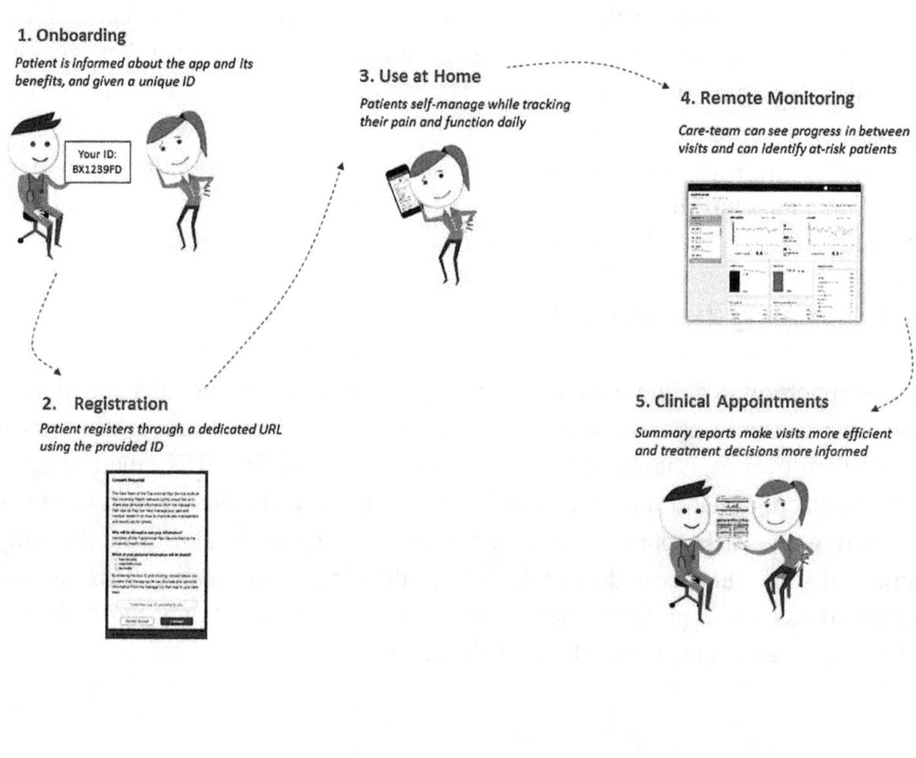

Measuring the Clinical Impact of Implementing a Virtual Community

One of the challenges of implementation is measuring the impact of adding this virtual community to the standard clinical protocol. TPS researchers aim to evaluate whether engagement with MMP during post-surgical recovery improves patient outcomes. The hypothesis is that patients using MMP to share data with their pain management team after surgery will report less pain as well as less pain-related interference with daily activities at 6 months post-surgery when compared to a control group of patients who have not used the virtual community to communicate with their post-surgical pain specialists at TPS. In order to evaluate this outcome, TPS researchers will analyze matched cohorts of patients who participated in the virtual community versus those who did not. At the end of this project, researchers will also evaluate whether the virtual community improved patient and clinician satisfaction with care.

FURTHER INNOVATION AND FUTURE DIRECTIONS

The partnership between ManagingLife and the Transitional Pain Service at Toronto General Hospital has led to multiple innovations in the collection and communication of health information for pain patients. Further innovations under development include (1) a pioneering system of "clinician alerts" that pro-actively signal clinically relevant trends to the patient's care team and (2) the implementation of a peer-to-peer community in the future, in which patients living with pain will be able to connect, share, and support each other.

In Development: Clinician Alerts

When patient pain data is gathered electronically and shared remotely, there are new possibilities in terms of how data are utilized to guide medical care. Based on patient self-reported pain data, a cutting-edge system of clinician alerts has been designed that will proactively capture and flag clinically significant trends and alert the care team. For example, the TPS team is concerned about indicators of neuropathic pain – such as "electric-shock" like pain, tingling, numbness, and burning sensations (Jensen et al., 2011) – because patients who report neuropathic pain indicators acutely after surgery are at higher risk for persistent pain one year later (Hayes, Browne, Lantry, & Burstal, 2002). Therefore, when patients record notable signs of neuropathic pain, an alert will be sent to the care team to flag this patient for follow up. Multimodal interventions can then be offered, including first line medications for neuropathic pain (e.g., gabapentin) and psychological interventions (e.g., mindfulness and relaxation) to calm the nervous system. The goal here is to use the digital platform to facilitate early multidisciplinary intervention and effective preventative health care in order to avert pain, suffering and increased health care costs in the future. The cost savings from preventing even one case of persistent chronic pain after surgery are substantial, as Cousins, Power, & Smith (2000) explained: "The savings that would accrue from the early detection and treatment in the postoperative period of a 30 year old patient who would otherwise progress to develop a persistent chronic pain syndrome and become a permanent burden on the health care system might initially amount to as much as $100,000 and to $.05 to $1 million during the rest of that individual's life" (p. 6).

Future Directions: Peer-to-Peer Support Community

Currently, the MMP virtual community supports communication between people living with pain and health providers. In future, the MMP development team envisions adding a peer-to-peer community that will facilitate support among people living with pain. People living with persistent pain greatly appreciate the opportunity to connect with others like themselves: "It is very difficult for anyone to understand the depth of … pain and the effect it has on your life and your loved ones until they have been there" (Rodham, McCabe, & Blake, 2009, p. 625). In addition, many people living with pain report that they have become more isolated as they are less mobile and participate in fewer social activities (Rodham et al., 2009). An internet-based support network may be a more accessible way to receive support from peers. Furthermore, there is some initial evidence that internet-based peer support forums may lead to improved clinical outcomes, such as reduced pain intensity and increased activity engagement (Bender, Radhakrishnan, Diorio, Englesakis, & Jadad, 2011). Some have gone so far as to say that the very intimate, often anonymous, self-disclosures that occurs in these types of virtual communities "offer a form of peer support that cannot be achieved face to face, and hence may represent a new form of treatment rather than a new method of delivery" (Bender et al., 2011, p. 1748). By adding a peer-support network to the MMP application, the goal is to expand the virtual community to facilitate the benefits associated with peer support.

CONCLUSION

Individuals living with pain have been independently adopting and using the MMP digital platform to understand their pain and improve communication with their health care providers, demonstrating their self-started engagement with this virtual community. Now, with the collaboration between ManagingLife and the TPS at Toronto General Hospital, the virtual community is extending beyond individuals in pain to encompass the community of patients and providers who participate in this clinical service. The implementation of this virtual community as part of clinical care in the TPS has presented multiple challenges in implementation, as well as opportunities for growth and development. Even in the present age of digital supremacy, integrating a virtual community with digital data sharing into clinical care in a major hospital is a challenging and groundbreaking task. This endeavor showcases the leading-edge of eHealth advancement, and highlights the emerging role of virtual communities in the healthcare system.

DISCLOSURE

Dr. Aliza Weinrib, Ph.D., C.Psych, has served as the clinical psychology lead for the Transitional Pain Service since its inception in 2014. Dr. Weinrib received compensation for the development of original content for Manage My Pain through funding obtained from the Industrial Research Assistance Program (IRAP) of the National Research Council of Canada (NRC). Tahir Janmohamed is the founder and CEO of ManagingLife, Inc. Joel Katz and Hance Clarke are unpaid members of the ManagingLife Advisory Board, providing guidance on the product and the company's research initiatives.

ACKNOWLEDGMENT

The work described in this chapter was supported by the National Research Council of Canada (NRC) Industrial Research Assistance Program (IRAP) Small Project Grant (Project #868245) and Business Innovation Access Program (BIAP; Project #845829), as well as an Ontario Centres of Excellence award (Project #23905). Joel Katz is supported by a Canadian Institutes of Health Research Canada Research Chair in Health Psychology held at York University. Hance Clarke is supported by a Merit Award from the Department of Anesthesia, University of Toronto. Muhammad Abid Azam is supported by a Canadian Institutes of Health Research Canada Graduate Scholarship.

REFERENCES

Accenture. (2013). *Losing patience: Why healthcare providers need to up their mobile game*. Retrieved from https://www.accenture.com/t20160629T221243__w__/us-en/_acnmedia/PDF-24/Accenture-Losing-Patience.pdf#zoom=50

Acceptance and Commitment Therapy EST Status for Chronic or Persistent Pain: Strong Research Support. Society of Clinical Psychology (Division 12). (2013). Retrieved June 1, 2015, from http://www.div12.org/psychological-treatments/disorders/chronic-or- persistent-pain/acceptance-and-commitment-therapy-for-chronic-pain/

Ariely, D. (1998). Combining experiences over time: The effects of duration, intensity changes and on-line measurements on retrospective pain evaluations. *Journal of Behavioral Decision Making*, *11*(1), 19–45. doi:10.1002/(SICI)1099-0771(199803)11:1<19::AID-BDM277>3.0.CO;2-B

Arnow, B. A., Hunkeler, E. M., Blasey, C. M., Lee, J., Constantino, M. J., Fireman, B., & Hayward, C. et al. (2006). Comorbid depression, chronic pain, and disability in primary care. *Psychosomatic Medicine*, *68*(2), 262–268. doi:10.1097/01.psy.0000204851.15499.fc PMID:16554392

Azam, M. A., Weinrib, A. Z., Montbriand, J., Burns, L. C., McMillan, K., Clarke, H., & Katz, J. (2017). Acceptance and Commitment Therapy to manage pain and opioid use after major surgery: Preliminary outcomes from the Toronto General Hospital Transitional Pain Service. *Canadian Journal of Pain*, *1*(1), 37–49. http://www.tandfonline.com/doi/full/10.1080/24740527.2017.1325317

Ballantyne, J. C., & Sullivan, M. D. (2015). Intensity of chronic pain — The wrong metric? *The New England Journal of Medicine*, *373*(22), 2098–2099. doi:10.1056/NEJMp1507136 PMID:26605926

Bender, J. L., Radhakrishnan, A., Diorio, C., Englesakis, M., & Jadad, A. R. (2011). Can pain be managed through the Internet? A systematic review of randomized controlled trials. *Pain*, *152*(8), 1740–1750. doi:10.1016/j.pain.2011.02.012 PMID:21565446

Breivik, H., Eisenberg, E., & OBrien, T. (2013). The individual and societal burden of chronic pain in Europe: The case for strategic prioritisation and action to improve knowledge and availability of appropriate care. *BMC Public Health*, *13*(1), 1229. doi:10.1186/1471-2458-13-1229 PMID:24365383

Chapman, R. R. (2009). Predictability of painful stimulation modulates subjective and physiological responses. *The Journal of Pain*, *11*(3), 239–246. doi:10.1016/j.jpain.2009.07.009 PMID:19853519

Cleeland, C. S., & Ryan, K. M. (1994). Pain assessment: Global use of the Brief Pain Inventory. *Annals of the Academy of Medicine, Singapore*, *23*(2), 129–138. PMID:8080219

Coalition, C. P. (2014). *The painful truth: The truth of pain management in Canada*. Retrieved from http://www.canadianpaincoalition.ca/media/painful_truth_report.pdf

Cousins, M. J., Power, I., & Smith, G. (2000). 1996 Labat lecture: Pain—a persistent problem. *Regional Anesthesia and Pain Medicine*, *25*(1), 6–21. PMID:10660235

Dewar, A., White, M., Posade, S. T., & Dillon, W. (2003). Using nominal group technique to assess chronic pain, patients perceived challenges and needs in a community health region. *Health Expectations*, *6*(1), 44–52. doi:10.1046/j.1369-6513.2003.00208.x PMID:12603627

Dewar, A. L., Gregg, K., White, M. I., & Lander, J. (2009). Navigating the health care system: Perceptions of patients with chronic pain. *Chronic Diseases in Canada*, *29*(4), 162–168. PMID:19804680

Dworkin, R. H., Turk, D. C., Wyrwich, K. W., Beaton, D., Cleeland, C. S., Farrar, J. T., & Ader, D. N. et al. (2008). Interpreting the clinical importance of treatment outcomes in chronic pain clinical trials: IMMPACT recommendations. *The Journal of Pain*, *9*(2), 105–121. doi:10.1016/j.jpain.2007.09.005 PMID:18055266

Eich, E., Reeves, J. L., Jaeger, B., & Graff-Radford, S. B. (1985). Memory for pain: Relation between past and present pain intensity. *Pain*, *23*(4), 375–380. doi:10.1016/0304-3959(85)90007-7 PMID:4088698

El Morr, C. (2010). Health Care Virtual Communities: Challenges and Opportunities. In C.-C. Maria Manuela, J. T. Antonio, & S. Ricardo (Eds.), *Handbook of Research on Developments in E-Health and Telemedicine: Technological and Social Perspectives* (pp. 278–298). Hershey, PA: IGI Global. doi:10.4018/978-1-61520-670-4.ch013

El Morr, C., & Kawash, J. (2007). Mobile virtual communities research: A synthesis of current trends and a look at future perspectives. *International Journal for Web Based Communities*, *3*(4), 386–403. doi:10.1504/IJWBC.2007.015865

Fashler, S. R., Cooper, L. K., Oosenbrug, E. D., Burns, L. C., Razavi, S., Goldberg, L., & Katz, J. (2016). Systematic review of multidisciplinary chronic pain treatment facilities. *Pain Research & Management, 2016*, 1–19. doi:10.1155/2016/5960987 PMID:27445618

Gatchel, R. J., & Okifuji, A. (2006). Evidence-based scientific data documenting the treatment and cost-effectiveness of comprehensive pain programs for chronic nonmalignant pain. *The Journal of Pain*, *7*(11), 779–793. doi:10.1016/j.jpain.2006.08.005 PMID:17074616

Goldberg, D. S., & McGee, S. J. (2011). Pain as a global public health priority. *BMC Public Health*, *11*(1), 770. doi:10.1186/1471-2458-11-770 PMID:21978149

Guo, X., Han, X., Zhang, X., Dang, Y., & Chen, C. (2015). Investigating m-health acceptance from a protection motivation theory perspective: Gender and age differences. *Telemedicine Journal and e-Health*, *21*(8), 661–669. doi:10.1089/tmj.2014.0166 PMID:25919800

Hausmann, L. R. M., Parks, A., Youk, A. O., & Kwoh, C. K. (2014). Reduction of bodily pain in response to an online positive activities intervention. *The Journal of Pain*, *15*(5), 560–567. doi:10.1016/j.jpain.2014.02.004 PMID:24568751

Hayes, C., Browne, S., Lantry, G., & Burstal, R. (2002). Neuropathic pain in the acute pain service: A prospective survey. *Acute Pain*, *4*(2), 45–48. doi:10.1016/S1366-0071(02)00026-8

Hayes, S. C., Strosahl, K. D., & Wilson, K. G. (2011). Acceptance and Commitment Therapy: The process and practice of mindful change. Guilford Press. New York, NY: Guilford Press. Retrieved from https://contextualscience.org/ACT_Randomized_Controlled_Trials

Hogan, M.-E., Taddio, A., Katz, J., Shah, V., & Krahn, M. (2016a). Health utilities in people with chronic pain using a population-level survey and linked healthcare administrative data. *Pain*. doi:10.1097/j.pain.0000000000000776

Hogan, M.-E., Taddio, A., Katz, J., Shah, V., & Krahn, M. (2016b). Incremental healthcare costs for chronic pain in Ontario, Canada – a population-based matched cohort study of adolescents and adults using administrative data. *Pain*, *157*, 1. doi:10.1097/j.pain.0000000000000561 PMID:26447708

Jamison, R. N., Raymond, S. A., Levine, J. G., Slawsby, E. A., Nedeljkovic, S. S., & Katz, N. P. (2001). Electronic diaries for monitoring chronic pain: 1-year validation study. *Pain*, *91*(3), 277–285. doi:10.1016/S0304-3959(00)00450-4 PMID:11275385

Jensen, T. S., Baron, R., Haanpää, M., Kalso, E., Loeser, J. D., Rice, A. S. C., & Treede, R.-D. (2011). A new definition of neuropathic pain. *Pain*, *152*(10), 2204–2205. doi:10.1016/j.pain.2011.06.017 PMID:21764514

Katz, J., Pagé, M. G., Fashler, S., Rosenbloom, B. N., & Asmundson, G. J. G. (2014). Chronic pain and the anxiety disorders: Epidemiology, mechanisms and models of comorbidity, and treatment. In *Mental Health and Pain* (pp. 119–155). Springer. doi:10.1007/978-2-8178-0414-9_8

Katz, J., Rosenbloom, B. N., & Fashler, S. (2015). Chronic pain, psychopathology, and DSM-5 somatic symptom disorder. *Canadian Journal of Psychiatry*, *60*(4), 160–167. doi:10.1177/070674371506000402 PMID:26174215

Katz, J., & Seltzer, Z. (2009). Transition from acute to chronic postsurgical pain: Risk factors and protective factors. *Expert Review of Neurotherapeutics*, *9*(5), 723–744. doi:10.1586/ern.09.20 PMID:19402781

Katz, J., Weinrib, A., Fashler, S. R., Katznelzon, R., Shah, B. R., Ladak, S. S., … Clarke, H. (2015). The Toronto General Hospital Transitional Pain Service: Development and implementation of a multidisciplinary program to prevent chronic postsurgical pain. Journal of Pain Research, 8, 695–702. doi:10.2147/JPR.S91924

Kehlet, H., Jensen, T. S., & Woolf, C. J. (2006). Persistent postsurgical pain: Risk factors and prevention. *Lancet*, *367*(9522), 1618–1625. doi:10.1016/S0140-6736(06)68700-X PMID:16698416

Klasnja, P., & Pratt, W. (2012). Healthcare in the pocket: Mapping the space of mobile-phone health interventions. *Journal of Biomedical Informatics*, *45*(1), 184–198. doi:10.1016/j.jbi.2011.08.017 PMID:21925288

ManagingLife. (2012). *Cindy's coming to terms with chronic pain*. Retrieved from https://www.managinglife.com/cindy

ManagingLife. (2016). *Manage My Pain (Version 2.63)* [Mobile Application Software]. Retrieved from https://play.google.com/store/apps/details?id=com.lcs.mmp.full&hl=en#details-reviews

Marco Leimeister, J., Schweizer, K., Leimeister, S., & Krcmar, H. (2008). Do virtual communities matter for the social support of patients? Antecedents and effects of virtual relationships in online communities. *Information Technology & People*, *21*(4), 350–374. doi:10.1108/09593840810919671

Moulin, D. E., Clark, A. J., Speechley, M., & Morley-Forster, P. K. (2002). Chronic pain in Canada-prevalence, treatment, impact and the role of opioid analgesia. *Pain Research & Management*, *7*(4), 179–184. doi:10.1155/2002/323085 PMID:12518174

Newton, B. J., Southall, J. L., Raphael, J. H., Ashford, R. L., & LeMarchand, K. (2013). A narrative review of the impact of disbelief in chronic pain. *Pain Management Nursing*, *14*(3), 161–171. doi:10.1016/j.pmn.2010.09.001 PMID:23972867

Organization, W. H. (2000). World Health Organization disabilty assessment schedule: WHODAS II. Phase 2 field trials. *Health Services Research.*

Polk, K., Schoendorff, B., Webster, M., & Olaz, F. (2016). *The Essential Guide to the ACT Matrix: A Step-by-Step Approach to Using the ACT Matrix Model in Clinical Practice*. Oakland, CA: New Harbinger Publications, Inc.

Preece, J. (2000). *Online communities: Designing usability supporting sociability.* New York: John Wiley & Sons Ltd.

Rahman, Q. A., Pirbaglou, M., Janmohamed, T., Ritvo, P., Heffernan, D., Clarke, H., & Katz, J. (2017). *Data mining to determine patterns of user engagement with Manage My Pain, an mHealth App for Chronic Pain.* Manuscript submitted.

Redelmeier, D. A., Katz, J., & Kahneman, D. (2003). Memories of colonoscopy: A randomized trial. *Pain*, *104*(1), 187–194. doi:10.1016/S0304-3959(03)00003-4 PMID:12855328

Rodham, K., McCabe, C., & Blake, D. (2009). Seeking support: An interpretative phenomenological analysis of an Internet message board for people with Complex Regional Pain Syndrome. *Psychology & Health*, *24*(6), 619–634. doi:10.1080/08870440802563245 PMID:20205016

Rubin, J., & Chisnell, D. (2008). *Handbook of usability testing: how to plan, design and conduct effective tests*. Hoboken, NJ: John Wiley & Sons.

Scascighini, L., Toma, V., & Sprott, H. (2008). *Multidisciplinary treatment for chronic pain: A systematic review of interventions and outcomes*. 10.1093/rheumatology/ken021

Schopflocher, D., Taenzer, P., & Jovey, R. (2011). The prevalence of chronic pain in Canada. *Pain Research & Management: The Journal of the Canadian Pain Society = Journal de La Société Canadienne Pour Le Traitement de La Douleur, 16*(6), 445–50. Retrieved from http://www.pubmedcentral.nih.gov/articlerender.fcgi?artid=3298051&tool=pmcentrez&rendertype=abstract

Siddall, P. J., & Cousins, M. (2004). *Persistent pain as a disease entity: Implications for clinical management.* 10.1213/01.ANE.0000133383.17666.3A

The National Academies Press. (2011). *Relieving Pain in America: A Blueprint for Transforming Prevention, Care, Education, and Research.* Washington, DC: The National Academies Press.

Tracey, I., & Bushnell, M. C. (2009). How neuroimaging studies have challenged us to rethink: Is chronic pain a disease? *The Journal of Pain, 10*(11), 1113–1120. doi:10.1016/j.jpain.2009.09.001 PMID:19878862

Treede, R., Rief, W., Barke, A., Aziz, Q., Bennett, M. I., Benoliel, R., … Wang, S. (2015). *A classification of chronic pain for ICD-11.* Academic Press.

Turk, D. C., Dworkin, R. H., Allen, R. R., Bellamy, N., Brandenburg, N., Carr, D. B., & Galer, B. S. et al. (2003). Core outcome domains for chronic pain clinical trials: IMMPACT recommendations. *Pain, 106*(3), 337–345. doi:10.1016/j.pain.2003.08.001 PMID:14659516

Usability of consumer products and products for public use - Part 2: Summative test method. (1998). Retrieved from https://www.iso.org/obp/ui/#iso:std:iso:ts:20282:-2:ed-2:v1:en

Vowles, K. E., Fink, B. C., & Cohen, L. L. (2014). Acceptance and Commitment Therapy for chronic pain: A diary study of treatment process in relation to reliable change in disability. *Journal of Contextual Behavioral Science, 3*(2), 74–80. doi:10.1016/j.jcbs.2014.04.003 PMID:27818931

Wall, P. D., & Jones, M. (1991). Defeating pain: The war against a silent epidemic. New York: Plenum Press.

Weinrib, A. (2016). *Manage My Pain.* Retrieved from https://www.managinglife.com/faq?id=9

Weinrib, A. Z., Azam, M. A., Birnie, K., Burns, L. C., Clarke, H., & Katz, J. (2017). (in press). The psychology of persisting post-surgical pain: New frontiers in risk factor identification, prevention, and management. *British Journal of Pain.*

Zhang, X., Guo, X., Lai, K. H., Guo, F., & Li, C. (2014). Understanding gender differences in m-health adoption: A modified theory of reasoned action model. *Telemedicine Journal and e-Health, 20*(1), 39–46. doi:10.1089/tmj.2013.0092 PMID:24161004

KEY TERMS AND DEFINITIONS

Acute Pain: A type of pain that typically lasts for a short duration (i.e. less than 3 months).

Chronic Pain: A type of pain that lasts for 3 or more months, outlasting the usual healing process. This pain can reoccur intermittently, get progressively worse, and can cause significant psychological and emotional suffering as well as disability.

Chronic Postsurgical Pain: Chronic pain resulting from a surgical procedure that lasts beyond the expected postsurgical healing period (2 – 3 months), and excludes other sources of pain and pre-existing pain.

Manage My Pain (MMP): A digital platform consisting of a mobile and web application used by sufferers of chronic pain to record, track, and analyze their pain information with the goal of helping them and their healthcare team better understand their symptoms and conditions.

ManagingLife: A software company that has developed the Manage My Pain digital platform.

Neuropathic Pain: Pain that is caused by damage or a disease in the somatosensory nervous system.

Pain: An unpleasant sensory or emotional experience associated with actual or potential tissue damage.

Toronto General Hospital (TGH): The Toronto General Hospital is part of the University Health Network as a major teaching hospital in downtown Toronto, and among the largest surgical centers in Canada.

Transitional Pain Service (TPS): A multidisciplinary clinical service developed within the Toronto General Hospital (Toronto, Canada) with the mission of preventing and managing chronic postsurgical pain and supporting opioid tapering. The TPS consists of anesthesiologists, pain physicians, nurse-practitioners, a psychologist, and a physiotherapist who are able to see patients before and after major surgeries.

University Health Network (UHN): The University Health Network is a healthcare and research organization in Toronto, Ontario, Canada. It is one of the largest such research organizations in Canada and North America.

Chapter 5
Effective Use of Virtual Communities for Health-Purposes in the Elderly

Elisabeth Beaunoyer
Laval University, Canada

Matthieu J. Guitton
Laval University, Canada

ABSTRACT

New strategies must be developed to adequately answer the growing health needs of the elderly. Virtual communities targeted to older adults may represent interesting tools, ranging from providing health-related information to operating preventive programs, or simply reducing social isolation and thus increasing the quality of life of the elderly. Besides generic issues shared with any eHealth virtual community (e.g., user engagement, participation, acceptance), the use of virtual communities by the elderly also bears some specific challenges, including limitations related to access to care or the presence of individuals with (age-related) disability. This Chapter describes some of the factors which should be taken into consideration when designing eHealth strategies aiming at developing or supporting virtual communities targeted to elderly population, and emphases the importance of integrating health-oriented senior-targeted virtual communities into holistic approach to allow for the communities to optimally develop and consolidate, and reach its goal in terms of health benefits.

DOI: 10.4018/978-1-5225-2958-3.ch005

INTRODUCTION

With the well-documented aging of the population, senior citizens represent an increasing proportion of the demographic pyramid of Western societies. From a public health point of view, this situation leads to major concerns. Indeed, an aging population has higher needs in terms of health, particularly a higher vulnerability to chronic diseases and associated co-morbidities. Furthermore, as people age, they typically require more social support, while being at the same time subjected to more social isolation. Therefore, this aging of the population imposes a growing burden on public health systems – a burden which is likely to grow even heavier in the coming decades. In a global context of limited resources, a major challenge to address this issue is to develop innovative solutions in order to assist this specific demographic population while taking into consideration its special needs.

In this context, the use of virtual communities targeted to elderly may represent an interesting health promotion tool. Online health-related communities might have several implications for clinical practice, enabling collaboration, in terms of exchanging experiences and sharing knowledge, between interdisciplinary health professionals from various institutions (van der Eijk, Faber, Aarts, Kremer, Munneke & Bloem, 2013). These tools can be useful to enhance the expertise of health professional, which in turn have a positive impact on patients themselves. Virtual communities are also created to be used directly by elderly patients. Indeed, Internet-based communities can be used to provide health-related information, to implement and operate preventive programs, or simply to reduce social isolation and thus increase the quality of life of the elderly. Over the last two decades, numerous studies have explored the association between Internet use among elderly people and well-being. For example, Internet use decreases loneliness and increases social contacts in assisted and independent living communities (Cotton et al., 2013). Internet use might affect well-being directly, or through its benefits toward other social variables such as loneliness and social support, and may differ according to living settings. Other studies focused more on physical health in creating online programs for various specific pathologies such as lung cancer (Brown-Johnson, Berrean & Cataldo, 2015), chronic pain (Berman, Iris, Bode & Drengenberg, 2009) or specific pathologies that are more frequent with increase of age such as cognitive impairment (Gigler, Blomeke, Shatil, Weintraub & Reber, 2013). Interventions aiming at encouraging the adoption of healthy life habits have been the object of a few studies again focusing on specific behaviors toward prevention of specific pathologies, such as sun protection (White, Starfelt, Young, Hawkes, Cleary, Leske, & Wihardjo, 2015) or more general health related-habits such as physical activity

(Mouton & Cloes 2015). Other senior-targeted online based-interventions, such as learning modules regarding hip fracture prevention (Nahm, Resnick, DeGrezia, & Brotemarkle, 2009) or Internet-mediated walking program that aims to enhance average daily steps, (Richardson et al., 2010), includes virtual community features, such as moderated discussion broad in their design, in which participants can exchange about their experiences. However, using virtual health promotion tools for this particular population poses a series of unique challenges. Among them is the problem of reduced technological literacy present in older individuals – an issue we will be discussing extensively later on in this Chapter. Few examples of online health communities have been documented. The ParkinsonNet community is a website where patients and professionals can interact with each other through various virtual communication technologies (van der Eijk et al., 2013). The Health and Welfare Information Portal is another online health community that includes a secured messaging system and a shared electronic health record for frail elderly, their informal caregivers and their health professionals (Makai et al., 2014). Although few attempts have been made to use virtual communities specifically targeted to elderly users – or more generally to develop eHealth or mHealth applications for this population, most of the projects so far have been exploratory in nature, and based on trial-error strategies rather than on a unified theoretical approach.

The main objective of this Chapter is to propose a reflection on the current situation and future directions of aged population-targeted virtual communities and to suggest elements to rationalize the development of health-oriented virtual community tools and approaches aimed at the elderly. Based on the most recent research in eHealth on the one hand, and studies of virtual communities on the other, this Chapter analyzes some of the different factors which can impact the effectiveness of senior-targeted health-related virtual communities, including the degree of synchronicity, the degree of anonymity, the degree of supervision of the community, and the characteristics of the interface. This Chapter also analyzes some of the specific advantages and disadvantages of different types of virtual communities. Such analyses unveil the fact that not all types of virtual communities are suitable or optimal to reach older populations. We will then discuss with a practical point of view the problem of evaluation, particularly in the context online environments, including the difficult issues of measuring the quality of online information, and health and technological literacy in target populations. Finally, some of the ethical aspects related to eHealth-oriented virtual communities targeted at the elderly will be discussed.

FACTORS POTENTIALLY AFFECTING THE EFFECTIVENESS OF SENIOR-TARGETED HEALTH-RELATED VIRTUAL COMMUNITIES

From both a theoretical and a practical point of view, the chance of survival of a virtual community depends upon a plethora of factors. Indeed, numerous elements need to be considered in order to design interfaces which could support the optimal development of virtual communities able to provide appropriate social support and health-related information for the elderly. Globally, these factors could be roughly divided into three categories: 1) general characteristics of the mode of communication, 2) generic challenges common to any eHealth virtual community, and 3) challenges specific to the aged populations. Of note, while we focus here on interfaces specifically developed to support health-related virtual communities targeting aged populations, what we describe also apply for spontaneously emerging virtual communities.

General Characteristics

The first set of factors which must be taken into consideration when dealing with interface designed to support the emergence – and the continuity of activity – of virtual communities are factors directly related to the specificity of the interface – what could be referred to as technical factors. The three main factors which should come in mind when designing any interface aiming at supporting a virtual community are the degree of synchronicity, the degree of anonymity, and the intrinsic characteristics of the interface. The degree of synchronicity refers to the time-scale in which the inter-individual interactions take place. Interactions can be synchronous (taking place simultaneously or in a very short temporal sequence, like in the case in chatrooms), or asynchronous (taking place with long intervals between interactions, like in the case of forums). These two opposites of the temporal continuum support very different styles of communication. Synchronous interfaces provide the advantages – and inconveniencies – of immediacy. Instantaneous feedback can be a major asset when it comes to immediate social support, but can also favour erroneous or unverified information. In contrast, asynchronous interfaces provide more time for users to develop their answer and provide meaningful information, but the delay of response might be problematic for people seeking for immediate support. However, older adults found asynchronous communication tools (e.g. discussion broads) especially helpful to support self-management (Stellefson et al., 2014). The degree of anonymity refers to the distance between the real-life identity of the users and the identity of the avatar used inside the virtual community. Anonymity can be total (all users are anonymous), or partial – and for partial anonymity, the situation can greatly vary between avatars displaying only a unique name as its identity, to interface proposing to link information of the user such as the gender, age, and geographical location to the avatar. The characteristics of the interface are all the technical aspects (ranging from the functionality to the external appearance) which practically define the interface. The more complex an interface is, the less likely it is to attract a wide base of users. Interfaces supporting virtual communities should find a good equilibrium between intuitive use and functionality in order to reach an optimal efficiency for the users. In the context of senior-targeted health-related virtual communities, an additional factor which can impact the effectiveness is the degree of supervision of the community, i.e., how much supervision is present in the community, whether this supervision is external (for instance, health specialists verifying the information or answering patients' queries) or internal (e.g., presence of moderator within the community). While this is actually true for any virtual community, this factor is central for the actualisation of virtual communities involving older populations.

Generic Challenges Common to Any eHealth Virtual Community

With the degree of the supervision of the community, we are touching directly to the second set of factors which can impact the effectiveness of senior-targeted health-related virtual communities: the factors related to eHealth applications. An essential factor, in fact a double factor, is more related to the nature of the information shared rather than the users themselves: the factual veracity of the information, and its perception, therefore, the degree of trust. Quite obviously, the degree of supervision of a community clearly impacts the degree of trust (perceived quality of information) and of veracity (real quality of information). Given the very personal topics discussed among members of a health-related virtual community, this factor is critical – that is especially the case when it comes to older people who might be more reluctant to trust information coming from uncertain sources in a new media environment. Of note, given the important self-regulation mechanisms which take place in virtual community, health-oriented virtual communities might have a participatory form of control of the quality of information, and even unsupervised communities might provide but a small amount of incorrect information. Nonetheless, the long-term engagement of users may become problematic if the perception of the quality of the information is low, given the fact that mistrust has been identify as a barrier to internet use among older adults (Gatto & Tak, 2008).

Following factors of this category are concerned by the impact that individual behaviour can have on the community. While user's engagement toward the community, user's participation, and user's acceptance of the interface are three factors which are important for any virtual community, they become determining when it comes to health-oriented communities. Indeed, the very reason for such virtual communities to be developed and implemented (or for that matter, to spontaneously emerge if they are not part of an integrated eHealth initiative) is to make sure the users stay within the community, and ideally stay active. Therefore, to ensure sustainability of the online community, there is a need for mutual exchange of personal information and for support fallowing the mention of personal problems instead of off topic conversations which tend to precede a decrease in the level of activity, notably among elderly (Pfeil, Zaphiris, & Wilson, 2010). The frequency of Internet use is also an important factor to consider since the sense of community level seems to be higher among frequent older Internet users (Sum, Mathews, Pourghasem, & Hughes, 2009). In order to optimise the engagement of the participants, the specific characteristics of the typical users will have to be considered at the very first stages of the community design. Another important factor to consider for developing eHealth virtual communities is the time issues. Development process should include a consideration for the time-consuming factor in the elaboration of the intervention, since it could seriously affect participant's engagement toward the community. Whereas one could think that older adult, often retired, might have more time to spend to use these tools, results of several studies suggested that time-consuming issue was a barrier to the use of online health interventions or associated with negative experience (Berman et al., 2009; Gatto & Tak, 2008).

Challenges Specific to the Aged Populations

So far, and despite the suggestion of specific adjustments to answer the needs of elderly populations, the factors we have raised are common to any virtual community-supporting interface. However, in addition to the technical issues (technical factors) and topic-related issues (eHealth factors) mentioned above, a third set of factors are coming from the population itself (population-specific factors). Indeed, as noted a few times already, older people have both different needs in terms of health care than the general population, and different perception of technology. Virtual communities used by the elderly need to adjust to the potential limitations related to access to care or the presence of individuals with (age-related) disability. Obviously, people having cognitive issues (for instance dementia or Alzheimer disease) will have more difficulties to interact in the context of a virtual community. For this reason, a direct contact, remote contact or social structure, could be helpful for cognitive impaired patients to encourage adherence to the program. More contact with the other participants or the researcher increase the odds of completing the program and might potentially benefits more cognitively to the patient (Gigler et al., 2013). Contacts can take place either through a phone conversation or a personal conversation on a communication tool, or could be achieve by organizing group sessions. Similarly, patients suffering from Parkinson disease are likely to not be able to optimally type on a keyboard – something considered as an obvious pre-requisite when using most interfaces.

The second of the two population-specific factors when it comes to older people is the global issue of the relation to the technology. This encompasses not only the general problem of technological literacy, but also the more pragmatic problem of the accessibility of the users to the technology. Using eHealth tools for elderly population always bear the risk of facing a generational problem, the issue of reduced technological literacy of some older individuals compared to younger people. This issue of technological literacy is however more complex, as a lot of sociodemographical factors can influence it. In addition, it is important to remember that to participate into a virtual community, one first need to have access to the Internet, i.e., to be able to find a point to "enter" into the virtual spaces. While this might sound mundane for young users who are likely to all have at least a smart phone or at least one mobile device, the situation might be quite different for older users. Finally, attrition is an important issue whatever the medical intervention envisioned (and, of note, whatever the target population considered). While this issue is obviously critical in a research context, it is also of central importance as a barrier to the implementation of health-related virtual communities as medical-aid tools. Indeed, even if a program might lead to positive health outcomes for the users, it won't be relevant if people don't use it. This is particularly true for older adults since, as mentioned above, they face specific difficulties compared to younger populations when it comes to their relation to technology. Attrition has already been demonstrated to be a problem in older adults' eHealth actual interventions (Berman et al., 2009; Stellefson et al., 2014). The issue of attrition can strongly affect the evaluation of eHealth intervention by adding an important population-based bias. Online community features can help reduce attrition, especially among population with low social support (Richardson et al., 2010). Interestingly, since the virtual community might increase social support even though this was not its original purpose, participants, already experiencing positive outcomes, may be even more motivated to engage in the program. Thus, in contrast to some other eHealth interventions based on individuals instead of communities, health-oriented virtual communities could be self-nurturing when it comes to retaining its participants.

While these different elements are taking place on different levels, they all should be strongly taken into consideration when deciphering which factors might predict the success – or the failure – of a virtual community-based intervention in this population. They also provide a general reading grid to evaluate the potential impact that an interface can have in supporting a health-related virtual community targeted to aged people. In this view, all virtual communities are not equal, as we will see in the next part of this Chapter.

ADVANTAGES AND DISADVANTAGES OF DIFFERENT TYPES OF VIRTUAL COMMUNITIES

Basically, a virtual community is a group of people sharing similar interests through virtual spaces. However, the reality is quite more complex than this simplistic definition, and not all virtual communities are equivalent when it comes to supporting seniors' health. Not all virtual communities can be considered as isomorphic. The characteristics of the interface which will support the community will strongly impact the degree of appropriateness of a virtual community for eHealth purposes in elderly population. Indeed, and quite obviously, a virtual community based on social media would not be the same than a community of user of a specific health application. In terms of complexity of the avatar – the primary vector through which users will enter interact with others to get into the community – one extremity of the virtual communities' continuum will be provided by communities using minimal avatar features, such as forums. At the other end of the spectrum, we will find communities emerging from and in 3D avatar-based immersive virtual worlds. In the following paragraphs, we will analyze some of the specific advantages and disadvantages of different types of virtual communities.

Forums

Historically one of the very first types of virtual communities supported by the Internet, forums are still a major tool to support health-related topics in the cyberspace. Forums cumulate the advantages of anonymity and asynchronous communication with the possibility to support long exchanges, thus allowing to explore topics with a reasonable degree of depth. Adding a forum broad to a healthy behaviors promotion website can enhance the learning experience of most older adults users by offering supportive comments to others and sharing helpful and practical information (Nahm, Resnick, DeGrezia, & Brotemarkle, 2009). However, among the major inconveniencies of such virtual communities are the issues related to the lack of supervision. Of course, most forums can be (and are) moderated. However, this might clearly not be enough in terms of control. Like for any other forum or social media, bullying may happen (Guitton, 2014). Another point resulting for the relative lack of control of what is published in forums, is the issues of medical accuracy of the information provided. Not only some information can be erroneous, but some can even be dangerous. While observational studies have demonstrated that the occurrence of dangerous information on health-related forums was lower than what could be feared, this can nonetheless represent a problem (Arsenault, Blouin & Guitton, 2016). Evidence that medical moderators or other users claiming to have some degree of professional health training really have such qualifications in real life are quasi-systematically impossible to verify, and users rely on the information (often sparse) provided on other users' profiles (including their history of activity in the forum) to assess the veracity of the information provided.

Social Media Networks

Social media have a very high potential when it comes to support the emergence and the continuity of virtual communities. They are characterised by the speed and intensity of the exchanges they can support, making the exchanges almost synchronous even in asynchronous settings. Social media allow to reach large amount of people in very short time with limited efforts, and in this regards, they represent the best tool in terms of cost/benefits when it comes to conveying simple messages. Since social network sites are systems used on a voluntary basis, free of charge, and accessible to older adults, they represent for older adults a media *a priori* easier to use than other virtual communities (Braun, 2013). The interconnectivity of the different social media also make them quite appropriate to enhance redundancy of the information, making it more likely to be considered as relevant by the targeted population. While already mentioned in the context of forums, bullying in social media is an even more acute issue, and can take very quickly uncontrollable proportions (Guitton, 2014). Given the fact that people belonging to an health-related virtual community might be at more risk of psychological distress, cyberbullying might have more dramatic consequences. The fact of belonging to a specific virtual community can provide a certain level of protection by the community against bullying attempts from outsiders, but nonetheless social media are part of interconnected networks, and the borders of a social media-based virtual community are more porous than those of other virtual communities. Once again, the lack of control of the quality of the information might be an issue for social media. However, given the speed and the amount of interactions taking place in such settings, dangerous or erroneous information are likely to get corrected pretty fast. In contrast to forums where information can be described in length, providing more complete pictures and potentially more social support (Arsenault et al., 2016), social media tend to focus on very short messages and interactions, and may be limited in the actual informational support they might provide regarding complex and multifactorial health issues such as the ones aged people are experiencing. Another problem related to social media-supported virtual communities is the heavy use social media are making of visual material, such as self-representing pictures. Young adults, more frequent users of *Facebook* than older adults, are more socially fulfilled by using it but they also experience more negative body image (Hayes, van Stolk-Cooke & Muench, 2015).While this is part of the codes of young users, this might come with some reticence for older people, particularly when their health status is associated with physical limitations, and might compromise the optimal involvement of the population in the virtual community. One of the keys to engage older adults when using social network sites is to focus on the usefulness and the relative safety of the application, which can be done by highlighting features that are most useful for them and for which they don't already have a clue how to use (Braun, 2013).

3D Avatar-Based Immersive Virtual Worlds

The virtual worlds based on 3D avatars, for which Second Life has been both a precursor, a prototype, and a model, obviously represent a considerable complexification of the avatar. In this type of setting, users are invited to freely navigate into extremely large virtual spaces through three-dimensional avatars primarily human-looking. Through their avatars, users can perform almost all actions possible for a human being and can interact with their (virtual) environment in extremely varied ways. When it comes to health applications, the advantages of such interfaces are obvious and numerous. Interacting through a 3D avatar allows one to act without caring of stigma associated with his or her real physical identity – sex, gender, race, physical appearance, socio-economical status, visible stigma of illnesses or handicap are all erased in virtual worlds, and one can presents an idealised image via the avatar. Removing the stigma can strongly promote the ease to interact with others, something further helped by the fact that possibilities of movements and "physical" interactions with other avatars are almost unlimited (Lomanowska & Guitton, 2014). Indeed, platforms such as Second Life have been the target of intense interest for programs targeting people with physical limitations. Another interesting characteristic of such settings is that they combine 3D avatars with instant messaging and other asynchronous features (such as group notices, or simply the possibility to interact with the environment in a way providing information, e.g., clicking on a sign resulting in the delivery of a notecard with relevant information). This leads to a major potential when it comes to optimally deliver health-related information to targeted population, who would not necessarily want to directly interact with health specialists (Lomanowska & Guitton, 2014). However, 3D avatar-based virtual worlds also bear a few issues when it comes to supporting virtual communities of older people. The first issue resides in the difficulty to manoeuver the avatar. While people used to play video or online games will find avatar commands to be quite intuitive, this can be quite more complex for people with limited technological literacy. Another issue is that these interfaces are not solely focusing on the avatar; indeed, the aforementioned density of communication media in such settings can become difficult to manage in terms of attentional resources, and simply overwhelming for people presenting some form of cognitive decline – a condition sadly enough often experienced, at least to some extend, by senior populations. Another issue lies not in the avatars themselves, but in the use that people make of the platforms. Indeed, when given the possibility to create infinite spaces, people tend to do so. In other world, a danger for eHealth application developers interested in using these virtual worlds is to create considerably more virtual space that can be inhabited by the avatars. This might result in a form of isolation: avatars would have to "walk" or at least explore a large amount of virtual space before actually meeting another avatar. If that would be done without using specific tools embedded in the interface (such as a radar or an avatar localiser – devices with which old people might not be familiar or comfortable), the odds of finding others might be quite reduced, therefore loosing some of the potential interest of the settings as a social interface. In order to maintain adequate levels of inter-individual communication – something which would be required for a community to survive this state of avatar-driven isolation – the members of the community have to develop multimdodal processes of redundancy of the information, e.g., massive use of group notices in addition to direct avatar-to-avatar interactions (Guitton, 2015a). While this is possible and has been evidenced in some communities in Second Life, this is nonetheless unlikely to be optimal in the case of senior-targeted virtual community as it requires (at least for a group of key members) important attentional resources and efforts in order to diffuse the relevant and community-building information across the community (Guitton 2015a). Therefore, and while once again such kind of 3D avatar-supported virtual communities are clearly of major interest for a lot of populations with various pathological conditions, they might not represent the ideal vector for elderly population.

Integrating Different Interfaces to Support Virtual Communities

The logic we have been adopted so far is to consider that a given virtual community is based upon a single media and format – whether a forum, a virtual world, a social media, etc. However, considering that the community is identical to the media would be a mistake. In the context of externally designed virtual communities (which would likely be the case for a therapeutic-oriented health community), it might be reasonable to think that the community would be first triggered via a single media (for instance a forum moderated by health professionals). However, the community could extend over other media – for instance, through some Twitter interactions. In any case, even when designing a specific virtual community for health purpose, redundancy of connections through various media is a strategy which has to be considered (Guitton, 2015a).

While the analyses so far have clearly unveiled that not all types of virtual communities are suitable or optimal to reach older populations, the information presented so far are more following a case-by-case logic rather than a systematic approach. Indeed, while factors can be identified, and while advantages and inconveniencies of specific types of communities can be mentioned, one of the issues with new technologies, is that they are indeed new, given no guaranties it will benefits the targeted population. Therefore, rather than trying to predict how a given virtual community would perform regarding health-oriented goals for elderly population, a better approach is to focus on an effective and complete evaluation of the virtual community. This is an essential aspect of the development process of senior-targeted health-related virtual communities to ensure its validity as an eHealth tool for older adults. However, several research challenges arise regarding notably evaluation and ethical and privacy issues. The next part of this Chapter will give a portrait of some of these research challenges.

THE ISSUE OF EVALUATION

While virtual communities can obviously have a positive impact, a central issue is to make sure that the resources allocation is optimal. Developing, and maintaining efficient health-oriented virtual communities is a valid public health strategy only if the costs and resources associated are less than what would be allocated to obtain the same effect with conventional strategies. In other words, in the context of limited resources, the cost/benefit ratio of virtual communities should be more advantageous than for conventional interventions. In this view, the key concept is the concept of evaluation – both in terms of evaluating the capacity of the community to attract and retain new members (so that the initial group of users grow to become an actual community), and evaluating the impact of the virtual community on the health status of its members. Actual studies on eHealth interventions targeting elderly, some of them having no virtual community features, used strategies to evaluate their health-oriented online intervention, mostly using patient health outcomes, patient use and satisfaction (Berman et al., 2009; Irvine Gelatt, Seeley, Macfarlane & Gau, 2013). Whereas those studies show positive outcomes, they target a specific elderly population and a specific health problem. The positives outcomes of general eHealth intervention for older adults are harder to demonstrate. For instance, a promising online health community intervention aimed to facilitate multidisciplinary communication among health care professionals failed to show health improvements among frail elderly (Makai et al., 2014). While the idea of an efficient evaluation is great in theory, the actual process is relatively hard and often not complete.

Before evaluating the effectiveness of the platform or intervention itself, the potentiality of engagement in the virtual community by the elderly population should be considered. Using virtual health promotion tools for this particular population poses a series of unique challenges in terms of physical and mental limitations, as mentioned above, and reduced technological literacy present in older individuals who did not grow up with information technologies, but who are instead what is referred to as digital immigrants. Older adults' health literacy levels affect their acceptance of the material since its incomprehension can be an important barrier while using the tool. As conventional health resources are limited, so are numeric resources (in terms of development power) and, more importantly, attentional resources of the elderly, who by being exposed to too many (sometimes poorly developed) applications might reduce their willingness to actively engage in new ones. Furthermore, the objective of the health-oriented virtual community must be clearly identified during the development process to ensure an adequate evaluation of the material. According to Mouton and Cloes (2015), a web-based intervention with virtual community feature was more likely to increase awareness toward physical activity than to induce significant behavior changes. Therefore, health prevention and health promotion seems to be more appropriate health-oriented virtual communities' goals than specific health behavior changes. Appropriate evaluations strategies should be implemented, and ideally as early as in the design steps, to ensure that the resources engaged are used efficiently, for the greatest benefit of a highly vulnerable population. This would also contribute in convincing policy makers of the necessity to support such initiatives at larger scales.

To effectively evaluate the impact of an online health intervention, multiple factors are currently being assessed (Veldel, Akhlaghpour, Vaghefi, Bergman, & Lapointe, 2013). First, the patient's health outcomes must obviously be assessed, including long-term follow-up measures. Furthermore, since participants could change their behaviors only because of the sensibilization caused by the exposure to the questionnaire – as experienced by some researchers (Irvine et al., 2013) – the evaluation process must include a control group that considers that possible bias. As not every program shows significant behaviors changes, they should be accompanied with an assessment of participant's beliefs and attitudes about their health, especially for preventive programs. Second, the clinical processes, such as a better documentation of patient's health status, are outcomes of interest (Veldel et al., 2013). They are essentials to assess the impact of health-oriented virtual communities on clinical care setting, and therefore to justify their integration in the care system. Third, the clinician's and patient's satisfaction are also valuable outcomes variables that are assess (Berman et al., 2009). These factors can influence the acceptability of the tool, hence the possibility of positive outcomes for both the patient and the clinician through the clinical process. Indeed, a health-oriented virtual community can help increase the engagement and empowerment of patients toward their own health care process and can help clinicians stay current about the medical advances in the field by sharing experiences, knowledge and disease-specific expertise (van der Eijk et al., 2013). This is especially true in the context of chronic disease, which are frequent among older adults, since the health care needs are complex and may differ from one patient to another. Fourth, the productivity, efficiency and costs factors are of importance to decision makers, and facilitate the integration of those programs in the clinical settings. A few other factors could be considered when it comes to the evaluation of online-oriented virtual communities. Particularly, the material should be pilot tested with a small group of older adults in order to see if an improvement of the technical aspects can be done to facilitate use of the platform and adherence to the program. Interventions often benefits from small changes to the interface such as the navigation links and reducing amount of text in pages (Berman et al., 2009), especially with an aging population. Finally, the process must include the evaluation of the online material itself. Such a process must include both quantitative, among which a variety of tools should be used (readability, sentiment analysis and understandability tools) and qualitative methods (Beaunoyer, Arsenault, Lomanowska & Guitton, 2016). Indeed, instead of using those tools as part of the evaluation process, they should be used in the development of online health intervention itself as well as other strategies mentioned above. Of note, the five strategies (see **Figure 1**) proposed are important to include in the online health intervention's evaluation if applicable to the content.

Figure 1. Factors to consider for the evaluation of an online health intervention

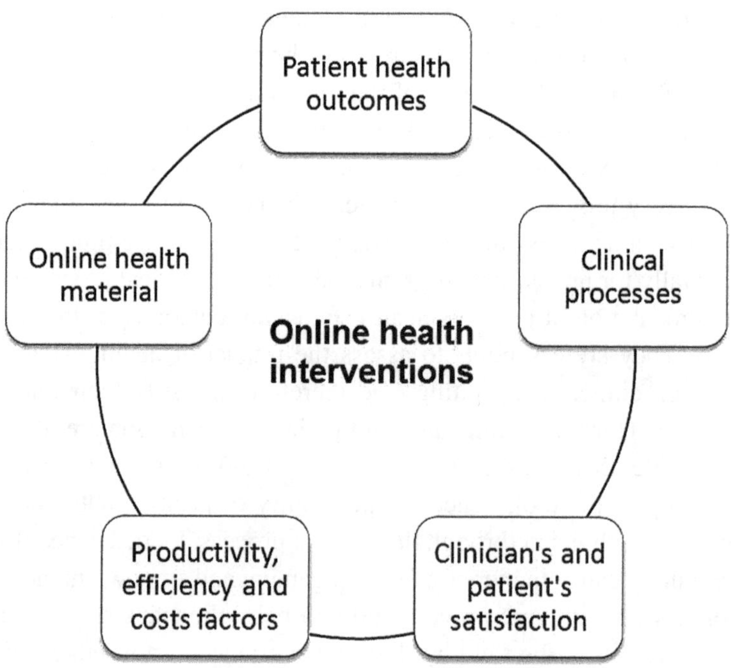

ETHICAL ISSUES

Besides potential cost savings, using eHealth allows greater access to treatment and increase communication options (Hilgart et al., 2012), which is more convenient for some elderly patients with disabilities. While health-oriented virtual communities can potentially present major benefits for patients, clinicians and care systems, they come with a several ethical challenges. These ethical challenges can roughly be divided between challenges arising from the virtual community itself, and issues related to aspects surrounding the technological setting – particularly issues of privacy and confidentiality.

Several problems can occur when dealing with health-related virtual communities, and taking these issues into consideration is part of a proper ethical reflection while designing applications or programs taking advantage of virtual communities for health purposes. When interacting through a virtual community, participants might be exposed to risks of problematic social comparison – the natural tendency to compare to others. However, and while this tendency is in the human nature, social comparison – either upward comparison (comparison with someone perceived as better) or downward comparison (comparison with someone perceived as worse) is usually not profitable in the context of health-oriented virtual communities, and could be in fact quite deleterious for the patients, either by affecting self-esteem or adherence to treatment (Guitton, 2015b). Such comparisons can also produce some level of anxiety can also appear due to trouble participants might have using the community, reducing its potential as a therapeutic tool.

Another ethical challenge for participants concerns the aspects related to privacy and confidentiality. Although these issues are central for a lot of virtual communities, these problems get somehow exacerbated in the case of elder people, who, due to their limited technological literacy compared to younger population, are more vulnerable to the dangers related to break of privacy. This is true both in terms of behavior within the community – for instance when displaying potentially unsafe self-disclosure behavior – and in terms of technical misuse – not adapted interactions with the interfaces, such as partial use of privacy features or confidentiality choices due to a limited understanding of the technical aspects of the settings. While a break of privacy due to unnecessary disclosure from participants is likely to happen in peer-to-peer online interactions (Guitton, 2015b), people not fully familiar with the socio-cultural codes of virtual communities and virtual spaces are more likely to fall in these involuntary trap. Most young adults, used to manage various social media account, and prompted regularly on the danger of cyberstalking, cyberbullying, and so on, are usually quite familiar with the ways to protect at least minimally their identity in virtual spaces. This is obviously not the case of elderly, who might act in a relatively naïve way in some situations involving self-disclosure of potentially critical information. The ethical – and practical – challenges related to privacy surrounding the virtual community can also be coming from the general technological problems related to security issues. When dealing with a health-related community, these issues are even more problematic, due to the very nature of the data exchanged and stored. This is particularly true when it comes to the interactions between online health community and electronics health records. While a health-oriented virtual community need to establish bases supporting joining the group – which might include giving health information when registering in order to ensure legitimacy of participants- limited information given by the user might not be valid information. Therefore, linking the virtual community registration to electronics health records constitute an alternative, but it bears rather obviously others major ethical and security considerations, such as the access to the database and possibilities of leak between health-oriented virtual community and electronics health records (Guitton, 2015b). Once again, given the fact that elder people generally have a lower technological literacy, they might have more trouble to understand the implication of their participation in such a virtual community. Therefore, the issue of informed consent is greater with that population, not to mention with those having cognition difficulties. Of note, this in turn might again generate some additional psychological stress for people trying to join or participate in the community – which would be contrary to the initial goal of the health-oriented community which is to provide help to patients.

CONCLUSION

As a concluding remark, it is interesting to note that most of the studies so far have focused on a single aspect of health in the elderly (for instance social support, information regarding a specific pathology or chronic disease, etc.), instead of considering health as a global process. Therefore, most senior-targeted eHealth applications focus on a specific and identifiable goal, rather than considering an enhancement of health more globally. However, once the initial objective is fulfilled (e.g., reduce temporarily loneliness), the tool might become obsolete for this given population. While it might still be working for new users, this clearly compromises the continuity of the virtual community itself as the turn-over of its members would be too fast. Also, users might get tired of writing about the same problematic while the ties with other community members get stronger. Since virtual communities need time to develop and consolidate, designing health-oriented virtual communities should be done with a holistic approach in mind in order to optimise the resources and efforts when trying to develop such type of virtual communities.

Research on health-related virtual communities is but a specific case of research on virtual communities. Therefore, the future directions of virtual community research also apply here. Among the questions researchers in the field will have to answer in the coming years or decades, are how one joins a given virtual community, how people get involved in the community and stays there, how information get optimally transferred across the community, and what are the mechanisms supporting the transformation of online-triggered behavioral patterns into real life actions. Another future challenge in this field of health-related virtual communities will be to be able to make the positive effects of belonging to the community go beyond a single dimension. Indeed, a health-oriented virtual community targeting aged people should not only try to reduce loneliness, but also have benefit for several health domains such as physical activity, hydration, healthy food consumption, treatment adherence, etc. In other words, further research directions on the development of senior-targeted eHealth applications should investigate how to efficiently include multiples health related objectives in the single virtual community design. Designers of eHealth applications should also consider users' needs for the characteristics of the application as well as the content. Health-oriented virtual communities, when adequately developed and evaluated, constitute an interesting approach for older adults whose are subject to more social isolation and health problems than younger populations.

REFERENCES

Arsenault, M., Blouin, M. J., & Guitton, M. J. (2012). Information quality and dynamics of patients interactions on tonsillectomy web resources. *Internet Interventions*, *4*, 99–104. doi:10.1016/j.invent.2016.05.002

Beaunoyer, E., Arsenault, M., Lomanowska, A. M., & Guitton, M. J. (2016). Understanding Online Health Information: Evaluation, Tools, and Strategies. *Patient Education and Counseling*. doi:10.1016/j.pec.2016.08.028 PMID:27595436

Berman, R. L. H., Iris, M. A., Bode, R., & Drengenberg, C. (2009). The Effectiveness of an Online Mind-Body Intervention for Older Adults with Chronic Pain. *The Journal of Pain*, *10*(1), 68–79. doi:10.1016/j.jpain.2008.07.006 PMID:18774342

Braun, M. T. (2013). Obstacles to social networking website use among older adults. *Computers in Human Behavior*, *29*(3), 673–680. doi:10.1016/j.chb.2012.12.004

Brown-Johnson, C. G., Berrean, B., & Cataldo, J. K. (2015). Development and usability evaluation of the mHealth Tool for Lung Cancer (mHealth TLC): A virtual world health game for lung cancer patients. *Patient Education and Counseling*, *98*(4), 506–511. doi:10.1016/j.pec.2014.12.006 PMID:25620075

Gigler, K. L., Blomeke, K., Shatil, E., Weintraub, S., & Reber, P. J. (2013). Preliminary evidence for the feasibility of at-home online cognitive training with older adults. *Gerontotechnology*, *12*(1), 26–35. doi:10.4017/gt.2013.12.1.007.00 PMID:26778939

Guitton, M. J. (2014). The importance of studying the dark side of social networks. *Computers in Human Behavior*, *31*, 355. doi:10.1016/j.chb.2013.10.055

Guitton, M. J. (2015a). Swimming with mermaids: Communication and social density in the Second Life merfolk community. *Computers in Human Behavior*, *48*, 226–235. doi:10.1016/j.chb.2015.02.004

Guitton, M. J. (2015b). Ethical challenges in online health games. In D. Novak, B. Tulu, & H. Brendryen (Eds.), *Holistic Perspectives in Gamification for Clinical Practice* (pp. 1–9). IGI Global; doi:10.4018/978-1-4666-9522-1.ch001

Hayes, M., van Stolk-Cooke, K., & Muench, F. (2015). Understanding Facebook use and the psychological affects of use across generations. *Computers in Human Behavior*, *49*, 507–511. doi:10.1016/j.chb.2015.03.040

Hilgart, M., Thorndike, F. P., Pardo, J., & Ritterband, L. M. (2012). 12 Ethical Issues of Web-Based Interventions and Online Therapy. The Oxford handbook of international psychological ethics, 161.

Irvine, I. B., Gelatt, V. A., Seeley, J. R., Macfarlane, P., & Gau, J. M. (2013). Web-based Intervention to Promote Physical Activity by Sedentary Older Adults: Randomized Controlled Trial. *Journal of Medical Internet Research*, *15*(2), e19. doi:10.2196/jmir.2158 PMID:23470322

Lomanowska, A. M., & Guitton, M. J. (2014). My avatar is pregnant! Representation of pregnancy, birth, and maternity in a virtual world. *Computers in Human Behavior*, *31*, 322–331. doi:10.1016/j.chb.2013.10.058

Makai, P., Perry, M., Robben, S. H., Schers, H. J., Heinen, M. M., Rikkert, M. G. O., & Melis, R. F. (2014). Evaluation of an eHealth intervention in chronic care for frail older people: Why adherence is the first target. *Journal of Medical Internet Research*, *16*(6), e156. doi:10.2196/jmir.3057 PMID:24966146

Mouton, A., & Cloes, M. (2015). Efficacy of a web-based, center-based or combined physical activity intervention among older adults. *Health Education Research, 30*(3), 422–435. doi:10.1093/her/cyv012 PMID:25772974

Nahm, E. S., Resnick, B., DeGrezia, M., & Brotemarkle, R. (2009). Use of discussion boards in a theory-based health web site for older adults. *Nursing Research, 58*(6), 419–426. doi:10.1097/NNR.0b013e3181bee6c4 PMID:19918152

Pfeil, U., Zaphiris, P., & Wilson, S. (2010). The role of message-sequences in the sustainability of an online support community for older people. *Journal of Computer-Mediated Communication, 15*(2), 336–363. doi:10.1111/j.1083-6101.2010.01523.x

Richardson, C. R., Buis, L. R., Janney, A. W., Goodrich, D. E., Sen, A., Hess, M. L., & Strecher, V. J. et al. (2010). An online community improves adherence in an internet-mediated walking program. Part 1: Results of a randomized controlled trial. *Journal of Medical Internet Research, 12*(4), e71. doi:10.2196/jmir.1338 PMID:21169160

Stellefson, M., Chaney, B., Barry, A. E., Chavarria, E., Tennant, B., Walsh-Childers, K., & Zagora, J. et al. (2013). Web 2.0 chronic disease self-management for older adults: A systematic review. *Journal of Medical Internet Research, 15*(2), e35. doi:10.2196/jmir.2439 PMID:23410671

Sum, S., Mathews, R. M., Pourghasem, M., & Hughes, I. (2009). Internet use as a predictor of sense of community in older people. *Cyberpsychology & Behavior, 12*(2), 235–239. doi:10.1089/cpb.2008.0150 PMID:19250013

van der Eijk, M., Faber, M. J., Aarts, J. W., Kremer, J. A., Munneke, M., & Bloem, B. R. (2013). Using online health communities to deliver patient-centered care to people with chronic conditions. *Journal of Medical Internet Research, 15*(6), e115. doi:10.2196/jmir.2476 PMID:23803284

Veldel, I., Akhlaghpour, S., Vaghefi, I., Bergman, H., & Lapointe, L. (2013). Health information technologies in geriatrics and gerontology: A mixed systematic review. *Journal of the American Medical Informatics Association, 20*(6), 1109–1119. doi:10.1136/amiajnl-2013-001705 PMID:23666776

White, K. M., Starfelt, L. C., Young, R. M., Hawkes, A. L., Cleary, C., Leske, S., & Wihardjo, K. (2015). A randomised controlled trial of an online theory-based intervention to improve adult Australians sun-protective behaviours. *Preventive Medicine, 72*, 19–22. doi:10.1016/j.ypmed.2014.12.025 PMID:25572618

KEY TERMS AND DEFINITIONS

Attrition: Process in which participants disengage in a treatment after they began participating.

Digital Immigrant: Person who did not grow up with digital technologies, but instead discovered and adopted them once already adult (in contrast to digital natives).

Empowerment: Process in which a person feel gaining control over his own actions.

Health Literacy: The degree to which individuals have the capacity to obtain, process, and understand basic health information and services needed to make appropriate health decisions.

Population Targeting: Design strategies aiming at targeting a specific segment of the population,

Social Support: Perception and impression to be cared for by others.

Technological Literacy: The degree to which individuals have the capacity to obtain, process, and understand basic technological information needed to use adequately computers, Internet, and mobile devices and applications.

Section 2
Innovation and Future Directions

Chapter 6
Virtual Community Engagement to Advance Interoperability in Digital Health

Gina DeBenedetti
Canada Health Infoway, Canada

Kelly Kuru
Canada Health Infoway, Canada

Peter Picton
Canada Health Infoway, Canada

Linda Monico
Canada Health Infoway, Canada

Tasha Shaw-Verbic
Canada Health Infoway, Canada

ABSTRACT

This chapter will provide an overview of InfoCentral, a virtual community platform launched for advancing digital health information in Canada. Developed and hosted by Canada Health Infoway, InfoCentral has become a hub and resource for stakeholders in digital health to discuss, consider, and evaluate common challenges among digital health system compatibility across the country (i.e., interoperability). A synopsis of the role Infoway contributes toward advancing Canadian digital health, the background and considerations for InfoCentral, along with a series of three flourishing virtual community case studies will be examined. Critical success factors and lessons learned in establishing, supporting and growing productive virtual communities conclude this chapter.

DOI: 10.4018/978-1-5225-2958-3.ch006

INTRODUCTION

Canada faces a unique challenge in the area of digital health. With the delivery of health care primarily the responsibility of Canada's provinces and territories, it falls under their individual mandates to support health care providers with information technology solutions that enable the effective sharing of information across care settings. Although each region shares the same goal of providing quality health care supported by effective digital health solutions, they may differ in prioritizing, procuring and implementing solutions. This variance has often led to incompatibility among systems, regions and provinces. Though there has been progress in proliferating digital health systems across the country, the connectivity, information flow and standardization, often referred to as interoperability, remains a significant challenge. With this challenge in mind, an initiative has been underway in Canada to bring together the vast array of players in digital health to ensure these issues are addressed. Under the guidance of the Digital Health Alliance managed by Canada Health Infoway, stakeholders representing provincial, territorial and regional governments, digital health vendors, clinicians and citizens have convened collaboration efforts primarily coordinated through an online platform called InfoCentral.

This chapter will provide an overview and rationale of this unique application of virtual community engagement as it applies to the digital health landscape of health care delivery in Canada. This chapter will include background information about Canada Health Infoway, its role in digital health development in Canada, and the launch of the Clinical Interoperability Action Plan in 2015. An overview of the InfoCentral collaboration environment will be provided, along with a discussion of the engagement tactics and critical success factors to moving collaboration forward on the platform. Finally, this chapter will discuss three case studies representing communities and working groups hosted on InfoCentral, citing key success factors impacting this online community.

BACKGROUND

About Canada Health Infoway

Canada Health Infoway's purpose is to realize the vision of healthier Canadians through innovative digital health solutions. Through targeted investments, Infoway helps deliver better quality and access to care and more efficient delivery of health services for patients and clinicians as a product of collaborative relationships with federal, provincial and territorial governments, clinicians, industry and Canadians.

In September 2000, Canada's Health Ministers made a commitment to "work together to strengthen a Canada-wide health infostructure to improve quality, access and timeliness of health care for Canadians." In response to this commitment, Infoway was created in 2001 to accelerate the development and implementation of electronic health information systems across the country, partnering with each province and territory in pursuit of a common goal.

A creation of Canada's federal government, Canada Health Infoway was established as an independent, not-for-profit corporation. The organization is accountable to the 14 Deputy Ministers of Health of the federal, provincial and territorial governments, known as the Members of the Corporation. In addition to these members, Infoway also has an independent Board of Directors, which is made up of leaders from Canada's public, health, legal, financial and technology sectors.

At the time of Infoway's creation, there was no common vision in place for digital health in Canada. The country lacked a strategy, architecture and plan to pursue the goal of a common electronic health record. National health information standards were not in place to support the construction of this infrastructure, and the privacy and security approaches and practices varied across the country. In terms of funding, the levels of provincial and territorial investment in health information technology differed considerably, and in most cases supporting strategies had yet to be developed. In short, the basic business case for health information technology along with an accompanying benefits evaluation framework had not been established.

Other countries faced similar challenges with their information and communication technology initiatives. Like Canada, they also lacked a solid understanding of the immensity and complexity of the task at hand. The following reference echoes this position with a review of health information exchanges established as a priority in seven nations with varying active clinical data exchange recognized in the observations (Jha, Doolan, Grandt, Scott, Bates, June 2008).

Infoway's original mandate was "to foster and accelerate the implementation of a Canadian Electronic Health Record (EHR) network, in order to manage Canadian health information from coast to coast to coast." Over the years, the mandate has evolved and is now referred to as the "three waves of digital health innovation."

During the first wave, Infoway focused on the building blocks, or foundational elements of digital health, and acted as a "strategic investor" by co-investing with the jurisdictions in projects throughout the country. The primary focus was on building six core systems: patient and provider registries; laboratory information systems; drug information systems; diagnostic imaging in hospitals; and clinical reports or immunizations.

During the second wave, the organization focused on increasing the use of digital tools by clinicians, such as electronic medical records systems for physicians (referred to as electronic health records in the U.S.). During this wave, progress was also made in the areas of telehealth and public health surveillance.

Currently in its third wave of digital health innovation, Infoway is focused on patient empowerment. The established vision of healthier Canadians through innovative digital health solutions, guides Infoway as it brings Canadian attention to the Triple Aim objectives of improving the patient experience (including quality and satisfaction), improving the health of populations and unlocking value for the health care system (Canada Health Infoway, 2017i).

Infoway is pursuing digital health solutions and services to: empower patients to take control of and manage their health; improve access and support seamless care coordination, communication, and collaboration between patients and their health care team; and enable clinical and system-level decision making to support new business models, improvements in care quality and health system efficiency.

Infoway addresses stakeholders' needs through: leveraging existing and pursuing new joint investment opportunities; purposeful stakeholder engagement, including convening partnerships, both public and private; creating and disseminating knowledge, standards and best practices; and providing pan-Canadian services and strategies.

Since inception, all of Infoway's funding has come from the federal government, through Health Canada. As of February 2017, Infoway had received a total of $2.15 billion through several grants, all based on agreements specifying mutual obligations.

The Solution: The Vision of Accelerating Interoperability

For the past decade, the Canadian health sector has invested considerable time, energy and funding establishing the necessary digital health systems and solutions to enable clinicians to access the vital clinical data they need to provide the best care possible to their patients.

After a decade's worth of this work establishing the foundation of electronic health information repositories, the next obstacle included developing the pathway to share the information across various locations and care providers. To clinicians, this information sharing, (clinical interoperability), means having access to usable clinical content from diverse sources without having to do extra or unnecessary work. To be successful in this aim, the core value proposition for clinicians remains, "access to clinical information with minimal disruption in workflow." In short, clinical interoperability is an essential prerequisite for high quality health care.

Over the course of 2013-2014, Infoway conducted a series of interviews and five regional forums designed to solicit stakeholder insights into the current and future states of clinical interoperability in Canada. Clinicians, digital health program leaders, vendors and others indicated that not everyone who needs to be involved in the broader discussion about clinical interoperability is always involved. They underlined the importance of having an overarching, effective governance structure to drive clinical interoperability and to coordinate, communicate and foster collaboration.

Driven from stakeholder insights on the elements required to accelerate the pace of clinical interoperability, Infoway drafted the Clinical Interoperability Strategy Framework, which includes five perspectives under an overarching multi-stakeholder engagement. Stakeholders indicated that achieving clinical interoperability in Canada would require significant and collaborative progress across each of these five perspectives. See Figure 1.

The five key areas/perspectives include:

- **Clinical Leadership:** Establish a clear vision for the clinician to contribute to the acceleration of interoperability, through real-world provider and patient experiences to create a sense of urgency in the need for interoperability for improved patient care and outcomes
- **Awareness, Promotion, Adoption of Interoperability Specifications:** Raise awareness and understanding, through stakeholder education, about interoperability specifications, (ie, recipes) including how they are used in implementation and testing, creating an inventory of common sets of specifications that may be leveraged and adopted across the country in clinical priority areas, creating value propositions for stakeholders to adopt
- **Simple, Open Technical Solutions**: Enable and support the rapid development of solution interoperability through open Application Programming Interface (API) processes for vendors to develop rapid development of digital health solutions; encourage solution portability through promotion of re-use to avoid costly customizations and delays and employ the use of national testing and certifications, especially in the areas of privacy and security
- **Health Information Exchange (HIE) best Practices**: Identify, educate through demonstration(s) and encourage adoption of HIE best practices and establish operational funding to support sustainable HIE interoperability services
- **Stakeholder Engagement**: Identify and engage key stakeholder groups (clinicians, patients, representatives of regional/national digital health programs, vendors, implementers of digital solutions to achieve a common vision and strategy for accelerating interoperability; enable an online environment to improve access and enhance the collaboration considering geography, timing and availability; share leading best practices in a timely manner

Figure 1. Clinical Interoperability Strategy Framework Perspectives (Canada Health Infoway, 2014)

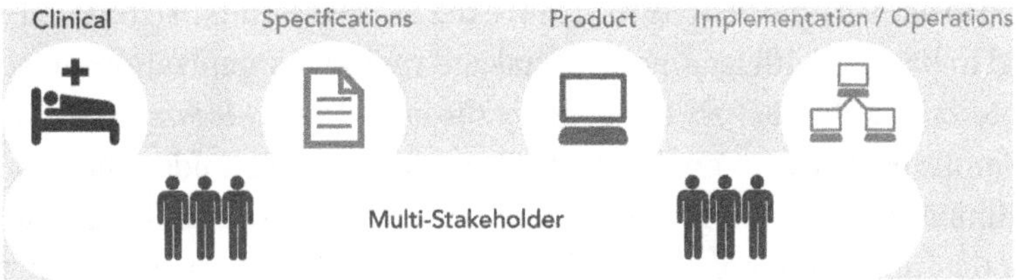

As a result of the consultation process, Infoway also developed an action plan referred to as *Accelerating Clinical Interoperability in Canada: The Path Forward* (Canada Health Infoway, 2014). The document was published in October 2014. The path (see Figure 2) includes five key areas, or clinical interoperability "opportunities for action," to accelerate clinical interoperability in Canada.

As mentioned previously, insights gathered during Infoway's stakeholder interviews and regional forums, indicated that while significant progress has been made on increasing the adoption and use of digital health solutions in Canada, the full value of digital health will be realized only when health information systems

Figure 2. The Path Forward to Accelerating Clinical Interoperability in Canada (Canada Health Infoway, 2014)

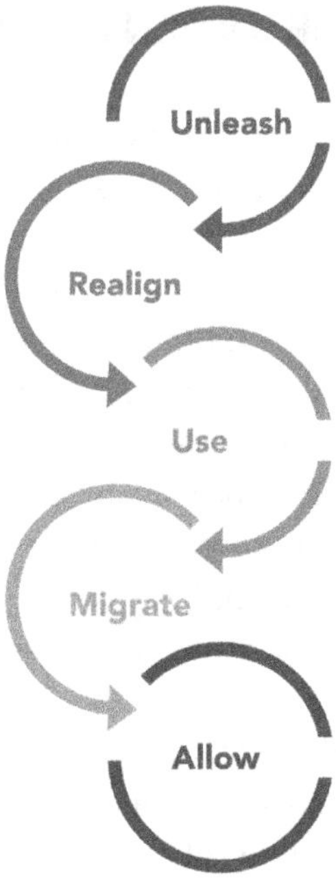

are connected and able to be easily accessed and shared by authorized clinicians. However, regions, clinicians and their representative associations, vendors and others need to actively participate to achieve the desired results. To this end, Infoway committed to partner with leading national and regional organizations to accelerate clinical interoperability across the country through *The Path Forward*. One output of this commitment was to ensure that all interested stakeholders have a voice in moving clinical interoperability forward. To satisfy this overarching tenet, and in support of the first four opportunities for action in *The Path Forward*, Infoway began development of a platform to facilitate collaboration and unite the health system's diverse set of stakeholders toward common goals. Overcoming the challenges of geography, time, and cost necessitated a virtual approach to collaboration, a platform to support online communication and activities and a host for virtual communities of interest to gather. These virtual communities, which can been defined as "an aggregation of individuals or business partners who interact around a shared interest, where the interaction is at least partially supported and/or mediated by technology and guided by some protocols or norms" (Porter, C. E., 2004), have been the primary reason for the platform to exist and thrive. Virtual communities provide a "means for knowledge to cross boundaries, generate and manage a body of knowledge for members to draw on, promote standardisation of practice, and innovate and create breakthrough ideas, knowledge, and practices" (Ranmuthugala, Plumb, Cunningham, Georgiou, Westbrook and Braithwaite, 2011).

INFOCENTRAL: AN ENVIRONMENT FOR COLLABORATION

To facilitate collaboration among stakeholders to achieve the goals set out by the Clinical Interoperability Action Plan (Pan-Canadian Clinical Interoperability Steering Committee, 2015), Infoway developed InfoCentral and launched it in January 2015. InfoCentral is a virtual community platform that is unique in providing a mechanism for clinicians, e-health representatives, vendors, developers and others to collaborate in the effort to accelerate clinical information sharing across Canada, spanning an holistic ecosystem of stakeholders (Canada Health Infoway, 2017c). It facilitates this collaboration by providing a space for knowledge sharing, best practices through community forums, document repository and virtual meetings. Further, the platform serves as a national source for developer and standards tools/resources. InfoCentral facilitates the collective identification and addressing of real issues or challenges in digital health.

InfoCentral has experienced tremendous growth over the past two years. The number of communities at the time of launch, January 2015, included 23, as of May 2017, the number of communities has grown to 40. It has evolved to support a varied group of collaborative efforts, and provide a number of tools that further support those working in e-health throughout Canada. The platform has enabled communities and working groups to apply their collective thinking to the current interoperability challenges facing the country across a number of vastly different clinical areas. The following offers an overview of the structure and features provided by the InfoCentral platform.

Communities and Working Groups

Virtual collaborative groups on InfoCentral are hosted under two categories: Communities and Working Groups (Figure 3). Communities are intended to include dialogue and ongoing collaboration by like-minded individuals on interoperability topics. They foster open, inclusive participation and encourage diverse perspectives. These groups are primarily intended for knowledge sharing and networking, where news and relevant reports can be shared, and discussions may be hosted. Communities may be domain specific, such as Diagnostic Imaging, or may relate to a specific technology area such as SNOMED CT (Systematized Nomenclature of Medicine – Clinical Terms) which is a comprehensive health care terminology standard used in many health information systems around the world (SNOMED International, 2017). Communities are formed by request from stakeholders, as a result of an identified need; while other groups were established in response to identified priorities arising from the Clinical Interoperability Action Plan, including: Clinician Engagement, Public Health Surveillance, Medication Management and Coordination of Care.

Figure 3. InfoCentral Communities and Working Groups (Canada Health Infoway, 2017d)

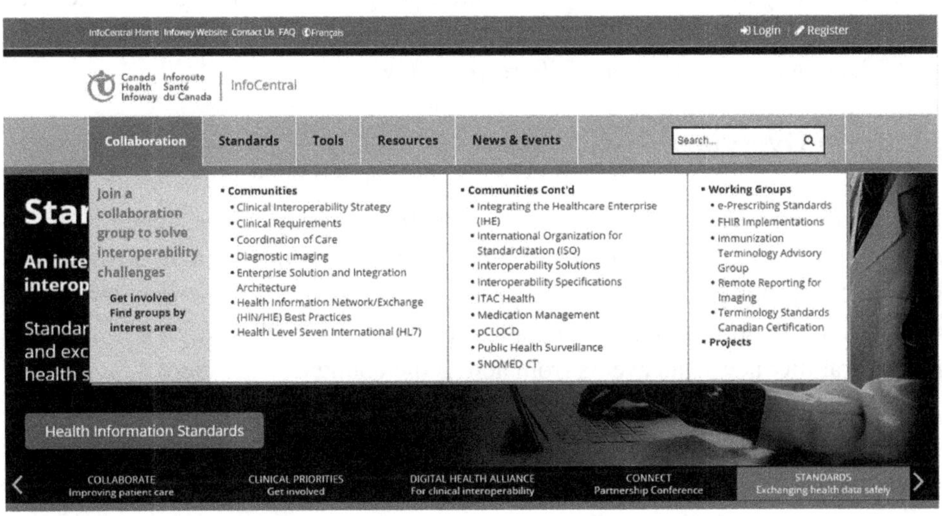

Working groups are established with specific goals in mind, (i.e., developing material for a specific project, collecting national insights to move a project forward). These working groups may be developed out of projects sponsored by Infoway, or from efforts that have been initiated through discussions among stakeholders. Other working groups have been created from existing committees whose mandates align with the goals set forth by the Action Plan, and most recently, to support projects or teams with a means of collaboration in digital health. In some of the communities, if the discussion trajectory in the group changes from knowledge-sharing to a goal oriented, time-sensitive outcome driven one, community members or those identifying with that goal may choose to open a working group to meet separately under the project. The working group may be associated with a community in a nested manner or operate completely independent. An example of this development was demonstrated with within the Medication Management Community. During a period, active discussions around the need for clinical requirements when embarking on large-scale services as in the case of e-Prescribing. Seizing the opportunity to align with work already underway on PrescribeIT™ (Canada Health Infoway, 2017g), Infoway's national electronic prescription service, the e-Prescribing Standards Working Group was established. This focused working group commented on a set of clinical requirements used as guiding document and ultimately worked toward the development of Canadian Clinical Drug Data Set, a national drug terminology, sponsored by Health Canada and hosted on InfoCentral as the release centre.

Steady growth in the number of users has been a significant contributor to InfoCentral's success. The platform was fortunate to have launched with several communities migrating from existing (non-virtual) groups. With a foundation to draw upon as the platform went live, InfoCentral has experienced a 73% increase in total users since its baseline launch; growing from 10,513 total users in 2015 to 18,220 users by the end of 2016. The number of groups has also grown since the launch, as of May, 2017 the combined number of communities and working groups is at 50, an increase of 65% and 30% respectively.

Platform Overview

InfoCentral enables access to many collaboration opportunities, features, tools and resources to address interoperability challenges within a group's respective project. The community and working group collaborative structure provides access to health information standards, tools and resources, as well as digital health and interoperability news and events from across the country.

Each Community and Working Group has a uniform presentation of features on its home page (see Figure 4). The tabs on each home page provide access to an About page, the document manager, the events calendar, as well as other features such as a Member listing and the Forum. A web conferencing tool is also available to members, along with a repository of relevant videos. A task manager is available within each community, although most have relied on more traditional methods, (e.g., a shared document). The virtual community includes a calendar function that enables a combined calendar (community-specific event calendars, in addition to the public events available to the entire InfoCentral platform). The document management functionality is an important customized feature on InfoCentral based on the needs of the communities. Each community or working group has its own document space, along with the capability to add sub-folders, facilitating effective knowledge sharing.

Features and functionality have been built into and enabled on InfoCentral to serve its user community. For example, the official languages for Canada are English and French and the corporate policy for Infoway requires that we conduct business in both languages. Users may select their preference for English or French on all Infoway websites, including InfoCentral. Figure 4 demonstrates a link for "Français" at the top of the screen, which enables users to toggle between the English and French environments. Although forum content provided by members is presented in the language it is posted, the navigation menus, news articles, reports and other content are available in French. Another significant feature is a single-sign-on between the Infoway corporate website, InfoCentral and many other valuable Infoway tools and resources accessed by users for background and/or education.

Figure 4.Community home page – Coordination of Care (Canada Health Infoway, 2017a)

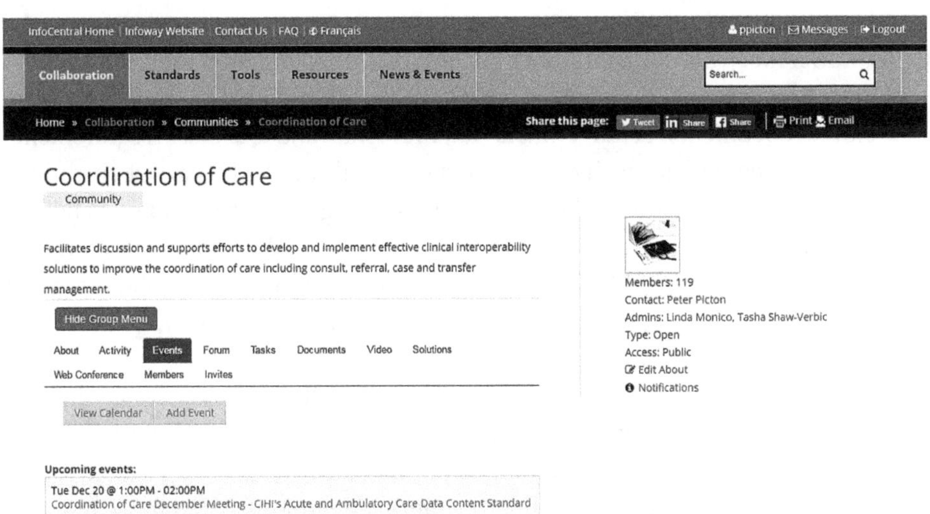

Tools and Additional Resources

As has been previously indicated, work in interoperability in the health care space most often involves the collaborative development and implementation of messaging and terminology standards. One of the key resources required by digital health solution implementers includes the latest standards releases and repositories. Infoway serves as the National Release Centre for these health information standards. To further support implementation efforts, Infoway has developed a number of related online tools (launched from InfoCentral) that may be accessed and used by developers and implementers of digital health solutions across the country, including:

- **Message Builder:** A core application and Application Program Interface (API) that facilitates the creation, population and access to HL7v3 messages and Clinical Document Architecture (CDA) documents. This tool enables the developer to focus on the business end of an application rather than on the detailed work of accessing and building the messages (Canada Health Infoway, 2017f).
- **Terminology Gateway:** A web-based solution that enables the distribution and sharing of terminology concepts, subsets and concept maps. Making this terminology, especially Canadian-specific content, available through the browser and via download, has delivered significant support for those working on interoperability projects (Canada Health Infoway, 2017j).
- **Terminology Service API, and the Fast Healthcare Interoperability Resources (FHIR) Terminology Service API:** provides developers access to the terminology libraries programmatically rather than through the browser, thereby providing further options to access these important assets (Canada Health Infoway, 2017j).
- **InfoScribe:** This collaboration tool provides the foundation for the Standards Selection Framework, which hosts published digital health solutions. These online documents detail clinical requirements and business requirements (e.g., use cases and business rules), along with the technical specifications for the interoperability solution (e.g., messaging and terminology standards used in connecting the associated systems). InfoScribe contains customized templates for these publications which provide a number of collaboration and online editing and publishing features (Canada Health Infoway, 2017e).

Though these tools generally exist independently, they are accessible directly through the InfoCentral menus, and have been branded as InfoCentral tools. Use of the tools in relation to the collaborative efforts can be discussed in the relevant community or working group. An Interoperability Solutions community has also been established to discuss specific features or details of the tools themselves, and to highlight work using these and other tools. InfoCentral also supports users by incorporating links to external supportive tools and standards libraries as appropriate. Providing this "one-stop shop" for work in digital health has been a key driver of engaging clinicians and implementers from across the country in the renewed effort to accelerate clinical interoperability.

VIRTUAL COMMUNITY CASE STUDIES

As described, InfoCentral hosts an array of virtual communities and working groups. This platform provides an opportunity for a comparative review of these groups as virtual communities. To identify aspects that influence engagement and the ultimate value in forming communities, this evaluation will consider the characteristics of each group, relative to membership as well as purpose. Further discussion will focus on the activities and related strategies used by the group, and the results achieved. Although at the time of writing, InfoCentral hosts a total of 50 communities of interest (public and private), a small group of communities has been selected to demonstrate the application and demonstration of how the five perspectives identified in the Clinical Interoperability Framework has supported the acceleration of Interoperability in Canada. Each of the communities of interest identified and discussed has played critical roles in moving the interoperability agenda in Canada. This review will examine the following InfoCentral working group and communities:

- Immunization Interoperability Working Group
- Diagnostic Imaging Community
- Coordination of Care Community

Immunization Interoperability Working Group

- **Purpose:** The Immunization Interoperability Working Group (IIWG) was established in August 2015 specifically to advance efforts in the sharing of immunization information, a key goal relating to the aforementioned Clinical Interoperability Action Plan under the priority area of Communicable Disease Management. Initial engagement on the topic of immunization took place in the Public Health Surveillance Community, a larger open community focused on knowledge sharing. The purpose of this community was identified as "building knowledge and collaborating on public health solutions to improve the electronic sharing and use of immunization and communicable disease information." (Canada Health Infoway, 2017h) As activities in this group progressed, work initiated with other levels of government to initiate projects focused on developing technology that would allow for the sharing of immunization records between health information systems. The IIWG was formed to focus decision making on developing interoperability standards through a collective effort. While the community is focused on knowledge sharing, the working group has a specific mandate of tasks including decisions revolving around the technical elements that would serve as the foundation for the effective sharing of electronic immunization records across the country. The contrast illustrates the inherent difference between a community of interest and a goal-oriented and timeline driven group. As such, the membership and activities of these groups were managed differently – as was the original intention in the development of the Community and Working Group classifications.

- **Membership:** Membership in the IIWG has reached 78 individuals to date. Thirty-five of the members originated from the Public Health Surveillance Community, a previously established non-virtual community. The remaining 43 were largely technical representatives from government and vendor communities who had a stake in the working group endeavours, but may not have deemed interaction in the larger Public Health Surveillance Community to be of interest to them. Overall, the IIWG was largely made up of health and policy representatives from Canada's regional government offices, as well as related federal agencies. The vendor and clinical communities were also represented – important stakeholders that were vital in providing insights and expertise to the process. It was important to engage this diverse group, both from the public as well as the private sector, as the success of the work was dependent upon adoption of the developed standards in practice.
- **Activities and Engagement Strategies:** Engagement of community members occurred through two main channels: forum discussion and web conferences. Though some topics were brought up and reviewed through the IIWG's forum on InfoCentral, the large majority of shared decision-making took place through web conferences to enable efficient real-time discussion. Approximately 30 of the Working Group's members became regular attendees at biweekly web conferences to discuss work items. Web conferences were often attended by 10-25 members, depending on the topic. Though most discussion occurred through the web conferences, the community platform provided an effective outlet for the dissemination of information – primarily

meeting notes and project outputs shared in the community document manager resulted in 250 downloads, and hosted follow-up discussion and planning. As well, continued membership in the working group made it possible to effectively inform interested parties about upcoming meeting details.

- **Outcomes:** The IIWG concluded its efforts in August 2016, one year after it was originally established. The group developed a national consensus on immunization data elements and these assets are informing immunization projects across several Canadian provinces. Prominent contributors to the working group effort from one province are now using these artifacts to help develop the digital health solutions that will enable clinicians and individual citizens to submit immunization records to the provincial repository.

Diagnostic Imaging Community

- **Purpose:** The Diagnostic Imaging Community was established along with the launch of InfoCentral in early 2015. Infoway previously managed several Working Groups focused on standards development in various medical domains, one of which was dedicated to Diagnostic Imaging. The new environment on InfoCentral enabled renewed discussions within this group, as well as opening up the discussion to other clinical, government and industry partners from across the country. The stated purpose of the community was established as "exploring Diagnostic Imaging topics to accelerate interoperability, such as Foreign Exam Management, Remote Reading and Radiology Synoptic Reporting."(Canada Health Infoway, 2017b)
- **Membership:** As of February 2017, there were 107 members of the Diagnostic Imaging Community. Though members of the formerly established Working Group provided the initial membership, the open nature of the community has provided the opportunity for more interested parties to participate in discussions. This particular community is unique in comparison to others, in that many members are more commonly in contact off-line. This community meets regularly in face-to-face opportunities such as medical imaging conferences. Collaboration within this community may have been more easily demonstrated because there was already an established sense of community among a number of the members. A sense of community or belonging has often been cited as a valuable aspect in priming engagement in virtual communities (Blanchard & Markus, 2004; Blanchard 2007).
- **Activities and Engagement Strategies:** As identified in the community's purpose, an aim of the community has been to accelerate interoperability for

the purpose of Remote Reading. In Diagnostic Imaging, this concept refers to "the practice of having medical images interpreted (read) by a reading specialist who is not present at the site where the diagnostic imaging study was acquired." Further, "the reading specialist is not reporting using the local Picture Archiving and Communication System (PACS) and dictation system at the acquiring site." (Reed, Larwood, Lindop, Macerola, & Picton, 2016) This topic became a focus of group meeting discussions and it was determined that a good starting point for tangible work would be the development of Clinical Requirements. In August 2015, a Clinical Requirements workshop was conducted as an in-person event to discuss the needs for "Cross Enterprise Remote Reading" from a clinical perspective. The small group convened for the workshop included lead representatives from industry, the public sector and the clinical community. A Clinical Requirements document created and served as the basis for further discussion conducted on the community forum and through bi-weekly web conferences hosted within the InfoCentral community (Reed, Larwood, Lindop, Macerola, & Picton, 2016). These activities provided a key input for the development of an Integrating the Healthcare Enterprise (IHE) Profile for "Remote Reporting for Imaging (TeleRadiology)." IHE Profiles are defined as follows:

IHE Profiles organize and leverage the integration capabilities that can be achieved by coordinated implementation of communication standards… They provide precise definitions of how standards can be implemented to meet specific clinical needs. (Integrating the Healthcare Enterprise, 2017)

Collaborative efforts to further utilize IHE profile and other related Diagnostic Imaging topics are ongoing within the community.

- **Outcomes:** The collaboration opportunities on the InfoCentral platform provided a foundational element to enabling the success of the Diagnostic Imaging Community. Efforts by members of the Diagnostic Imaging Community, facilitated by InfoCentral's discussion forum and virtual meetings, resulted in a Remote Reading profile being developed and most recently, sanctioned by Integrating the Healthcare Enterprise (IHE), an international organization supporting the coordinated use of health information standards. The value of this work will be realized as vendors begin to integrate its identified requirements in their products and add this functionality to new and existing health information systems. As this profile developed organically from discussions of its members, rather than through a mandated priority, it demonstrates the potential for such an online community to have collaboration lead to real world solutions. The existing cohesion of this community, combined with a clear mandate and desired outcome can be attributed to this group's ability to move such a valuable endeavour forward.

Coordination of Care Community

- **Purpose:** Along with Communicable Disease Management and Medication Management, Coordination of Care was identified as a priority of the Clinical Interoperability Action Plan. Across Canada, there have been some excellent examples of how sharing clinical information among health organizations and clinicians has improved the coordination of care for patients. Nevertheless, much work needs to be done to improve clinician capabilities of sharing health information electronically with their colleagues and patients to improve the delivery of care, through effective transitions of care among providers. Since its inception (April 2015), the purpose of the Coordination of Care Community has been to "facilitate discussion and support efforts to develop and implement effective clinical interoperability solutions to improve the coordination of care including consult, referral, case and transfer management." The Coordination of Care Community has taken a holistic approach and has involved discussions relating to various aspects of these digital health solutions (including messaging and terminology standards).
- **Membership:** At its onset, the Coordination of Care Community recruited members from its predecessor Working Group in the Standards community. As the community progressed, a more diverse membership developed. The Community now has 121 members and is one of the largest communities on InfoCentral. Almost half of the members are affiliated with federal or provincial governments or related agencies. A number have health care or IT related backgrounds, including subject matter experts in health care messaging and terminology standards, while some have translated their experience in clinical areas to leadership and strategy development roles in government. Approximately 15% identify themselves as either Healthcare Providers and Administrators, or as being affiliated with Research or Academia. A similar number work for Health Information System vendors or in related consulting firms. This combination of backgrounds and roles brings valuable diversity of knowledge and experience to the community.
- **Activities and Engagement Strategies:** Unlike other groups, which have had ongoing collaborative efforts, the Coordination of Care Community has focused on knowledge sharing. One of the key engagement activities has been a monthly webinar series that has featured presentations relating primarily to

ongoing coordination of care implementation projects across Canada. Topics have included patient portals, electronic referral and electronic consult, along with other systems that require the transfer of complex health information from system to system to support effective care coordination. Webinars have consistently drawn attendance of 20-45 members, with one webinar drawing more than 80 attendees, as it was cross-promoted by the presenters to interested parties outside the membership of the community. The forum and document space for the community has been an excellent resource for members as it has been used to post presentation materials and provide members with an opportunity to pose follow-up questions. Finally, increased efforts have been made to raise awareness about the topic areas and successes of respective implementations in news articles and editorial content on InfoCentral.

- **Outcomes:** As a knowledge sharing community, the Coordination of Care Community has achieved a considerable engagement. Leaders from the community have indicated that this community, predominantly dedicated to knowledge sharing, relative to the work being done across the country and the technologies used in these initiatives has enabled members to appreciate the approach and processes required in their respective regions. By cultivating continued interest in Coordination of Care through the knowledge sharing webinar series and forum activity, a foundation has been established for a representative national network and productive collaboration.

LESSONS LEARNED

Through our experiences with the collaboration communities and our evaluation of the metrics, previously shared in this chapter associated with InfoCentral engagement (ie, users), we offer the following "lessons learned" or critical success factors to best support virtual communities.

Mandate, Clarity and Purpose Determine the Level of Engagement and Activity

The old adage, "if you build it – they will come," (Lawrence, Lawrence & Robinson, 1989) is not always the principle upon which a collaborative community environment should be built. Acknowledgement of these opportunities has created a stronger framework to encourage and support participation. However, many potential participants have competing priorities during the business day so there is an expectation of receiving instant value from the interactions in which they invest their time. With that in mind, the impetus has been on InfoCentral's communities and working groups to provide useful, timely and valuable content and opportunities to attract and retain users.

Audience Needs, Ease of Access and Integration With Host Technology Determine the Frequency With Which Communities Engage

Soon after launch, evaluation solicited from communities indicated that there were elements, which could be improved to continue to attract new communities and members. Specifically, navigation, the wireframe, access to the community pages as well as tools and resources were referenced. As with any evaluation process, the development team re-evaluated the road map for future development and expedited the plan to make the required edits to facilitate an improved user experience.

A federated (single) sign-on was completed, enabling communities to navigate between community forum and out to the tools and resources section. Changes were made to the wireframe so the standards, tools and resources were more easily found and accessed. As well, we increased the promotion of the work done within the communities, made refinements to the enhanced features within the communities, and added the social media feed to the collaboration hub main page so it was easier to navigate and engage with a more vibrant and active community. We also assigned an Infoway employee to each community to act as an ambassador to navigate the platform's features and functionality. These employees also act as stewards to collect timely feedback for continual promotion and enhanced community engagement. As a result of these actions, an increase in traffic and participation on the site has been demonstrated, as measured by traffic and an increase in the number of groups, growth of 73% in users and 55% in groups.

One Size Does Not Fit All When Establishing Community Measures for Success

The communities and working groups using InfoCentral as a collaboration hub have been established and continue to exist for many reasons. Some are reinventions of a former structure, while others are entirely new. The importance of this distinction may enable community or working group leaders to assess the viability of new groups and determine appropriate measurements for success.

These measurements of success include:

- **Growth:** Evaluate growth in users, consumption of content and material (downloads, pageviews), usage of tools, growth of groups (number, size groups), traffic sources (direct, email, referrals, social).
- **Engagement:** Assess frequency of meetings, number of deliverables, achievements of specific goals, and forum posts with calls to action.
- **Integrated and Useful User Experience:** Gather feedback from users in order to identify opportunities to evolve user interface and ensure quality of functionality, while building a road map for future developments and enhancements.

Consideration should be given to the willingness of the group, and the circumstances of why or how the group shifted, changed direction or refocused the medium for collaboration. The motivation for the group to come together is an integral part of the group purpose and should be built into the metrics for success. In some cases, a reinvented group may be able to accelerate its progress based on the fact members have established relationships, norms and a culture to rely on, and in other cases, the history may impact the progress in a negative capacity.

Marketing and Promotion Efforts Enhance the Engagement and Grow the Virtual Community Footprint

InfoCentral has recognized the value of engagement resources as a mechanism to enhance the dissemination of messages, news and events that support and in some cases initiate interoperability-related dialogue. Additionally, marketing and engagement efforts are focused on raising the profile of work that has been initiated cross-country through and across the various communities. A news and events area displays upcoming community events, implementation projects and ongoing work and serves to initiate dialogue in topics and/or thought leadership areas. Editorials, also referred to as "spotlights" on InfoCentral, share insights on work, the stakeholders involved and the lessons learned. Together, news, spotlights and editorials assisted in reaching a wider audience (16% growth in monthly newsletter subscribers, from 1,315 in 2015 to 1,523 in 2016, which is in addition to other users reading these articles on InfoCentral directly). These articles are aimed at driving interest and participation in communities and working groups and inspiring a recognition for the platform as the place to collaborate and access valuable information.

In addition, the use of purposeful social medial outreach to engage a broader community has facilitated the generation of additional interest in virtual communities, contributing to the accelerated growth trajectory for InfoCentral. Since the launch of the platform, there has been a significant increase in number of visits from traffic sources such as referrals and social media. Referrals grew from 4,712 visits in 2015 to 8,266 visits in 2016, a 75% increase. Visits from social media also saw a growth of 82%, from 696 visits in 2015 to 1272 visits in 2016, with LinkedIn as the greatest source of return.

Evaluation and Continual Feedback Critical for Continued Support

A commitment to collect feedback, evaluate the changes required and remain nimble to ensure modifications are made in an efficient manner demonstrates support for community engagement. InfoCentral, as a collaboration platform, predominantly seeks to be user-centric and was built for a very niche market. As such, there is very little in the way of comparison we might offer at this time. The team responsible for operations, outreach and engagement continues to work with partners, stakeholders and internal Infoway team to explore the need to improve upon the platform, including capabilities, metrics for analyses and measures.

Delivering quality to users through the collaborative communities, in addition to the tools and resources available on the platform, enables the InfoCentral team to curate a needs-based road map of enhancements. The operations team meets regularly to review comments and requests delivered through the request for change tool on the platform and determine the timing associated with the modifications against the activities planned within and for each community.

Continuous efforts are applied to evaluate the needs of each audience on the platform. Given the area of digital health, there are virtual communities representing the following variety: technical, standards, implementers, developers, clinicians, government representatives, policy makers, vendors and health information technology executives. There are communities and working groups that are more uniform in audience, which makes capturing the needs relatively uncomplicated. Increasingly however, there are virtual communities that are drawing upon a variety of audiences. While this is the ultimate measure of success -- communities of purpose that bring together multiple views -- it is also more challenging to audit and make recommendations for an entire ecosystem of virtual communities.

Evaluation, open communication and active feedback to the communities, in a timely manner, have been critical imperatives to growing the platform and the virtual communities it serves. As time passes and Infoway's mandate continues to evolve, we anticipate that InfoCentral, its virtual communities and working groups will continue to be valuable and productive resources for people who work to advance digital health in Canada.

REFERENCES

Blanchard, A. L. (2007). Developing a Sense of Virtual Community Measure. *Cyberpsychology & Behavior, 10*(6), 827–830. doi:10.1089/cpb.2007.9946 PMID:18085972

Blanchard, A. L., & Markus, M. L. (2004). The Experienced Sense of a Virtual Community: Characteristics and Processes. *SIGMIS Database, 35*(1), 64–79. doi:10.1145/968464.968470

Canada Health Infoway. (2014). *The Path Forward: Accelerating Clinical Interoperability in Canada.* Retrieved February 28, 2017, from https://ic.infoway-inforoute.ca/en/resources/docs/cistratdocs/40-the-path-forward

Canada Health Infoway. (2017). *Summary Corporate Plan 2017-2018.* Toronto, Canada: Canada Health Infoway.

Canada Health Infoway. (2017a). *Coordination of Care.* Retrieved February 28, 2017, from https://ic.infoway-inforoute.ca/en/collaboration/communities/coordination-of-care

Canada Health Infoway. (2017b). *Diagnostic Imaging Community.* Retrieved February 28, 2017, from https://ic.infoway-inforoute.ca/en/collaboration/communities/diagnostic-imaging

Canada Health Infoway. (2017c). *InfoCentral.* Retrieved February 28, 2017, from https://www.infoway-inforoute.ca/en/communities/infocentral

Canada Health Infoway. (2017d). *InfoCentral Home.* Retrieved February 28, 2017, from https://ic.infoway-inforoute.ca/en/

Canada Health Infoway. (2017e). *InfoScribe Home.* Retrieved February 28, 2017, from https://infoscribe.infoway-inforoute.ca/display/IH/InfoScribe

Canada Health Infoway. (2017f). *Message Builder.* Retrieved February 28, 2017, from https://ic.infoway-inforoute.ca/en/tools/developer-tools/message-builder

Canada Health Infoway. (2017g). *PrescribeIT: Canada's Electronic Prescription Service.* Retrieved February 28, 2017, from https://www.infoway-inforoute.ca/en/solutions/e-prescribing/prescribeit

Canada Health Infoway. (2017h). *Public Health Surveillance Community.* Retrieved February 28, 2017, from https://ic.infoway-inforoute.ca/en/collaboration/communities-2/public-health-surveillance

Canada Health Infoway. (2017i). *Summary Corporate Plan 2017-2018*. Toronto, Canada: Canada Health Infoway.

Canada Health Infoway. (2017j). *Terminology Gateway*. Retrieved February 28, 2017, from https://tgateway.infoway-inforoute.ca/

Integrating the Healthcare Enterprise. (2017). *Profiles*. Retrieved February 28, 2017, from http://ihe.net/profiles/

Jha, A. K., Doolan, D., Grandt, D., Scott, T., & Bates, D. W. (2008, December). The Use of Health Information Technology in Seven Nations. *International Journal of Medical Informatics*, *77*(12), 848–854. doi:10.1016/j.ijmedinf.2008.06.007 PMID:18657471

Lawrence, G., Lawrence, C. (Producers), & Robinson, P. (Director). (1989). *Field of Dreams*. [Motion Picture]. Universal Pictures.

Pan-Canadian Clinical Interoperability Steering Committee. (2015). *Clinical Interoperability Action Plan & Notes May 2015*. Retrieved February 28, 2017, from https://ic.infoway-inforoute.ca/en/resources/docs/cistratdocs/254-clinical-interoperability-action-plan-notes-may-2015/file

Porter, C. E. (2004). A Typology of Virtual Communities: A Multi-Disciplinary Foundation for Future Research. *Journal of Computer-Mediated Communication*.

Ranmuthugala, Plumb, Cunningham, Georgiou, Westbrook, & Braithwaite. (2011). How and why are communities of practice established in the healthcare sector? A systematic review of the literature. *BMC Health Services Research, 11*(273).

Reed, M., Larwood, D., Lindop, C., Macerola, B., & Picton, P. (2016). *Cross Enterprise Remote Reading Clinical Requirements*. Retrieved February 28, 2017, from https://ic.infoway-inforoute.ca/en/resources/docs/imagingdocs/736-cross-enterprise-remote-reading-clinical-requirements-26aug15

SNOMED International. (2017). *What is SNOMED CT?*. Retrieved February 28, 2017, from http://www.snomed.org/snomed-ct/what-is-snomed-ct

KEY TERMS AND DEFINITIONS

Digital Health: The use of information technology and electronic processes to enhance the delivery of health care services or to facilitate better health. Digital health is often used interchangeably with the term eHealth.

Electronic Medical Record (EMR): The medical record accumulated for an individual within one health care provider's facility. The term is often used to refer to the system that stores and manages these records.

Electronic Health Record (EHR): An integrated collection of a person's encounters with the health care system that provides a health history often accumulated from multiple health information systems.

Infostructure: The organizational structures and technology that supports the collection and distribution of information.

Interoperability: The ability of electronic systems to exchange information and make use of this shared data. Clinical interoperability refers to this capability in the context of health information systems used by health care providers and patients.

Chapter 7
Exploring Healthy Connection:
Communication, Social Networks, and Wellbeing

Jessica L. Moore
Butler University, USA

ABSTRACT

Virtual social connection has become a way of life for many people. The continued implementation of new technologies in social interaction presents an ever-escalating need for researchers and practitioners to understand the implications of mediated interaction and virtual communities on human health and wellbeing. Accordingly, this chapter presents research on the salience of communication and social bonds in relation to human health and wellbeing, explores ways in which individual as well as relational health and wellbeing are affected by the use of social network sites, and argues a case for research on the health-related functions of expressive narratives in virtual settings such as online social networks. Considerations and future directions for research of these issues conclude this chapter.

INTRODUCTION

Establishing healthy social connections can buffer stress and help people cope with a variety of expected and unexpected events in life. And more than ever people are turning to virtual spaces in order to make social connections. This chapter explores the research related to establishing and maintaining social connections as well as the communicative processes that hinder and enhance health and wellbeing. Towards that end, this chapter establishes the salience of communication and social bonds in

DOI: 10.4018/978-1-5225-2958-3.ch007

relation to human health and wellbeing, explores ways in which individual as well as relational health and wellbeing are affected by the use of social network sites, and presents a case for theoretical and applied research on the health-related functions of expressive communication in virtual settings such as online social networks. Additionally, this chapter pays special attention to the function of social support. Issues, controversies, and problems that face researchers are offered for consideration, as are directions for future research. The ultimate goal of this chapter is to build upon the existing body of work in the field by considering how communication that unfolds in social networks impacts human health and wellbeing.

Background

The structure and content of our social worlds support our health, wellbeing, and general quality of life. Researchers have developed a significant body of scholarship that focuses on identifying and supporting the cognitive and communicative processes that enhance our individual, relational, and socio-cultural welfare. Critical, humanistic, and social scientific researchers alike have pursued an understanding of human symbolic exchange, and growing numbers of researchers are uniquely interested in making contributions to a body of scholarship central to healthy lives, relationships, and communities.

Underlying this chapter is an understanding that health and wellbeing are not simply characterized by the lack of mental or physical illness, but the *presence* of factors that sustain and enhance our psychological and physiological wellness. Affection, inclusion, and control, for example, are fundamental human needs that are often given and received through the social connections we make with others. What's more, the fulfillment of these needs via interaction with people with whom we have formed relationships is a necessity for humans to function normally (Baumeister & Leary, 1995). The quality of our social ties, it is argued, contributes directly to the quality of physical and mental wellbeing.

Research on the relationship between social connection and physiological health, for example, establishes a positive association between social support and cardiovascular, endocrine, neuroendocrine, and immune system functioning (Uchino, Cacioppo, & Kiercolt-Glaser, 1996). Stress exposure weakens immune system functioning and, thus, physical health; however, social support has been shown to buffer the damage inflicted by stress on biological functions (Uchino, 2004). Studies reveal that the break-up of a close relationship such as a marriage can elevate blood pressure and weaken the immune system, but these effects may be inhibited by the prevalence of other positive social connections (Russek & Schwartz, 1997; Albrecht & Goldsmith, 2003). It seems that direct positive social ties cushion people from the potentially negative impact of hardships on physical health (Ryff & Singer, 2008). In addition to the direct effects of social connections on physical health, research indicates that social ties may also have indirect effects on health and wellbeing by providing health protective social environments or pathways to health information and resources. For instance, social groups have the ability to provide people with attitudinal and behavioral support systems that inhibit members from engaging in harmful behaviors such as smoking or substance abuse while also encouraging members toward health protective behaviors such as physical activity, safe sex practices, and mammograms or cancer screenings (Albrecht & Goldsmith, 2003). Ultimately, the physiological impact of maintaining positive social ties is conclusive—people who establish and preserve close relationships have better physical health than those who do not maintain such quality ties.

Beyond physical health and wellbeing, research also indicates that social connection can provide important mental health benefits. For example, people who are habitually socially isolated are likely to experience psychosocial distress whereas people with quality strong-tie networks, such as friends, family, significant others, are likely to reap psychosocial benefits (Hefner & Eisenberg, 2009). Fletcher and Fitness (1990) note that the presence of positive feelings about close relationships has been linked to psychological wellbeing, which lends credence to the notion that is the *quality* of social ties that supports mental health and not merely the existence of social interactions. People who are in stable committed intimate relationships, for instance, are happier than people who are not in such relationships (Diner, Gohm, Suh, & Oishi, 2000). And on the flip side, research indicates that people with low quality social ties are more susceptible to alcoholism, eating disorders, schizophrenia, and depression, among other mental health disorders than people with strong social ties and support networks (Segrin, 1998). Notably, a lack of social support is found to have a stronger relationship with psychological distress than poverty (Caron, Latimer, & Tousignant, 2007). What's more, social connection is important across a lifespan. Levula, Wilson, and Harre (2015) report social connections to be important determinants of mental health outcomes across three life stages—adolescence, adulthood, and seniors.

It is important to recognize that physical health and mental health are not mutually exclusive. Physical health and illness can certainly have an impact on one's state of mind, and mental health and illness can influence physiological functioning. In fact, some researchers and integrated medicine experts might argue that both forms of wellness are part of a larger system that ought not be treated independently. Despite potential differences in approach, researchers agree that the quality of our social connections contributes significantly and profoundly to our overall physiological and psychological heath and wellbeing.

COMMUNICATION, SOCIAL NETWORKS, AND WELLBEING

The widespread use of online social networks is one of the fastest growing worldwide communication trends to emerge in the 21st century. Thus, virtual communities have a profound influence on the ways people seek, develop, maintain, and even dissolve relationships. Researchers and practitioners alike are interested in understanding the ways in physical and mental health and wellbeing are influenced by online social spaces. What is clear is that communication via computer-mediated channels (e.g., computers, tablets, smart phones) is a common and consistent practice in the lives of many Americans. Hence, this chapter explores several areas of contemporary scholarship on virtual communities, paying special attention to the role of communication in social networks and how it shapes human health and wellbeing.

Social Support

Social connection and communication are central to improving the wellbeing of people in need. Burleson and MacGeorge (2002) define *supportive communication* as "verbal and nonverbal behavior produced with the intention of providing assistance to others perceived as needing that aid" (p. 374). Research indicates that supportive communication promotes both physical and psychological health by providing health-relevant information, motivating healthy behavior, promoting self-esteem and self-care, and reducing emotional distress (MacGeorge, Feng, and Burleson, 2011), among other functions. Researchers most often conceptualize supportive communication as *social support*, which encompasses the general comfort, assistance, advice, or assurance that people experience (i.e., give and take) as a function of social relationships. Practically speaking, social support stands to provide protection for people who need to be encouraged, tangible assistance for people in times of need, and/or personal advice about life experiences when people need direction (Moore & Craig, 2009). Accordingly, social support enables people to cope with an amalgamation of individual, relational, or social stressors that ultimately have an impact on physical and mental wellbeing (Burleson & MacGeorge, 2002; High & Solomon, 2011).

Social support is needed throughout multiple stages of life (Pecchioni, Wright, & Nussbaum, 2005), provides buffers from stressful life events (Cohen & Wills, 1985), and importantly, is *enacted through communication with others* (Goldsmith, 2004). Social support has been categorized in a variety of ways, yet a communicative perspective on social support tends to focus on the centrality of symbolic exchange of messages or meaning made between people. Communication scholars commonly recognize several types of social support including *emotional support* (e.g., expressions of empathy, care, and acceptance), *informational support* (e.g., sharing information, offering advice), *instrumental support* (e.g., assisting with tasks), *esteem support* (e.g., affirming identities, expressing value, enhancing self-worth), *network support* (e.g., providing new support contacts, expanding support resources), *tangible support* (e.g., practical material aid), and *appraisal support* (e.g., offering new perspectives or ideas), among others (Burleson & MacGeorge, 2002; Goldsmith & Albrecht, 2011; Xu & Burleson, 2001). Additionally, social support may vary in the degree to which messages are *person-centered*, which is the extent to which message content reflects an awareness of and adaptation to the affective, subjective, and relational elements of communication contexts (Burleson, 1982). According to High and Solomon (2011), high person-centered messages are "sophisticated utterances because they acknowledge several different factors, including the distressed person, the social situation, the process of communication, and people's emotional and cognitive states" (p. 121). Whether providing people with emotional support in order to promote a positive affective experience or offering informational support to help people solve problems, scholars recognize that there are a variety of ways in which people communication social support and, to that end, that there are a variety of ways that social support benefits health and wellbeing.

Social Support and Social Networks

This chapter opened with an exploration of the physical and psychological benefits of social ties and turned to explain the various forms of communication that often underlie social support processes. In the section that follows, the discussion will extend to the role of virtual communities and, in particular, social network sites in providing avenues through which social support can be enacted and sustained.

Scholars agree that traditional conceptions of social support often consist of family members, friends, and significant others, also known at *strong tie* networks (Albrecht & Goldsmith, 2003). However, *weak tie* networks are also able to provide social support that can be equally useful (Wright, 2002); weak ties simply refers to "a wide range of potential supporters who lie beyond the primary network of family and friends" (Adelman, Parks, & Albrecht, 1987, p. 126). Though it is most common for people to depend upon people with whom they are close to support them through difficult times, weak tie networks play an important role in helping people manage uncertainty and find much-needed support. In fact, it has been argued that weak tie support is sometimes perceived as more useful than strong tie support because it offers multifaceted information and diverse points of view, involves less social risk when disclosing information, offers more objective feedback, and necessitates less role obligations than does interaction with strong tie networks (Wright & Miller, 2010). What's more, weak tie networks can be particularly beneficial for people who are coping with similar life stressors or health issues that carry a burden of social stigma. Wright and Bell (2003) argue that in certain situations weak ties may provide more effective social support than close family and friends due to the fact that weak tie support can often be shared without the risks of damaging close personal relationships.

One of the most prolific forms of weak tie support can be found in virtual communities. Researchers acknowledge that a variety of relationship types can and do form online (Bugeja, 2005; McKenna, 2008; Schneiderman, 2003). And researchers note that, "computer-mediated communication coexists with face-to-face interaction as the prominent modes of for giving and receiving social support" (High & Solomon, 2011, p. 132). Virtual communities increasingly act as developmental conduits through which individuals can seek, discover, and form social ties with others (Moore & Craig, 2009). Social network environments, in particular, provide communication contexts that influence the provision of weak tie social support. For example, virtual communities connect users with otherwise physically and socially "distant" other with whom they can openly engage in dialogue about similar topics of interest, provide and request information about risk-laden issues, and generally provide support in times of need.

As researchers note, *similarity*, *risk*, and *availability* are three significant reasons that people turn to social networks to seek and give social support (High & Solomon, 2011; Moore & Craig, 2009; Wright & Muhtaseb, 2011). Ridings and Gefen (2004) argue that virtual communities are ideal contexts to engage in mediated communication given the multifaceted and varied platforms that exists where people can socially connect with relative strangers. In fact, researchers posit that one major benefit of social networks is the ability to connect based on shared *similarity*. Similarity might be based on personal or identity characteristics such as single parenthood, sexual identity, or race, but similarity may also be found in the specific content or topic of the virtual community such as grief and loss, post-traumatic stress disorder, or breast cancer. It is also possible that support found in virtual communities such as social networks is intersectional in nature, thereby crossing issues of identity and purpose. Wright (2002) argues that similarity to others online or similar experiences are two of the major advantages of utilizing online support. The ability to establish social ties and hear from people going through similar challenges helps people normalize their own experiences and receive much needed validation for what they are feeling. Yamasaki (2016) notes that sharing social support based on similarities helps people gain a sense of belonging, realize that they are not alone, and feel better about themselves as a byproduct of reciprocating support for other members of the network community. In addition to shared similarities, social networks can be particularly beneficial for people who are managing *risk*, particularly risks associated with stigmatized physical or psychological health conditions. Wright and Bell (2003) state, "Stigma refers to the sense of shame, disgrace or taboo associated with a particular illness/condition, usually stemming from fears and prejudices surrounding cultural conceptions of a health issue" (p. 42). Research indicates that weak tie social networks are particularly popular for people contending with stigmatized conditions such as eating disorders, sexually transmitted diseases, substance abuse, or mental health issues. People often feel less inhibited when communicating about sensitive issues in virtual environments, particularly confidential or anonymous environments, thereby avoiding the guilt or shame that often accompanies a particular situation or condition (Wright & Muhtaseb, 2011). This research supports the aforementioned idea that virtual communities provide users with important social networks among whom they may openly seek and express views (e.g., appraisal support), request information (e.g., informational support), suggest solutions (e.g., instrumental support), and communicate about feelings (e.g., emotional support) with minimal risk (Herring, 1996). Beyond similarity and risk, simple *availability* is also a commonly cited benefit of online social networks that is linked to health and wellbeing. Simply stated, people like knowing that someone will "be there for them" in times of need. While family members, friends, and significant others may be physically proximate, they are not always physically or emotionally available for people *where* and *when* people are in need of support. While it is true that most people experience some degree of social support from these strong tie relationships, research is also clear that weak tie relationships play a valuable role in enacting social support (Goldsmith & Albrecht, 2011; MacGeorge et al., 2011). A study conducted by Dunham, Hurshman, Litwin, Gusella, Ellsworth, and Dodd (1998) offers a glimpse in to the importance of social availability in virtual communities. Researchers provided new single mothers unlimited access for six months to an online social support community. Many of these single mothers reported being isolated from their normal social network of friends due to the responsibilities of a new baby. Significantly, this study found that the lonelier the mother, the more likely she was to seek support from the online social network. And, over time, the more frequently mothers engaged with others in the social network the more likely their sense of belonging to the group increased and the less likely they were to experience parental stress. Social network communities not only provide people with the ability to establish simple connections with others, but afford access to others during times of loneliness, enhance feelings of connectedness, reduce stress, and potentially regain or enhance one's overall sense of wellbeing.

Researchers agree that there are a plethora of benefits associated with establishing social connections via online social networks (High & Solomon, 2011; Moore & Craig, 2009; Wright & Muhtaseb, 2011; Yamasaki, 2016). A few of those benefits have been articulated herein, but the benefits discussed are not exhaustive and are arguably not mutually exclusive in function. Also, as will be noted later in this chapter, the benefits of virtual connections are not without limitations. Nonetheless, there is ample evidence that online social networks can be significant in helping people manage uncertainty, establish and maintain social connections, and deal with difficult *emotions* during stressful times.

Expressive Communication, Social Networks, and Wellbeing

People who cope well with life's stressors tend to be people who enlist social support (Veroff, Kulka, & Douvan, 1981), and effectively coping with stressors is critical in maintaining health and wellbeing (Albada & Moore, 2012; Levula et al., 2016; Ryff & Singer, 2008). This chapter opened with an exploration of the physical and mental health benefits of social ties and turned to examine the various forms of social support as well as how that support is enacted in virtual communities such as online social networks. While the case has been established that receiving social support (e.g., emotional support, esteem support) is important to health and wellbeing, less has been stated about the function of affective expression in support processes. In the following section, research on expressive (i.e., emotional, affective) communication is presented. Specifically, this section of the chapter presents research on the efficacy of the expressive writing paradigm in managing physical and mental health and explore how expressive writing studies might inform novel research and practice on social support in social networks.

Expressive (i.e., emotional) writing is a useful tool for physical and psychological health recovery and management. Pennebaker (1999) argues that the act of constructing narratives via expressive writing is a natural human process that allows people to understand their experiences as well as themselves. Putting thoughts into story-like form, he argues, seems to assist people with maintaining a sense of predictability and control over their lives (Pennebaker, 1999; Pennebaker & Seagal, 1999). When people are able to put their emotional experiences into narrative form, particularly during times of uncertainty or affective tumult, physical and mental health typically improves (Albada & Moore, 2012). For example, expressive writing studies report positive health outcomes for several physiological functions including blood pressure, liver enzymes, lung function, and the immune system (Baikie & Wilhelm, 2005; Slatcher & Pennebaker, 2007). Expressive writing has also been tied to improvements in mental health, such as improvements in mood and overall psychological wellbeing (Park & Blumberg, 2002; Pennebaker, Kiecolt-Glaser, & Glaser, 1988). Research in the realm of expressive writing is robust and researchers suggest that is it an effective conduit for maintaining mental and physical health.

Researchers have also extended expressive writing studies to strong tie relationships such as romantic partners. Studies show that emotional communication supported by expressive writing helps partners develop empathic understanding and communicate difficult feelings (Snyder, Gordon, & Baucom, 2006). The act of writing about one's emotional experiences seems to help people identify, understand, organize, and effectively communicate emotions to others. Partners who experience stressful events such as infidelity, for example, report that expressive writing helps ameliorate anger, depression, and martial distress by providing a platform to process and document their cognitive, affective, and/or behavioral experiences and subsequently communicate those experiences more effectively to their significant other (Snyder et al., 2006). Thus, there is good evidence that expressive writing stands to contribute to positive relational effects in a manner that is not altogether different from the effects observed for physical or psychological health. Notably, researchers and practitioners alike have well-documented the interdependence of physical, mental, and relational health. For example, relational upheavals can lead to maladaptive health behaviors such as smoking, excessive drinking, poor eating habits, and disrupted sleep patterns. Such maladaptive behaviors then disrupt immune function, raise cortisol levels, and result in cardiovascular changes, among other biological markers of stress. In short, relational health stands to impact physical health. Likewise, mental health disorders such as depression, bi-polar disorder, and schizophrenia can lead to strain in close relationships as a result of dealing with the emotional and behavioral strains commonly associated with such conditions. And, the negative impact that breast cancer, prostate cancer, muscular dystrophy, HIV, and a host of other physical ailments can have on individuals, couples, and families is well-established. That is, both mental and physical health challenges commonly impact relationships. Accordingly, it is important for researchers to recognize the mutual and potentially synergistic effects that expressive writing and/or expressive communication might have on physiological, psychological, and relational health (Pennebaker & Chung, 2010).

Expressive writing shares some significant functions and characteristics with social support. Both have the potential to prompt situational appraisals, reduce stress, improve social relationships, and alter attitudes, beliefs, or behaviors that impact health outcomes. Also, *emotional support* has been characterized as communication of empathy, care, or affective support, whilst *expressive writing* has been associated with understanding and care for self and for others. Despite these commonalities, opportunities to examine symbolic exchange across contextual bounds remain. For instance, does *intra*personal emotional expression (e.g., expressive writing) and *inter*personal emotional expression (e.g., expressive written communication in a social network) differ in health outcomes? Does quality or quantity of expressive writing/communication impact the effects? Room remains to explore how expressive writing functions outside the methodological parameters often prescribed in lab studies. Traditional experimental expressive writing studies ask participants to write uninterrupted for 15 minutes with pencil and paper about their deepest emotions tied to a particular issue, experience, or trauma, and most often the writing is private or reviewed only by a researcher or clinician. This process is then often repeated at prescribed intervals-- usually three to four days over the course of a week or once a week for four to six weeks (Pennebaker, 1999; Pennebaker & Seagal, 1999). While results from expressive writing studies have been robust overall, there are a dearth of studies examining the impact of expressive writing in spaces where privacy is variable, such as virtual communities. While the expressive writing paradigm has proven successful in studies that maintain the confidentiality of participants' writing, a similar sort of confidentiality can be argued for certain virtual environments. In fact, selective exposure is one of the features that people generally find most attractive about mediated spaces—some social networks are open only to members and often times social networks allow users to make active choices about levels of privacy. Thus, it may be that expressive communication and exchange in online social networks serve a similar function as expressive writing completed in a lab. Given the temporal and economic limitations that may prevent many people from participating in clinician-supervised writing, understanding the potential similarities and differences between forms of affective expression should be of interest to researchers, clinicians, and lay persons alike.

CONSIDERATIONS AND FUTURE DIRECTIONS

As stated near the beginning of this chapter, virtual communities have a profound influence on the ways people seek, maintain, and dissolve relationships. Advances have been made toward understanding the communicative processes that unfold in these environments, but this progress has not been made without challenges. While a growing body of research exists analyzing the impact of social support, social networks, and human health and wellbeing, technical advances and user adoption rates have outpaced the work of scholars. Thus, this leaves much of the virtual world understudied with researchers responsible for generating theoretical explanations and practical solutions for constantly changing social practices. Researchers are truly only beginning to forward models that take into account the multifaceted and dynamic nature of human communication processes across developing social environments. This chapter now turns to offer considerations for the existing body of work as well as potential areas for future research.

This chapter began by communicating the importance of social bonds on human health and wellbeing. Information was presented on the importance of social connection in relation to both physical and mental health. Moreover, this chapter reemphasized that physical health and illness can have an impact on one's state of mind and mental health and illness can influence physiological functioning. Additionally, research on the importance of *social support* was presented that expressed the significance of communication in establishing and maintaining a sense of social wellbeing. Though research was offered that addressed some common ways that social support is enacted (e.g., informational support, emotional support, instrumental support), that body of research is sometimes lacking in explanatory power. This may be one area of research for scholars to pursue. Also, given the capacity for social support messages to be sent and received, it could be useful for scholars to understand the directional nuance of supportive messages. What one sends isn't always what one wants to receive, and yet people arguably show others how they want to be treated via their own behavior.

Additionally, one might question whether social support in traditional face-to-face environments operates similarly across mediated environments such as *social networks*. High and Solomon (2011) note McLuhan's (1964) claim that "the medium is the message" and argue that variations in features and functions of computer mediated environments influence the social support processes that unfold within them. The authors go on to provide some evidence that the characteristics of support messages themselves may determine the types of virtual spaces in which they are likely to occur, but more research is needed in this area to fully understand what High and Solomon (2011) characterized as the "interplay" between the medium and the message when it comes to social support in mediated environments. Given the ubiquity and growth of online social networks, this is one area of research that stands to inform both research and practice. Also, scholars must consider the implications of people utilizing virtual communities or social network sites as primary sources of social support. Social isolation and loneliness are increasing in their pervasiveness, and it behooves researchers to understand the social consequences that lay therein.

Lastly, this chapter explored research on *expressive writing* and documented its utility for physical and psychological health management. The interdependence of physical, mental, and relational health was noted, as were the potentially synergistic effects that expressive writing could have on physical, mental, and relational health and wellbeing. However, a gap was noted between expressive writing and social support paradigms. It is clear that virtual communities provide ripe environments for expressive writing (e.g., emotional communication) to naturally unfold, but more research is needed to understand the impact these practices might have on human health and wellbeing. Scholars are urged to purse these questions, among others, as they continue to explore research on human social ties and the impact they have on physical and mental health.

CONCLUSION

Virtual communities play an increasingly significant role in the processes through which people establish and maintain human connections. From impersonal relationships to close relationships and weak tie networks to strong tie networks, social networks are important to building social capital, exchanging social support, and maintaining health and wellbeing. Importantly, communication is central to this process and, as some have argued, social support may only be enacted through communication (Burleson & MacGeorge, 2002; MacGeorge et al., 2011). This chapter presents research on the salience of communication and social bonds on human health and wellbeing and explores the intersections of social support, expressive communication, and social networks. Additionally, consideration was offered to some of the challenges that face researchers interested in virtual communities, communication, and health, and some opportunities were provided for consideration for researchers and practitioners alike. It has been suggested that one of the more remarkable developments in modern society is the diffusion of new communication technologies from the organization into the sphere of social and personal relationships (O'Sullivan, 2000). This chapter reflects said development, and hopes to shed light on the communicative processes that enhance healthy connections in virtual communities and beyond.

REFERENCES

Adelman, M. B., Parks, M. R., & Albrecht, T. L. (1987). Beyond close relationships: Support in weak ties. In T. L. Albrecht & M. B. Adelman (Eds.), *Communicating social support* (pp. 105–125). Beverly Hills, CA: SAGE.

Albada, K., & Moore, J. L. (2013). Moving from positive thinking to positive talk: Implications for relational wellbeing. In M. J. Pitts & T. J. Socha (Eds.), *Positive communication in health and wellness* (pp. 117–132). New York: Peter Lang Publishers.

Albrecht, T. L., & Goldsmith, D. J. (2003). Social support, social networks, and health. In T. L. Thompson, A. M. Dorsey, K. I. Miller, & R. Parrott (Eds.), *Handbook of health communication* (pp. 263–284). Mahwah, NJ: Lawrence Erlbaum Associates.

Baikie, K., & Wilhelm, K. (2005). Emotional and physical health benefits of expressive writing. *Advances in Psychiatric Treatment*, *11*(5), 338–346. doi:10.1192/apt.11.5.338

Baumeister, R., & Leary, M. (1995). The need to belong: Desire for interpersonal attachments as a fundamental human motivation. *Psychological Bulletin*, *117*(3), 497–529. doi:10.1037/0033-2909.117.3.497 PMID:7777651

Bugeja, M. (2005). *Interpersonal divide: The search for community in a technological age*. New York: Oxford University Press.

Burleson, B. R., & MacGeorge, R. L. (2002). Supportive communication. In M. L. Knapp & J. A. Daly (Eds.), *Handbook of interpersonal communication* (pp. 374–424). Thousand Oaks, CA: SAGE.

Caron, J., Latimer, E., & Tousignant, M. (2007). Predictors of psychological distress in low-income populations of Montreal. *Canadian Journal of Public Health, 98*(Suppl. 1), S35–S44. PMID:18047159

Cohen, S., & Wills, T. A. (1985). Stress, social support, and the buffering hypothesis. *Psychological Bulletin, 98*(2), 310–357. doi:10.1037/0033-2909.98.2.310 PMID:3901065

Diener, E., Gohm, C. L., Suh, E., & Oishi, S. (2000). Similarities of the relations between marital status and subjective well-being across cultures. *Journal of Cross-Cultural Psychology, 31*(4), 419–436. doi:10.1177/0022022100031004001

Dunham, P. J., Hurshman, A., Litwin, E., Gusella, J., Ellsworth, C., & Dodd, P. W. D. (1998). Computer-mediated social support: Single young mothers as a model system. *American Journal of Community Psychology, 26*(2), 281–306. doi:10.1023/A:1022132720104 PMID:9693693

Fletcher, G. J. O., & Fitness, J. (1990). Occurrent social cognition in close relationship interaction: The role of proximal and distal variables. *Journal of Personality and Social Psychology, 59*(3), 464–474. doi:10.1037/0022-3514.59.3.464

Goldsmith, D. J. (2004). *Communicating social support*. New York, NY: Cambridge University Press. doi:10.1017/CBO9780511606984

Goldsmith, D. J., & Albrecht, T. L. (2003). Social support, social networks, and health: A guiding framework. In T. L. Thompson, R. Parrot, & J. F. Nusbaum (Eds.), *Handbook of health communication* (pp. 335–348). Mahwah, NJ: Routledge.

Hefner, J., & Eisenberg, D. (2009). Social support and mental health among college students. *The American Journal of Orthopsychiatry, 79*(4), 491–499. doi:10.1037/a0016918 PMID:20099940

Herring, S. C. (Ed.). (1996). *Computer-mediated communication: Linguistic, social and cross-cultural perspectives*. Philadelphia, PA: John Benjamins. doi:10.1075/pbns.39

High, A. C., & Solomon, D. H. (2011). Locating computer-mediated social support within online communication environments. In K. B. Wright & L. M. Webb (Eds.), *Computer-mediated communication in personal relationships*. New York: Peter Lang.

Levula, A., Wilson, A., & Harre, M. (2016). The association between social network factors and mental health at different life stages. *Quality of Life Research: An International Journal of Quality of Life Aspects of Treatment, Care and Rehabilitation*, *25*(7), 1725–1733. doi:10.1007/s11136-015-1200-7 PMID:26669317

MacGeorge, E. L., Feng, B., & Burleson, B. (2011). Supportive communication. In M. L. Knapp & J. A. Daly (Eds.), *Handbook of interpersonal communication* (4th ed.; pp. 317–354). Thousand Oaks, CA: Sage.

McKenna, K. Y. A. (2008). MySpace or your place: Relationship initiation and development in the wired and wireless world. In S. Sprechter, A. Wenzel, & J. Harvey (Eds.), *Handbook of Relationship Initiation* (pp. 235–248). New York: Psychology Press.

Meyerowitz, J. (1985). *No sense of place: The impact of electronic media on social behavior*. New York: Oxford University Press.

Moore, J. L., & Craig, E. A. (2009). Relationship development and maintenance in a wired world. In J. Park & E. Abels (Eds.), *Interpersonal relations and social patterns in communication technologies: Discourse norms, language structures and cultural variables*. Hershey, PA: IGI Global.

O'Sullivan, P. B. (2000). What you don't know won't hurt me: Impression management functions of communication channels in relationships. *Human Communication Research*, *26*, 403–431.

Pecchioni, L. L., Wright, K. B., & Nussbaum, J. F. (2005). *Life-span communication*. Mahwah, NJ: Lawrence Erlbaum Associates.

Pennebaker, J. W. (1999). Psychological factors influencing the reporting of physical symptoms. In A. Stone, J. Turkkan, C. Bachrach, J. Jobe, H. Kurtzman, & V. Cain (Eds.), *The science of self-report: Implications for research and practice* (pp. 299–316). Mahwah, NJ: Erlbaum.

Pennebaker, J. W., & Chung, C. K. (2010). Expressive writing, emotional upheavals, and health. In J. F. Evans (Ed.), *Wellness and writing connections: Writing for better physical, mental, and spiritual health*. Enumclaw, WA: Idyll Arbor, Inc.

Pennebaker, J. W., Kiecolt-Glaser, J. K., & Glaser, R. (1988). Disclosure of traumas and Narrative & Satisfaction, 16 immune function: Health implications for psychotherapy. *Journal of Consulting and Clinical Psychology*, *56*, 239–245. doi:10.1037/0022-006X.56.2.239 PMID:3372832

Pennebaker, J. W., & Seagal, J. D. (1999). Forming a story: The health benefits of narrative. *Journal of Clinical Psychology*, *55*(10), 1243–1254. doi:10.1002/(SICI)1097-4679(199910)55:10<1243::AID-JCLP6>3.0.CO;2-N PMID:11045774

Ridings, C. M., & Gefen, D. (2004). Virtual community attraction: Why people hang out online. *Journal of Computer-Mediated Communication*, *10*(1). Retrieved from http://jcmc.indiana.edu/vol10/issue1/ridings_gefen.html

Russek, L. G., & Schwartz, G. E. (1997). Feelings of parental caring predict health status in midlife: A 35-year follow-up of the Harvard Mastery Study of Stress. *Journal of Behavioral Medicine*, *30*(1), 1–13. doi:10.1023/A:1025525428213 PMID:9058175

Ryff, C. D., & Singer, B. H. (2008). Know thyself and become what you are: An eudemonic approach to psychological wellbieng. *Journal of Happiness Studies*, *9*(1), 13–39. doi:10.1007/s10902-006-9019-0

Schneiderman, B. (2003). *Leonardo's laptop: Human needs and the new computing technologies*. Cambridge, MA: The MIT Press.

Segrin, C. (1998). Disrupted interpersonal relationships and mental health problems. In B. H. Spitzberg & W. R. Cupach (Eds.), *The dark side of close relationships* (pp. 327–365). Mahwah, NJ: Erlbaum.

Slatcher, R. B., & Pennebaker, J. W. (2007). Emotional expression and health. In S. Ayers, A. Baum, C. McManus, S. Newman, K. Wallston, J. Weinman, & R. West (Eds.), *Cambridge Handbook of Psychology, Health & Medicine* (2nd ed.; pp. 84–86). Cambridge, UK: Cambridge University Press. doi:10.1017/CBO9780511543579.019

Snyder, D. K., Gordon, K., & Baucom, D. H. (2004). Treating affair couples. Extending the written disclosure paradigm to relationship trauma. *Clinical Psychology: Science and Practice*, *11*(2), 155–159. doi:10.1093/clipsy.bph066

Uchino, B. N. (2004). *Social support and physical health: Understanding the health consequences of relationships*. New Haven, CT: Yale University Press. doi:10.12987/yale/9780300102185.001.0001

Uchino, B. N., Cacioppo, J. T., & Kiercolt-Glaser, J. K. (1996). The relationship between social support and physiological processes: A review with emphasis on underlying mechanisms and implications for health. *Psychological Bulletin*, *119*(3), 488–531. doi:10.1037/0033-2909.119.3.488 PMID:8668748

Veroff, J., Kulka, R. A., & Douvan, E. (1981). *Mental health in America: Patterns of help-seeking from 1957-1976*. New York: Basic Books.

Wood, J. T. (2000). *Relational communication: Continuity and change in personal relationships*. Belmont, CA: Wadsworth.

Wright, K. B. (2002). Social support within an on-line cancer community: An assessment of emotional support, perceptions of advantages and disadvantages, and motives for using the community from a communication perspective. *Journal of Applied Communication Research*, *30*(3), 195–209. doi:10.1080/00909880216586

Wright, K. B. (2004). On-line relational maintenance strategies and perceptions of partners within exclusively internet-based and primarily internet-based relationships. *Communication Studies*, *55*(2), 239–253. doi:10.1080/10510970409388617

Wright, K. B., Bell, S. B., Wright, K. B., & Bell, S. B. (2003). Health-related support groups on the Internet: Linking empirical findings to social support and computer-mediated communication theory. *Journal of Health Psychology*, *8*(1), 39–54. doi:10.1177/1359105303008001429 PMID:22113899

Wright, K. B., & Miller, C. H. (2010). A measure of weak-tie / strong-tie support network preference. *Communication Monographs*, *77*(4), 502–520. doi:10.1080/03637751.2010.502538

Wright, K. B., & Muhtaseb, A. (2011). Personal relationships and computer mediated support groups. In K. B. Wright & L. M. Webb (Eds.), *Computer-mediated communication in personal relationships*. New York: Peter Lang.

Xu, Y., & Burleson, B. R. (2001). Effects of sex, culture, and support type on perceptions of spousal social support: An assessment of the support gap hypothesis in early marriage. *Human Communication Research*, *24*(4), 535–566. doi:10.1111/j.1468-2958.2001.tb00792.x

Yamasaki, J. (2016). Communicating health and connection in supportive communities. In J. Yamasaki, P. Geist-Martin, & B. F. Sharf (Eds.), *Storied health and illness: Communicating personal, cultural, and political complexities*. Long Grove, IL: Waveland Press.

KEY TERMS AND DEFINITIONS

Community Connectedness: A strong sense of identification with or feeling of belonging to a community.

Interpersonal Communication: Communication that occurs between two people within the context of their relationship and that, as it evolves, helps them to negotiate and define their relationship.

Message: Verbal and nonverbal elements of communication to which people give meaning.

Social Capital: Features of social life such as networks, norms, and trust, that facilitate cooperation and coordination for mutual benefit.

Social Network: A belief that one's own culture is superior to other cultures.

Social Support: Verbal or nonverbal assistance, comfort, or advise we seek or give to others.

Strong Tie Networks: Social networks made up of people with whom we have close relationships such as friends, family members, and significant others.

Weak Tie Networks: Social networks made up of people other than those with whom we have close relationships.

Chapter 8
Enablers and Facilitators for Sustainable Implementation of E-Services in Two-Sided Markets and Ecosystems

Vivian Vimarlund
Linköping University, Sweden

ABSTRACT

E-health innovations are globally described as one of the major driving forces to innovate health and social care because its potential contribution to improve quality, access to care, and to engage patients in decisions related to their own health and wellbeing .However, despite the increasing number of reports that indicate the potential savings and benefits that e-health services can bring to the sector, generic implementation of e-health services that contribute to develop and sustain new ways to deliver health and social care are not yet reported. In this chapter, we suggest enablers and facilitators for generic implementation of e-health services in two-sided markets as e-health.

INTRODUCTION

The impact of e-health innovations has been the object of academic study since the beginning of 2000 (Eysenbach, 2001; Pagliari et al, 2005). The first wave of innovations were focused on the micro level, and were introduced so as to reduce costly time-consuming errors associated with manual data entry, to increase system usability, to facilitate internal communication, and to stimulate good information

DOI: 10.4018/978-1-5225-2958-3.ch008

management practices for local work teams. These e-health innovations were also used to improve administrative issues: i.e., to keep records, order supplies, support the provision of basic services (for example, prescription renewal and the cancellation of appointments), and to facilitate one-way communication between stakeholders (namely, patients and practitioners) via the use of simple interfaces. E-health innovations, at this level, normally, did not allow for interaction with patients or an exchange of information with patients in real-time. Neither were there any automatic verification mechanisms available to confirm the receipt of a request. In some cases, an e-mail is sent to confirm a request, but such e-mails are not usually sent in real-time or automatically (Vimarlund & Koch; 2012; Vimarlund, Davoody & Koch 2013).

The increased use of the Internet has enabled the existence of a virtual global space which is characterized by 24/7 accessibility to information and services. Associated with this level of accessibility, we find an increased interest in the implementation of applications and innovations that change the way care professionals and patients interact with each other and within healthcare organizations. Consequently, the second wave of e-health innovation was expected to create a modern and flexible 'information exchange' along the entire chain of care delivery, thereby empowering end-users to actively use e-health innovations for communication and interaction purposes (Vimarlund et al, 2005).

This new organizational structure that emerged in association with e-health innovations (i) improves the internal- and external integration of actors, (ii) supports and enables the creation of integrated services (for example, allows for collaboration with pharmacies and social care actors), and (iii) develops virtual communities and intermediary platforms that further facilitates interaction between practitioners and patients (European Commission, 2012; Chiu, Hsu & Wang, 2006); for instance, in the establishment of 'net-doctors' or virtual doctor services, virtual care centres, children's virtual hospitals, and online tests. This second wave of e-health innovations placed a great deal of focus on how virtual communities could be used so as to bring healthcare providers, educators, patients, health professionals, and stakeholders together, so that they could exchange knowledge and information, and expand their knowledge capital (Vimarlund, Timpka & Patel, 1999) within and between organizations. Another result of this focus described above was that it facilitated the establishment of patient-centred approaches (McKinsey, 2015).

Today, E-health innovations, in a manner similar to market-oriented innovations, are globally described as one of the major driving forces behind the ongoing innovation of healthcare and social care organizations because of its potential to improve quality, to facilitate access to 24/7care, to engage patients in decisions related to their own health and wellbeing, and to develop new market structures where producers and consumers can interact with each other through intermediary platforms. For these reasons, countries across Europe have adopted strategies to create technical intermediary infrastructures, for example, portals that facilitate the transition to a patient-centred health system (WHO European Region, 2016; Vimarlund 2016). Furthermore, these infrastructures simultaneously contribute to (i) improved productivity, (ii) an increased digital presence which can support the new consumer, (iii) the provision of personalized care, and (iv)stimulation of the e-health market.

However, as e-health undergoes the digital transformation that has occurred in many other sectors of modern society (and the global economy), (Barrett, Davidson, Prahbu & Vargo, 2015) an important discussion must be held. The discussion centres around the implementation of intermediary infrastructures that will facilitate the meeting between suppliers and developers, on the one hand, and consumers on the other the issues or pre-requisites that they need to fulfil, and the impact these infrastructures will have on the market.

Previous research in the area of health informatics has shown that the introduction of IT-based innovations in e-health contexts has profound consequences for complex organizations, such as healthcare and social care organisations are. These include changes in the organizations' structure, changes in work processes, as well as changes in the nature of the interaction between practitioners, and between practitioners and patients (Eysenbach, 2001; Vimarlund, Davoody & Koch 2013). The outputs that are identified in this chapter should be of interest to leaders and stakeholders, at the moment when they are to make strategic decisions about the implementation of intermediary infrastructures that are aimed at attracting both sides of the market (Vimarlund, 2016).

DEFINITIONS

Implementation

The concept of 'implementation' is defined as "a specified set of activities designed to put into practice an activity or program of known dimensions" (Fixsen, Naoom, Blase, Friedman, & Wallace, 2005). According to this definition, implementation processes are purposeful and are described in sufficient detail so that independent observers can detect the presence and strength of the "specific set of activities" related to implementation. It is common to read about the 'implementation' of a program or practice as if it were an accomplished fact when the context of the statement makes it clear that some process (more or less clearly described) had been put in place to *attempt* the implementation of that program or practice. The concept of 'implementation', as defined above, seems to inevitably take different shapes and forms in different cultures and institutional settings. Most researchers agree that an implementation process means to 'carry out', 'accomplish', 'fulfil', 'produce', or 'complete' a given task (Durlak & DuPre, 2008; O'Toole, 2000; O'Toole, 2004), and that a specified set of activities designed to put into practice an activity or program of known dimensions has to be developed.

Furthermore, a difference between 'implementation research' and 'policy implementation' or 'implementation of IT-based innovations' is also usually made. This difference is based on the claim that they constitute different fields of research. While 'implementation research' has been defined as "the scientific study of methods to promote the uptake of research findings, and hence to reduce inappropriate effects of policies, programs or innovations, where the context, i.e. the social, cultural, economic, political, legal, and physical environment, as well as the institutional setting, comprising various stakeholders and their interactions, plays a central role", 'policy implementation' is defined as "what develops between an intention of the government to do something and its ultimate impact following action" (O'Toole, 2004). In this chapter, we define 'implementation' as "a specified set of activities designed to put into practice an innovation (program, system, technical application, or policy) of known dimensions in complex organizations, such as healthcare and social care, so as to achieve a specific end."

Two-Sided E-Health Markets

'Two-sided e-health markets' are defined in this study as "markets in which one or several virtual platforms take on the role of an 'intermediary' so as to enable interactions between stakeholders, producers, suppliers, and end-users (Vimarlund, 2016). In addition to this, such an intermediary serves to get the multiple sides that participate in the delivery of healthcare and social care services (i.e., pharmaceutical companies, healthcare and social care providers, professional groups, customers, patients, and citizens) "on board". Consequently, intermediaries develop virtual arenas for interaction and facilitate 'inter-operability' between the many sides of the e-health market. Further, these interactions are expected to allow users 24/7 access to resources while they are on the move. The more consumers join the market, the more suppliers are interested in offering products, and *vice versa*.

Virtual Communities

'Virtual communities' are defined as "social networks formed or facilitated through digital innovations where people with common interests and needs interact repeatedly within certain boundaries" (Demiris, 2006; Lee, Vogel & Limayem, 2003, Porter, 2004). Virtual communities are assumed to facilitate personal learning, enhance storytelling and the exchange of ideas, foster social relationships, enable an ongoing dialogue with customers, and provide a context for the development of products and services through collaboration with innovative users (20- Preece, 2000; Slevin, 2000; Wagner & Bolloju, 2005; Röll, 2004; Blanchard & Markus, 2004; Füller, Bartl, Ernst & Mühlbacher, 2006; Nambisan, 2002).

Research on virtual communities has been mainly focused on (i) knowledge exchange and individual learning, (ii) self-support groups and the exchange of ideas, and (iii) the provision of contexts for the development of products and services through collaboration with innovative users. In this chapter, we add a new dimension to the discussion of virtual communities as we explore the challenges that confront the development of sustainable two-sided markets in which technical platforms are used as "intermediaries" for the producers, consumers and suppliers of services in e-health contexts. This is done with the aim to (i) aggregate information on buyers, suppliers and products; (ii) facilitate the search for appropriate products; (iii) reduce information asymmetries; and (iv) match buyers and sellers for transactions.

Increased Interest in Implementation Studies in one Sided Markets

Research publications that focus on 'implementation' can be found since the 1970s. Such publications were found mainly in the USA during a period of growing concern about the effectiveness of public policy, especially its economic effectiveness. These studies often discussed policy formulation or how one might improve the analysis of the variables that could explain the impact of implementation processes, rather than the effectiveness of the implementation process or the relationship between implementation and outcomes (Durlak, A. & DuPre, 2008; Vimarlund, 2016). These studies were characterized as 'explorative', and were conducted intention of explaining the implementation gap, from the perspective of central government policy makers, using a top-down perspective.

In contrast to the top-down studies performed during the 1970s, studies performed during the 1980s were focused on the role of staff members as they put the policies into action, and the importance of the decisions that staff members made when delivering policies to individuals and organizations. Furthermore, the importance of implementing structures or networks was emphasised, as well as the interactions that occur between different actors with a bottom-up perspective (Vimarlund, 2016). Publications on implementation research emerged in the latter half of the 1980s focused on the significance of research methodology and on the importance of the sustainability of the results associated with the implementation process. Many of these studies, however, can be characterized as comparative case studies which were aimed at improving our understanding of implementation.

With respect to implementation studies, a large number of various topics have been the subject of debate. These have included, for example, top down *versus* bottom up approaches, an emphasis on policy content *versus* implementation of policy, and role of qualitative methods *versus* quantitative research methods. Numerous researchers, in their reviews of the literature on this field have stated, however, that interest in implementation studies decreased at the end of the 1900s, and the beginning of the 2000s (O'Toole, 2000). Notwithstanding this previous decrease, implementation research literature has grown significantly over the last few years. The number of relevant publications has increased in academic journals in education, health, social sciences, economic and/or environmental areas. This demonstrates that, today, implementation research has developed into a truly multidisciplinary research field.

The massive implementation of IT-based innovation and e-services in many sectors and the concomitant studies that have addressed the effects of institutional and inter-organizational relationships as a consequence of these IT-based innovations have emphasised the importance of issues of governance. In the discussion of the *values* of the implementation of IT-based innovations and e-services, issues concerning 'process reengineering', 'resource allocation', 'organizational issues', and 'individual behaviour and its consequences' are commonly mentioned; often as exogenous factors related to the use of a new IT system. Evaluation reports have, however, usually shown that the introduction of IT in complex organizations leads to failures, resistance against the use of the IT system, or to a non-optimal use of scarce resources (Leviss, Gugerty & Kaplan, 2010).). These reports are further focused on sustaining a one-sided market that derives most of its value from a single class of users. They are also mainly concerned with how the implementation of innovations should be performed and how these implementations are being received by organizations, users, consumers, and stakeholders, in real-life (Vimarlund & Keller, 2014).

Implementation research reports have not yet provided the knowledge that is needed for the successful implementation of e-health innovation as, for example, intermediary platforms, in *two-sided* e-health markets, where an increase in the number of users on one side of the market creates a rise on the other side, thereby giving rise to a cross-sided exchange benefit. Consequently, it has been difficult to generate general assumptions about key issues with respect to implementation (for example, rules and laws, norms and values that have to be taken into consideration in an implementation process); neither is it an easy task to develop a sustainable theoretical framework of the generic characteristics of implementation processes in cases where platforms are used as intermediaries between the two sides of the market.

INTERMEDIARY PLATFORMS IN TWO-SIDED E-HEALTH MARKETS

One of the most important issues related to the private sector becoming a part of the e-health market is the introduction of intermediary platforms for accelerating diffusion of innovation, for shortening cycle times, and for actively promoting alternative ideas and thinking. A major obstacle that is faced by the e-health market today is that many innovations have no defined end-point. Innovations in e-health are often incremental and form part of a continuous process that consists of numerous small-scale advances.

In addition to the obstacle mentioned above, the success of the implementation of intermediary platforms will depend on the manner in which they are incorporated and used by the two sides of the market, as well as on the mechanisms that are adopted so as to keep the actors connected to the platform. Nevertheless, the implementation of intermediary platforms that sustain the further development of the two-sided e-health market (in terms of the implementation of IT-based applications) remains complex, in many aspects. They are also aimed at facilitating the exchange of e-health services that have different goals, such as improving the exchange of information, providing services that transcend geographical barriers, or empowering and engaging patients. Note that they need to be developed in such a way so that they can serve two groups of users that, in most cases, share a common supplier; for example, specialists with a license to deliver health and social care. Further, they are expected to connect the different actors, either directly, through feedback from the healthcare community, or indirectly, by integrating them with regulatory or reimbursement mechanisms that stimulate actors to remain a part of the platform and/or to continuously use the offered e-health services over time (Vimarlund,2016).

The literature on the two-sided market has been, in general, industry specific and has focused on how to get the two sides of the market 'on board' with the implementation of innovations (Rysman, 2009; Schmalensee & Evans, 2007). Since e-health is dynamic in nature, it is constantly evolving, as alternatives and innovations emerge. In addition to taking into consideration traditional issues related to the implementation of IT-based innovations the implementation of intermediary platforms will need to persuade the two sides of the market to join this new paradigm, whilst avoiding market inefficiencies such as monopolies, cartels, or negative external effects. This must be done while following the rules, regulations, policies, of the healthcare system. Some examples of the most critical issues that need to be addressed (because they impact on the sustainability of the market) are: (a) ownership, (b) types of networks, (c) business models. These issues are described below:

Ownership of the Technical Infrastructure

The question of who will own the e-health platform is of importance in the context of attracting firms and organizations that are willing to produce and offer e-health innovations through an intermediary platform. Thus, it must be clearly indicated whether the platform will be owned by a public or by a private organization (for example, a county council, a healthcare unit, an insurance company, or a pharmaceutical company), or by private agents (for example, a patient organization, or by the company that produced the e-health service), or whether by a different ownership model that is based on a series of contractual arrangements and property rights for the e-health innovations that will be offered. In such cases, it will be necessary to identify who the owner is and the circumstances under which of the intermediary platform has the right to restrict access and use of the intermediary infrastructure, and whether it is necessary to restrict access to the virtual community that they support for safety or privacy reasons (for example, as in the case of the 'virtual doctors').

Single Home and Multi-Home Alternatives

In a market where consumer preferences are sufficiently homogenous (due the nature of the services offered) and given that providers are committed to guaranteeing quality, safely, and privacy, the possibility for the individuals to access several providers through the same platform can contribute to an increase in social welfare. If it is possible to access simultaneous platforms owned by different providers (so-called *multi-homing*), any intermediary platform that aims to support the further development of a two-sided e-health market needs to attract a higher number of stakeholders and consumers, to offer either redundancy or establish gateway services for an increased diversity of producers, consumers, and suppliers.

Different Kinds of Network Externalities

Network externalities are said to exist when consumer utility depends on the consumption of the same good or service by other agents and is affected by the specific price applied to that side. Network externalities exist in a two-sided market in which e-health innovations are offered. For example, in telemedicine services, a buyer will take into account the number of potential sellers using the same service as well as the kind of guarantees that the intermediary has applied in an effort to achieve balance and sustainability. Because intermediary infrastructures are expected to support both sides of the market, and, simultaneously create virtual communities for interaction, the development of networks that guarantee that the community created will fulfil the expectations of e-health markets, they will need to diminish risks and develop communities were all information can be transferred from all producers to all consumers in a structured, well defined, complete, and undistorted manner. To mitigate against adverse actors, the intermediary platform should guarantee the existence of the following networks:

- Knowledge networks to develop new ways of thinking, where security and safety issues that can be helpful in solving transnational problems can be discussed. Knowledge networks should further support knowledge creation around products, services, and goods, and disseminate ideas for further innovation in order to align developers and customers' needs in a realistic manner.
- Policy networks to create policies, even though they are not necessarily networks for government policy makers. Policy network activities should cover all the steps in the process (i.e., going beyond mere policy proposals). This would include agenda setting, policy formulation, rulemaking, coordination, implementation, and the development and evaluation of security policies and principles.
- Advocacy networks to change the agenda or policies of governments, corporations, or other institutions. An advocacy network challenges business leaders to rethink not only their business strategy, but also their larger purpose and role in the global marketplace. Such networks should contribute to the visualization of important issues in the e-health area.
- Watchdog networks to ensure business transparency; where intermediary platforms are scrutinized to ensure that they behave appropriately. Issues that are dealt with by these networks range from corruption and the environment, to financial services. The area for interaction that the intermediary offers should be characterized as transparent, prepared for developing a brand name or reputation that is sustainable over time, facilitates management systems, early warning systems, and the visualization of open source support systems, if any.

Payment and Reimbursement Models Used in The Two-Sided Market

Of special importance for the sustainability of a two-sided e-health market is the establishment of innovative payment and reimbursement models that encourage market actors, suppliers, and consumers to join the intermediary platform. In two-sided e-health markets, the challenge is to develop payment and reimbursement models that can be applied in communities in which a series of regulations and policies which are intended to stimulate the market co-exists. The price structure that is used, however, will depend greatly on cross-price elasticity mechanisms that can be used to subsidize groups of users, or on the use of price instruments. Such price instruments would be chosen depending on the range of options that is provided by the suppliers of services and on the differences and dependencies that exists between payment and reimbursements models, with respect to both the production and use of services. It is possible that the typical approach, of paying for the outcome, not for the actions *per se*, needs to be reviewed and/or changed because of the decrease in transaction costs (such as the cost of searching for buyers or sellers), and because the increase in competition between the different suppliers that the intermediary platform supports.

CONCLUSION

A market is two-sided if, at any point in time, there are: (i) two distinct groups of users; (ii) the value obtained by one type of user increases in correlation with an increase in the number of, or the quality of, the other type of user; and (iii) an intermediary platform is necessary to internalize the externalities that are created by one group for the other group. The implementation of intermediary platforms that sustain the further development of a two-sided e-health market is, nevertheless, similar to the implementation of IT-based applications. It is also complex, due to necessity of serving different groups of users with different aims and expectations (Durlak & DuPre, 2008; O'Toole, 2004; Vimarlund &Keller, 2014).

Previous studies on the implementation of IT-based innovations indicate that neither policies nor e-health innovations or services can be implemented on any useful scale without the support of political, financial, and human service systems, and that this support is important throughout every stage of the implementation process (Vimarlund &Keller, 2014). Previous research has also shown that the implementation of e-health innovations demands system re-engineering, organizational change, reallocation of resources, innovation of management and the existence of infrastructure that support the interaction between the different actors (Vimarlund &Keller, 2014).

The implementation of intermediaries that support two-sided e-health markets, specifically virtual communities' markets, implies the commitment of institutions and management engagement programs, as well as the existence of clear guidelines, at the administrative, managerial, and financial level, for both sides of the market and for the virtual community they interact with. Since the services and products that are exchanged via the intermediary platform are normally produced by industrial actors, it is rational to argue that all the groups should be engaged in the co-production of services and products, and be interested in sharing knowledge to build a body of evidence that can used attract additional healthcare users in joining the intermediary platform.

At present, no explicit models or methodological frameworks exist for the implementation of intermediary platforms that sustain the development of two-sided e-health markets. The development of implementation strategies that can be used in this new paradigm, and remain attractive to all the parties, demands that we consider past experiences of implementing IT-based innovations in single markets, and add to these experiences the issues that are presented in this chapter. Of special importance is to guarantee the existence of networks that control quality, privacy, safety, and security for both consumers and producers, whilst simultaneously establishing policies and guidelines that promote continuous innovation within the intermediary. It is also necessary to diminish the current degree of information asymmetry that exists between providers, developers, and consumers, and to facilitate trade by allowing the expansion, aggregation, and globalization of the market, as well as the customization of goods and services.

REFERENCES

Barrett, M., Davidson, E., Prahbu, J., & Vargo, S. L. (2015). Service innovation in the digital age: Key contributions and future directions. *Management Information Systems Quarterly*, *39*, 135–154.

Blanchard, A., & Markus, M. (2004). The experienced sense of a virtual community: Characteristics and processes. *The Data Base for Advances in Information Systems*, *35*(1), 65–79. doi:10.1145/968464.968470

Chiu, C.-M., Hsu, M.-H., & Wang, E. (2006). Understanding knowledge sharing in virtual communities: An integration of social capital and social cognitive theories. *Decision Support Systems*, *42*(3), 1872–1888. doi:10.1016/j.dss.2006.04.001

Demiris, G, (2006). The diffusion of virtual communities in health care: concepts and challenges. *Patient Educ Couns.*, *62*(2), 178-88.

Durlak, J. A., & DuPre, E. P. (2008). Implementation matters: A review of research on the influence of implementation on program outcomes and the factors affecting implementation. *American Journal of Community Psychology*, *41*(3-4), 327–350. doi:10.1007/s10464-008-9165-0 PMID:18322790

Durlak, J. A., & DuPre, E. P. (2008). Implementation matters: A review of research on the influence of implementation on program outcomes and the factors affecting implementation. *American Journal of Community Psychology*, *41*(3-4), 327–350. doi:10.1007/s10464-008-9165-0 PMID:18322790

European Commission. (2012). eHealth Action Plan 2012-2020 - Innovative healthcare for the 21st century. Report. Brussels: Author.

WHO European Region. (2016). *From innovation to implementation – eHealth in the WHO European Region.* Author.

Eysenbach, G. (2001). What is e-health? *Journal of Medical Internet Research*, *3*(2), e20. doi:10.2196/jmir.3.2.e20 PMID:11720962

Fixsen, D. L., Naoom, S. F., Blase, K. A., Friedman, R. M., & Wallace, F. (2005). Implementation Research: A Synthesis of the Literature. Tampa, FL: University of South Florida, Louis de la Parte Florida Mental Health Institute, The National Implementation Research Network (FMHI Publication #231).

Füller, J., Bartl, M., Ernst, H., & Mühlbacher, H. (2006). Community based innovation: How to integrate members of virtual communities into new product development. *Electronic Commerce Research*, *6*(1), 57–73. doi:10.1007/s10660-006-5988-7

Lee, F. S., Vogel, D., & Limayem, M. (2003). Virtual community informatics: A review and research agenda. *Journal of Information Technology Theory and Application*, *5*(1), 47–61.

Leviss, J., Gugerty, B., & Kaplan, B. (2010). *HIT or Miss: Lessons Learned from Health Information Technology Implementations* (2nd ed.). Chicago: AHIMA Press.

McKinsey. (2015) *The Internet ofThings: Mapping the value beyond the hype*. Author.

Nambisan, S. (2002). Designing virtual customer environments for new product development: Toward a theory. *Academy of Management Review*, *27*(3), 392–413.

OToole, L. J. (2000). Research on policy implementation: Assessment and prospects. *Journal of Public Administration: Research and Theory*, *10*(2), 263–288. doi:10.1093/oxfordjournals.jpart.a024270

OToole, L. J. (2004). The Theory-Practice Issue in Policy Implementation Research. *Public Administration*, *82*(2), 309–329. doi:10.1111/j.0033-3298.2004.00396.x

Pagliari, C., Sloan, D., Gregor, P., Sullivan, F., Detmer, D., Kahan, J. P., & MacGillivray, S. et al. (2005). What is e-Health. A Scoping Exercise to Map the Field. *Journal of Medical Internet Research*, *7*(1), e9. doi:10.2196/jmir.7.1.e9 PMID:15829481

Porter, C. (2004). A typology of virtual communities: A multi-disciplinary foundation for future research. *Journal of Computer-Mediated Communication*, *10*(1).

Preece, J. (2000). *Online Communities. Designing Usability, Supporting Sociability*. Chichester, UK: Wiley.

Röll, M. (2004). Distributed KM – improving knowledge worker's productivity and organizational knowledge sharing with weblog-based personal publishing. *BlogTalk 2.0 – The European Conference on Weblogs*. Retrieved from http://www.roell.net/publikationen/distributedkm.pdf

Rysman, M. (2009). The economics of two-sided markets. *The Journal of Economic Perspectives*, *23*(3), 125–144. doi:10.1257/jep.23.3.125

Schmalensee, R., & Evans, D. S. (2007). The industrial organization of two-sided platforms. *Competition Policy Int.*, *3*(1), 151–179.

Slevin, J. (2000). The Internet and Society. Cornwall, UK: Polity Press.

Vimarlund. (2011). *Att fånga nyttan av IT-investeringar inom vård och omsorg.En analysmodell för planering och uppföljning av IT-investeringar- ehälsonätverk.* Forskningsrapport. (in Swedish)

Vimarlund, V. (Ed.). (2016). E-Health Two-sided markets. Academic Press.

Vimarlund, V., Davoody, N., & Koch, S. (2013). Steps to consider for effective decision making when selecting and prioritizing eHealth services. *Studies in Health Technology and Informatics*, *192*, 239–243. PMID:23920552

Vimarlund, V., & Keller, C. (2014). The many faces of implementation. Vinnova Report 2014:06.

Vimarlund, V., & Koch, S. (2012). *Identifying where the values come from IT-innovations in health and social care.* Intelligent Information Management.

Vimarlund, V., Timpka, T., & Patel, V. (1999). Information Technology and Knowledge Exchange in Health-Care Organizations. *Proceedings of AMIA,* 632-636.

Wagner, C., & Bolloju, N. (2005). Supporting knowledge management in organizations with conversational technologies: Discussion forums, weblogs, and wikis. *Journal of Database Management*, *16*(2), 1–8.

KEY TERMS AND DEFINITIONS

Business Models: A business model describes the rationale of how organizations/ enterprises create, delivers and capture value. Business models include strategies, infrastructure, and organisational structure, trading practices, operational processes and policies.

E-**Health:** The term e-health refers to IT-based applications that are used to provide health services and health information.

Innovation: Innovation is the process of translating an idea or invention into a good or service that creates value. Innovations often result when ideas are applied by a company/enterprise in order to further satisfy the needs and expectation of the customers.

Intermediary Platforms: A IT-based solution that facilitates the interaction between the two- sided of the market bringing sellers, buyers and users together. .

Multi-Home: the possibility to be connected to multiple providers that offer similar products or services.

Patient-Centred System: A care system in which health care providers explain treatments and alternatives to patients to provide the necessary information for patient to active involve them in decision processes and medical decision making.

Sustainable: The development of something that meets the needs of the present without comprising the ability of future generation to meet their own needs.

Compilation of References

Accenture. (2013). *Losing patience: Why healthcare providers need to up their mobile game*. Retrieved from https://www.accenture.com/t20160629T221243__w__/us-en/_acnmedia/PDF-24/Accenture-Losing-Patience.pdf#zoom=50

Acceptance and Commitment Therapy EST Status for Chronic or Persistent Pain: Strong Research Support. Society of Clinical Psychology (Division 12). (2013). Retrieved June 1, 2015, from http://www.div12.org/psychological-treatments/disorders/chronic-or- persistent-pain/acceptance-and-commitment-therapy-for-chronic-pain/

Adelman, M. B., Parks, M. R., & Albrecht, T. L. (1987). Beyond close relationships: Support in weak ties. In T. L. Albrecht & M. B. Adelman (Eds.), *Communicating social support* (pp. 105–125). Beverly Hills, CA: SAGE.

Aikens, K. A., Astin, J., Pelletier, K. R., Levanovich, K., Baase, C. M., Park, Y. Y., & Bodnar, C. M. (2014). Mindfulness goes to work. *Journal of Occupational and Environmental Medicine*, *56*(7), 721–731. doi:10.1097/JOM.0000000000000209 PMID:24988100

Ajzen, I. (1991). The theory of planned behaviour. *Organizational Behavior and Human Decision Processes*, *50*(2), 179–211. doi:10.1016/0749-5978(91)90020-T

Albada, K., & Moore, J. L. (2013). Moving from positive thinking to positive talk: Implications for relational wellbeing. In M. J. Pitts & T. J. Socha (Eds.), *Positive communication in health and wellness* (pp. 117–132). New York: Peter Lang Publishers.

Albrecht, T. L., & Goldsmith, D. J. (2003). Social support, social networks, and health. In T. L. Thompson, A. M. Dorsey, K. I. Miller, & R. Parrott (Eds.), *Handbook of health communication* (pp. 263–284). Mahwah, NJ: Lawrence Erlbaum Associates.

Ali, K., Farrer, L., Gulliver, A., & Griffiths, K. M. (2015). Online Peer-to-Peer Support for Young People With Mental Health Problems: A Systematic Review. *JMIR Mental Health*, *2*(2), e19. doi:10.2196/mental.4418 PMID:26543923

Allen, D., Braithwaite, J., Sandall, J., & Waring, J. (2016). Towards a sociology of healthcare safety and quality. *Sociology of Health & Illness*, *38*(2), 181–197. doi:10.1111/1467-9566.12390 PMID:26679563

Allen, K. (2013). *Consumption of culture by older Canadians on the Internet.* Statistics Canada.

American College Health Association. (2013). *American College Health Association-National College Health Assessment II: Canadian Reference Group Data Report Spring 2013.* Hanover, MD: American College Health Association.

Argyle, M. (1969). *Social Interaction.* London: Methuen.

Ariely, D. (1998). Combining experiences over time: The effects of duration, intensity changes and on-line measurements on retrospective pain evaluations. *Journal of Behavioral Decision Making, 11*(1), 19–45. doi:10.1002/(SICI)1099-0771(199803)11:1<19::AID-BDM277>3.0.CO;2-B

Arnow, B. A., Hunkeler, E. M., Blasey, C. M., Lee, J., Constantino, M. J., Fireman, B., & Hayward, C. et al. (2006). Comorbid depression, chronic pain, and disability in primary care. *Psychosomatic Medicine, 68*(2), 262–268. doi:10.1097/01.psy.0000204851.15499.fc PMID:16554392

Arora, N. K., Finney Rutten, L. J., Gustafson, D. H., Moser, R., & Hawkins, R. P. (2007). Perceived helpfulness and impact of social support provided by family, friends, and health care providers to women newly diagnosed with breast cancer. *Psycho-Oncology, 16*(5), 474–486. doi:10.1002/pon.1084 PMID:16986172

Arroll, B., Elley, C. R., Fishman, T., Goodyear-Smith, F. A., Kenealy, T., Blashki, G., & MacGillivray, S. et al. (2009). Antidepressants versus placebo for depression in primary care. *Cochrane Database of Systematic Reviews,* (3): CD007954. PMID:19588448

Arsenault, M., Blouin, M. J., & Guitton, M. J. (2012). Information quality and dynamics of patients interactions on tonsillectomy web resources. *Internet Interventions, 4,* 99–104. doi:10.1016/j.invent.2016.05.002

Azam, M. A., Weinrib, A. Z., Montbriand, J., Burns, L. C., McMillan, K., Clarke, H., & Katz, J. (2017). Acceptance and Commitment Therapy to manage pain and opioid use after major surgery: Preliminary outcomes from the Toronto General Hospital Transitional Pain Service. *Canadian Journal of Pain, 1*(1), 37–49. http://www.tandfonline.com/doi/full/10.1080/24740527.2017.1325317

Baikie, K., & Wilhelm, K. (2005). Emotional and physical health benefits of expressive writing. *Advances in Psychiatric Treatment, 11*(5), 338–346. doi:10.1192/apt.11.5.338

Ballantyne, J. C., & Sullivan, M. D. (2015). Intensity of chronic pain — The wrong metric? *The New England Journal of Medicine, 373*(22), 2098–2099. doi:10.1056/NEJMp1507136 PMID:26605926

Barak, A., Boniel-Nissim, M., & Suler, J. (2008). Fostering empowerment in online support groups. *Computers in Human Behavior, 24*(5), 1867–1883. doi:10.1016/j.chb.2008.02.004

Barrett, M., Davidson, E., Prahbu, J., & Vargo, S. L. (2015). Service innovation in the digital age: Key contributions and future directions. *Management Information Systems Quarterly, 39,* 135–154.

Barry, M. J., & Edgman-Levitan, S. (2012). Shared decision making - The pinnacle of patient-centered care. *The New England Journal of Medicine*, *366*(9), 780–781. doi:10.1056/NEJMp1109283 PMID:22375967

Baumeister, R., & Leary, M. (1995). The need to belong: Desire for interpersonal attachments as a fundamental human motivation. *Psychological Bulletin*, *117*(3), 497–529. doi:10.1037/0033-2909.117.3.497 PMID:7777651

Baym, N. (1995). The emergence of community in computer-mediated communication. In S. Jones (Ed.), *Cybersociety* (pp. 35–68). Thousand Oaks, CA: SAGE.

Beaunoyer, E., Arsenault, M., Lomanowska, A. M., & Guitton, M. J. (2016). Understanding Online Health Information: Evaluation, Tools, and Strategies. *Patient Education and Counseling*. doi:10.1016/j.pec.2016.08.028 PMID:27595436

Beiter, R., Nash, R., McCrady, M., Rhoades, D., Linscomb, M., Clarahan, M., & Sammut, S. (2015). The prevalence and correlates of depression, anxiety, and stress in a sample of college students. *Journal of Affective Disorders*, *173*, 90–96. doi:10.1016/j.jad.2014.10.054 PMID:25462401

Béland, D., & Viriot Durandal, J.-P. (2013). Aging in France: Population Trends, Policy Issues, and Research Institutions. *The Gerontologist*, *53*(2), 191–197. doi:10.1093/geront/gns149 PMID:23220395

Bell, V. (2007). Online information, extreme communities, and Internet therapy: Is the Internet good for our mental health? *Journal of Mental Health (Abingdon, England)*, *16*(4), 445–457. doi:10.1080/09638230701482378

Bender, J., & Jiang, H. (2013). Online communities: Prevalence and predictors of use, and reasons for non-use. In Medicine 2.0. London: Medicine 2.0.

Bender, J., & Miller, A. (2016). Scoping review of virtual health communities as standalone or adjunct interventions. In *Proceedings of the 37th Annual Society of Behavioral Medicine Conference*. Washington, DC: Society of Behavioural Medicine.

Bender, J. L., Jimenez-Marroquin, M. C., Ferris, L. E., Katz, J., & Jadad, A. R. (2013). Online communities for breast cancer survivors: A review and analysis of their characteristics and levels of use. *Supportive Care in Cancer*, *21*(5), 1253–1263. doi:10.1007/s00520-012-1655-9 PMID:23179491

Bender, J. L., Jimenez-Marroquin, M. C., & Jadad, A. R. (2011). Seeking support on Facebook: A content analysis of breast cancer groups. *Journal of Medical Internet Research*, *13*(1), e16. doi:10.2196/jmir.1560 PMID:21371990

Bender, J. L., Katz, J., Ferris, L. E., & Jadad, A. R. (2013). What is the role of online support from the perspective of facilitators of face-to-face support groups? A multi-method study of the use of breast cancer online communities. *Patient Education and Counseling*, *93*(3), 472–479. doi:10.1016/j.pec.2013.07.009 PMID:23928354

Bender, J. L., O'Grady, L., & Jadad, A. R. (2008). Supporting cancer patients through the continuum of care: A view from the age of social networks and computer-mediated communication. *Current Oncology (Toronto, Ont.), 15*, S42–S47. PMID:18769582

Bender, J. L., Radhakrishnan, A., Diorio, C., Englesakis, M., & Jadad, A. R. (2011). Can pain be managed through the Internet? A systematic review of randomized controlled trials. *Pain, 152*(8), 1740–1750. doi:10.1016/j.pain.2011.02.012 PMID:21565446

Bender, J. L., Wiljer, D., Sawka, A. M., Tsang, R., Alkazaz, N., & Brierley, J. D. (2016). Thyroid cancer survivors perceptions of survivorship care follow-up options: A cross-sectional, mixed-methods survey. *Supportive Care in Cancer, 24*(5), 2007–2015. doi:10.1007/s00520-015-2981-5 PMID:26530226

Bender, J. L., Wiljer, D., To, M. J., Bedard, P. L., Chung, P., Jewett, M. A., & Gospodarowicz, M. et al. (2012). Testicular cancer survivors supportive care needs and use of online support: A cross-sectional survey. *Supportive Care in Cancer, 20*(11), 2737–2746. doi:10.1007/s00520-012-1395-x PMID:22382589

Beresford, P., Perring, R., Nettle, M., & Wallcraft, J. (2015). *From mental illness to a social model of madness and distress*. Retrieved on January 12, 2017 from http://www.shapingourlives.org.uk/wp-content/uploads/2016/05/FROM-MENTAL-ILLNESS-PDF-2.pdf

Berman, R. L. H., Iris, M. A., Bode, R., & Drengenberg, C. (2009). The Effectiveness of an Online Mind-Body Intervention for Older Adults with Chronic Pain. *The Journal of Pain, 10*(1), 68–79. doi:10.1016/j.jpain.2008.07.006 PMID:18774342

Blanchard, A. L. (2007). Developing a Sense of Virtual Community Measure. *Cyberpsychology & Behavior, 10*(6), 827–830. doi:10.1089/cpb.2007.9946 PMID:18085972

Blanchard, A. L. (2008). Testing a model of sense of virtual community. *Computers in Human Behavior, 24*(5), 2107–2123. doi:10.1016/j.chb.2007.10.002

Blanchard, A. L., & Markus, M. L. (2004). The Experienced Sense of a Virtual Community: Characteristics and Processes. *SIGMIS Database, 35*(1), 64–79. doi:10.1145/968464.968470

Blanchard, A. L., Welbourne, J. L., & Boughton, M. D. (2011). A model of online trust: The mediating role of norms and sense of virtual community. *Information Communication and Society, 14*(1), 76–106. doi:10.1080/13691181003739633

Blank, T. O., & Adams-Blodnieks, M. (2005). The who and the what of usage of two cancer online communities. *Computers in Human Behavior, 23*(3), 1249–1257. doi:10.1016/j.chb.2004.12.003

Blumer, J. G., & Katz, E. (1974). *The uses of mass communications: Current perspectives on gratifications research*. Beverly Hills, CA: Sage Publications.

Boettcher, J., Astrom, V., Pahlsson, D., Schenstrom, O., Andersson, G., & Carlbring, P. (2014). Internet-based mindfulness treatment for anxiety disorders: A randomized controlled trial. *Behavior Therapy, 45*(2), 241–253. doi:10.1016/j.beth.2013.11.003 PMID:24491199

Bogart, L., & Helgeson, V. S. (2000). Social comparisons among women with breast cancer: A longitudinal investigation. *Journal of Applied Social Psychology, 30*(3), 547–575. doi:10.1111/j.1559-1816.2000.tb02496.x

Bourdieu, P. (1983). The field of cultural production, or: The economic world reversed. *Poetics, 12*(4-5), 311–356. doi:10.1016/0304-422X(83)90012-8

Bourdieu, P. (1985). The genesis of the concepts of Habitus and of Field. *Sociocriticism, 2*, 11–24.

Bourdieu, P. (1990). *The logic of practice*. Cambridge, UK: Polity Press.

Boyatzis, R. E. (1998). *Transforming Qualitative Information*. London: Sage.

Boyde, D., & Ellison, N. (2008). Social network sites: Definition, history and scholarship. *Journal of Computer-Mediated Communication, 13*(1), 210–230. doi:10.1111/j.1083-6101.2007.00393.x

Braun, M. T. (2013). Obstacles to social networking website use among older adults. *Computers in Human Behavior, 29*(3), 673–680. doi:10.1016/j.chb.2012.12.004

Braun, V., & Clarke, V. (2006). Using thematic analysis in psychology. *Qualitative Research in Psychology, 3*(32), 77–101. doi:10.1191/1478088706qp063oa

Breivik, H., Eisenberg, E., & OBrien, T. (2013). The individual and societal burden of chronic pain in Europe: The case for strategic prioritisation and action to improve knowledge and availability of appropriate care. *BMC Public Health, 13*(1), 1229. doi:10.1186/1471-2458-13-1229 PMID:24365383

Broom, A. (2005). The eMale: Prostate cancer, masculinity, and online support as a challenge to medical expertise. *Journal of Sociology (Melbourne, Vic.), 41*(1), 87–104. doi:10.1177/1440783305050965

Broom, A. (2005). Virtually he@lthy: The impact of internet use on disease experience and the doctor-patient relationship. *Qualitative Health Research, 15*(3), 325–345. doi:10.1177/1049732304272916 PMID:15761103

Brown, B., Chalmers, M., Bell, M., Hall, M., MacColl, I., & Rudman, P. (2005). Sharing the square: Collaborative Leisure in the City Streets. In H. Gellersen, K. Schmidt, M. Beaudouin-Lafon, & W. Mackay (Eds.), *ECSCW 2005: Proceedings of the Ninth European Conference on Computer-Supported Cooperative Work* (pp. 427-447). Dordrecht, The Netherlands: Springer Netherlands. doi:10.1007/1-4020-4023-7_22

Brown-Johnson, C. G., Berrean, B., & Cataldo, J. K. (2015). Development and usability evaluation of the mHealth Tool for Lung Cancer (mHealth TLC): A virtual world health game for lung cancer patients. *Patient Education and Counseling, 98*(4), 506–511. doi:10.1016/j.pec.2014.12.006 PMID:25620075

Brown, P. R., & Calnan, M. W. (2016). Chains of (dis)trust: exploring the underpinnings of knowledge-sharing and quality care across mental health services. In *An Introduction to Social Constructionism*. London: Routledge. doi:10.1002/9781119276371.ch7

Bugeja, M. (2005). *Interpersonal divide: The search for community in a technological age*. New York: Oxford University Press.

Burg, M. A., Adorno, G., Lopez, E. D. S., Loerzel, V., Stein, K., Wallace, C., & Sharma, D. K. B. (2015). Current unmet needs of cancer survivors: Analysis of open-ended responses to the American Cancer Society Study of Cancer Survivors II. *Cancer*, *121*(4), 623–630. doi:10.1002/cncr.28951 PMID:25581252

Burke, M., & Kraut, R. E. (2016). The relationship between Facebook use and well-being depends on communication type and tie strength. *Journal of Computer-Mediated Communication*, *21*(4), 265–281. doi:10.1111/jcc4.12162

Burleson, B. R., & MacGeorge, R. L. (2002). Supportive communication. In M. L. Knapp & J. A. Daly (Eds.), *Handbook of interpersonal communication* (pp. 374–424). Thousand Oaks, CA: SAGE.

Butler, A. C., Chapman, J. E., Forman, E. M., & Beck, A. T. (2006). The empirical status of cognitive-behavioral therapy: A review of meta-analyses. *Clinical Psychology Review*, *26*(1), 17–31. doi:10.1016/j.cpr.2005.07.003 PMID:16199119

Buunk, B., Gibbons, F., & Reis-Bergan, M. (1997). Social comparison in health and illness - An overview. In B. Buunk, F. Gibbons, & M. Reis-Bergan (Eds.), *Health, coping and well-being*. Lawrence Erlbaum Associates.

Cairns, S. L., Massfeller, H. F., & Deeth, S. C. (2010). Why do postsecondary students seek counselling? *Canadian Journal of Counselling and Psychotherapy*, *44*(1), 34–50.

Calleja, G. (2010). Digital games and Escapism. *Games and Culture*, *5*(4), 335–353. doi:10.1177/1555412009360412

Canada Health Infoway. (2014). *The Path Forward: Accelerating Clinical Interoperability in Canada*. Retrieved February 28, 2017, from https://ic.infoway-inforoute.ca/en/resources/docs/cistratdocs/40-the-path-forward

Canada Health Infoway. (2017). *Summary Corporate Plan 2017-2018*. Toronto, Canada: Canada Health Infoway.

Canada Health Infoway. (2017a). *Coordination of Care*. Retrieved February 28, 2017, from https://ic.infoway-inforoute.ca/en/collaboration/communities/coordination-of-care

Canada Health Infoway. (2017b). *Diagnostic Imaging Community*. Retrieved February 28, 2017, from https://ic.infoway-inforoute.ca/en/collaboration/communities/diagnostic-imaging

Canada Health Infoway. (2017c). *InfoCentral*. Retrieved February 28, 2017, from https://www.infoway-inforoute.ca/en/communities/infocentral

Canada Health Infoway. (2017d). *InfoCentral Home*. Retrieved February 28, 2017, from https://ic.infoway-inforoute.ca/en/

Canada Health Infoway. (2017e). *InfoScribe Home*. Retrieved February 28, 2017, from https://infoscribe.infoway-inforoute.ca/display/IH/InfoScribe

Canada Health Infoway. (2017f). *Message Builder*. Retrieved February 28, 2017, from https://ic.infoway-inforoute.ca/en/tools/developer-tools/message-builder

Canada Health Infoway. (2017g). *PrescribeIT: Canada's Electronic Prescription Service*. Retrieved February 28, 2017, from https://www.infoway-inforoute.ca/en/solutions/e-prescribing/prescribeit

Canada Health Infoway. (2017h). *Public Health Surveillance Community*. Retrieved February 28, 2017, from https://ic.infoway-inforoute.ca/en/collaboration/communities-2/public-health-surveillance

Canada Health Infoway. (2017j). *Terminology Gateway*. Retrieved February 28, 2017, from https://tgateway.infoway-inforoute.ca/

Canadian Cancer Society (CCS). (2016). *Canadian Cancer Statistics 2016*. Author.

Canadian Medical Association (CMA). (2013). *Health and Health Care for an Aging Population: Policy Summary of The Canadian Medical Association*. Retrieved from https://www.cma.ca/Assets/assets-library/document/en/advocacy/policy-research/CMA_Policy_Health_and_Health_Care_for_an_Aging-Population_PD14-03-e.pdf

Canadian Medical Association (CMA). (2016). *The State of Seniors Health Care in Canada*. Retrieved from https://www.cma.ca/En/Lists/Medias/the-state-of-seniors-health-care-in-canada-september-2016.pdf

Caron, J., Latimer, E., & Tousignant, M. (2007). Predictors of psychological distress in low-income populations of Montreal. *Canadian Journal of Public Health*, *98*(Suppl. 1), S35–S44. PMID:18047159

Carroll, J. M. (2014). *The neighborhood in the Internet: Design research projects in community*. London: Routledge.

Carter, W., & Fisher, S. S. (2004). Mobile sound communities. *Proceedings of the 2004 ACM SIGCHI International Conference on Advances in Computer Entertainment Technology*. Retrieved from http://dl.acm.org/citation.cfm?doid=1067343.1067399

Cavanagh, K., Strauss, C., Cicconi, F., Griffiths, N., Wyper, A., & Jones, F. (2013). A randomised controlled trial of a brief online mindfulness-based intervention. *Behaviour Research and Therapy*, *51*(9), 573–578. doi:10.1016/j.brat.2013.06.003 PMID:23872699

Centres for Disease Control and Prevention. (2010). Current depression among adults --- United States, 2006 and 2008. *Morbidity and Mortality Weekly Report*, *59*(38), 1229–1235. PMID:20881934

Chambers, R., Schmid, M., & Birch-Jones, J. (2016). *Digital Healthcare: the essential guide*. Oxford, UK: Otmoor Publishing.

Chandler, A. (2016). *Self-Injury, Medicine and Society: Authentic Bodies*. London: Palgrave Macmillan. doi:10.1057/978-1-137-40528-9

Chang, T., Chopra, V., Zhang, C., & Woolford, S. J. (2013). The role of social media in online weight management: Systematic review. *Journal of Medical Internet Research*, *15*(11), e262. doi:10.2196/jmir.2852 PMID:24287455

Chapman, R. R. (2009). Predictability of painful stimulation modulates subjective and physiological responses. *The Journal of Pain*, *11*(3), 239–246. doi:10.1016/j.jpain.2009.07.009 PMID:19853519

Cheung, R., O'Donnell, S., Madi, N., & Goldner, E. (2017). Factors associated with delayed diagnosis of mood and/or anxiety disorders. *Health Promotion and Chronic Disease Prevention in Canada: Research. Policy & Practice*, *37*(5), 137–148.

Chi, M. J., Lee, C. Y., & Wu, S. C. (2011). The prevalence of chronic conditions and medical expenditures of the elderly by chronic condition indicator (CCI). *Archives of Gerontology and Geriatrics*, *52*(3), 284–289. doi:10.1016/j.archger.2010.04.017 PMID:20452688

Chiu, C.-M., Hsu, M.-H., & Wang, E. (2006). Understanding knowledge sharing in virtual communities: An integration of social capital and social cognitive theories. *Decision Support Systems*, *42*(3), 1872–1888. doi:10.1016/j.dss.2006.04.001

Chorbev, I., Sotirovska, M., & Mihajlov, D. (2011). Virtual communities for diabetes chronic disease healthcare. *International Journal of Telemedicine and Applications. Art.*, *721654*, e7.

Christensen, H., Batterham, P., Mackinnon, A., Griffiths, K. M., Kalia Hehir, K., Kenardy, J., & Bennett, K. et al. (2014). Prevention of generalized anxiety disorder using a web intervention, iChill: Randomized controlled trial. *Journal of Medical Internet Research*, *16*(9), e199. doi:10.2196/jmir.3507 PMID:25270886

Christensen, K., Doblhammer, G., Rau, R., & Vaupel, J. W. (2009). Ageing populations: The challenges ahead. *Lancet*, *374*(9696), 1196–1208. doi:10.1016/S0140-6736(09)61460-4 PMID:19801098

Cleeland, C. S., & Ryan, K. M. (1994). Pain assessment: Global use of the Brief Pain Inventory. *Annals of the Academy of Medicine, Singapore*, *23*(2), 129–138. PMID:8080219

Clement, S., Schauman, O., Graham, T., Maggioni, F., Evans-Lacko, S., Bezborodovs, N., & Thornicroft, G. et al. (2015). What is the impact of mental health-related stigma on help-seeking? A systematic review of quantitative and qualitative studies. *Psychological Medicine*, *45*(1), 11–27. doi:10.1017/S0033291714000129 PMID:24569086

Coalition, C. P. (2014). *The painful truth: The truth of pain management in Canada*. Retrieved from http://www.canadianpaincoalition.ca/media/painful_truth_report.pdf

Cohen, S., & Wills, T. A. (1985). Stress, social support, and the buffering hypothesis. *Psychological Bulletin, 98*(2), 310–357. doi:10.1037/0033-2909.98.2.310 PMID:3901065

Corrigan, P. W., Kerr, A., & Knudsen, L. (2005). The stigma of mental illness: Explanatory models and methods for change. *Applied & Preventive Psychology, 11*(3), 179–190. doi:10.1016/j.appsy.2005.07.001

Corry, P. (2008). *Stigma shout: service user and carer experiences of stigma and discrimination*. London: Time to Change.

Coulthard, K., Patel, D., Brizzolara, C., Morriss, R., & Watson, S. (2013). A feasibility study of expert patient and community mental health team led bipolar psychoeducation groups: Implementing an evidence based practice. *BMC Psychiatry, 13*(1), 301. doi:10.1186/1471-244X-13-301 PMID:24215655

Cousins, M. J., Power, I., & Smith, G. (2000). 1996 Labat lecture: Pain—a persistent problem. *Regional Anesthesia and Pain Medicine, 25*(1), 6–21. PMID:10660235

Crabtree, J. W., Haslam, S. A., Postmes, T., & Haslam, C. (2010). Mental Health Support Groups, Stigma, Self-Esteem: Positive and Negative Implications of Group Identification. *The Journal of Social Issues, 66*(3), 553–569. doi:10.1111/j.1540-4560.2010.01662.x

Creswell, J. D., Irwin, M. R., Burklund, L. J., Lieberman, M. D., Arevalo, J. M. G., Ma, J., & Cole, S. W. et al. (2012). Mindfulness-based stress reduction training reduces loneliness and pro-inflammatory gene expression in older adults: A small randomized controlled trial. *Brain, Behavior, and Immunity, 26*(7), 1095–1101. doi:10.1016/j.bbi.2012.07.006 PMID:22820409

Crocco, A. G., Villasis-Keever, M., & Jadad, A. R. (2002). Analysis of cases of harm associated with use of health information on the internet. *Journal of the American Medical Association, 287*(21), 2869–2871. doi:10.1001/jama.287.21.2869 PMID:12038937

Cruwys, T., Dingle, G. A., Haslam, C., Haslam, A. S., Jetten, J., & Morton, T. A. (2013). Social group memberships protect against future depression, alleviate depression symptoms and prevent depression relapse. *Social Science & Medicine, 98*, 179–186. doi:10.1016/j.socscimed.2013.09.013 PMID:24331897

Cuijpers, P. (2003). Examining the Effects of Prevention Programs on the Incidence of New Cases of Mental Disorders: The Lack of Statistical Power. *The American Journal of Psychiatry, 160*(8), 1385–1391. doi:10.1176/appi.ajp.160.8.1385 PMID:12900296

Cutrona Russell, D. C. (1990). Type of social support and specific stress: Toward a theory of optimal matching. In S. B. Sarason & G. Pierce (Ed.), Social support: An interactional view. New York: Wiley.

Daher, M. (2012). Cultural beliefs and values in cancer patients. *Annals of Oncology*, *23*(suppl 3), 66–69. doi:10.1093/annonc/mds091 PMID:22628419

Dahlin, M., Andersson, G., Magnusson, K., Johansson, T., Sjögren, J., Håkansson, A., & Carlbring, P. et al. (2016). Internet-delivered acceptance-based behaviour therapy for generalized anxiety disorder: A randomized controlled trial. *Behaviour Research and Therapy*, *77*, 86–95. doi:10.1016/j.brat.2015.12.007 PMID:26731173

Daine, K., Hawton, K., Singaravelu, V., Stewart, A., Simkin, S., & Montgomery, P. (2013). The power of the web: A systematic review of studies of the influence of the Internet on self-harm and suicide in young people. *PLoS ONE*, *8*(10), e77555. doi:10.1371/journal.pone.0077555 PMID:24204868

Das, A., & Faxvaag, A. (2014). What Influences Patient Participation in an Online Forum for Weight Loss Surgery? A Qualitative Case Study. *Interact J Med Res.*, *3*(1), e4. doi:10.2196/ijmr.2847 PMID:24509408

Davidson, L., Bellamy, C., Guy, K., & Miller, R. (2012). Peer support among persons with severe mental illnesses: A review of evidence and experience. *World Psychiatry; Official Journal of the World Psychiatric Association (WPA)*, *11*(2), 123–128. doi:10.1016/j.wpsyc.2012.05.009 PMID:22654945

Davis, F. D. (1989). Perceived usefulness, perceived ease of use, and user acceptance of information technology. *Management Information Science Quarterly*, *13*(3), 319–339.

Davison, K. P., Pennebaker, J. W., & Dickerson, S. S. (2000). Who talks? The social psychology of illness support groups. *The American Psychologist*, *55*(2), 205–217. doi:10.1037/0003-066X.55.2.205 PMID:10717968

Delanty, G. (2010). *Community*. London: Routledge.

Demiris, G, (2006). The diffusion of virtual communities in health care: concepts and challenges. *Patient Educ Couns.*, *62*(2), 178-88.

Demiris, G. (2005). Virtual Communities in Health Care. *Intelligent Paradigms for Healthcare Enterprises*, *184*, 121-137.

Department of Health. (2001). *The Expert Patient: A New Approach to Chronic Disease Management*. London: Department of Health.

Deshpande, A., & Jadad, A. (2006). Web 2.0: Could it help move the health care system in the 21st century? *Journal of Mens Health & Gender*, *3*(4), 332–336. doi:10.1016/j.jmhg.2006.09.004

Dewar, A. L., Gregg, K., White, M. I., & Lander, J. (2009). Navigating the health care system: Perceptions of patients with chronic pain. *Chronic Diseases in Canada*, *29*(4), 162–168. PMID:19804680

Dewar, A., White, M., Posade, S. T., & Dillon, W. (2003). Using nominal group technique to assess chronic pain, patients perceived challenges and needs in a community health region. *Health Expectations*, *6*(1), 44–52. doi:10.1046/j.1369-6513.2003.00208.x PMID:12603627

Dey, S., Nambiar, D., & Lakshmi, J. K. (2012). Health of the Elderly in India: Challenges of Access and Affordability. In National Research Council (US) Panel on Policy Research and Data Needs to Meet the Challenge of Aging in Asia. Aging in Asia: Findings From New and Emerging Data Initiatives (Vol. 15). Washington, DC: National Academies Press (US).

Diener, E., Gohm, C. L., Suh, E., & Oishi, S. (2000). Similarities of the relations between marital status and subjective well-being across cultures. *Journal of Cross-Cultural Psychology*, *31*(4), 419–436. doi:10.1177/0022022100031004001

Digital, N. H. S. (2017). *Hospital accident and emergency activity, 2015-16*. Retrieved on January 11, 2017, from http://www.content.digital.nhs.uk/catalogue/PUB23070

DiNucci, D. (1999, July). Fragmented future. *Print*, *53*(4), 32.

Drozd, F., Raeder, S., Kraft, P., & Bjørkli, C. A. (2013). Multilevel growth curve analyses of treatment effects of a Web-based intervention for stress reduction: Randomized controlled trial. *Journal of Medical Internet Research*, *15*(4), e84. doi:10.2196/jmir.2570 PMID:23607962

Dunham, P. J., Hurshman, A., Litwin, E., Gusella, J., Ellsworth, C., & Dodd, P. W. D. (1998). Computer-mediated social support: Single young mothers as a model system. *American Journal of Community Psychology*, *26*(2), 281–306. doi:10.1023/A:1022132720104 PMID:9693693

Durlak, J. A., & DuPre, E. P. (2008). Implementation matters: A review of research on the influence of implementation on program outcomes and the factors affecting implementation. *American Journal of Community Psychology*, *41*(3-4), 327–350. doi:10.1007/s10464-008-9165-0 PMID:18322790

Dworkin, R. H., Turk, D. C., Wyrwich, K. W., Beaton, D., Cleeland, C. S., Farrar, J. T., & Ader, D. N. et al. (2008). Interpreting the clinical importance of treatment outcomes in chronic pain clinical trials: IMMPACT recommendations. *The Journal of Pain*, *9*(2), 105–121. doi:10.1016/j.jpain.2007.09.005 PMID:18055266

Easterbrook, M., & Vignoles, V. L. (2013). What does it mean to belong? Interpersonal bonds and intragroup similarities as predictors of felt belonging in different types of groups. *European Journal of Social Psychology*, *43*(6), 455–462.

Eich, E., Reeves, J. L., Jaeger, B., & Graff-Radford, S. B. (1985). Memory for pain: Relation between past and present pain intensity. *Pain*, *23*(4), 375–380. doi:10.1016/0304-3959(85)90007-7 PMID:4088698

El Morr, C. (2007, May). *Mobile virtual communities in healthcare: Managed self care on the move*. Paper presented at the International Association of Science and Technology for Development – Telehealth Conference, Montreal, Canada.

El Morr, C. (2010). Health Care Virtual Communities: Challenges and Opportunities. In C.-C. Maria Manuela, J. T. Antonio, & S. Ricardo (Eds.), *Handbook of Research on Developments in E-Health and Telemedicine: Technological and Social Perspectives* (pp. 278–298). Hershey, PA: IGI Global. doi:10.4018/978-1-61520-670-4.ch013

El Morr, C. (2010b). Mobile Virtual Communities in Healthcare: The Chronic Disease Management Case. In S. Mohammed & J. Fiadi (Eds.), *Ubiquitous Health and Medical Informatics: The Ubiquity 2.0 Trend and Beyond* (pp. 258–258). IGI Global. doi:10.4018/978-1-61520-777-0.ch013

El Morr, C., Cole, C., & Perl, J. (2014). A health virtual community for patients with chronic kidney disease. *Procedia Computer Science*, *37*, 333–339. doi:10.1016/j.procs.2014.08.049

El Morr, C., & Kawash, J. (2007). Mobile virtual communities research: A synthesis of current trends and a look at future perspectives. *International Journal for Web Based Communities*, *3*(4), 386–403. doi:10.1504/IJWBC.2007.015865

El Morr, C., & Maret, P. (Eds.). (2012). *Virtual Community Building and the Information Society: Current and Future Directions*. Hershey, PA: Information Science Reference. doi:10.4018/978-1-60960-869-9

Esquivel, A., Meric-Bernstam, F., & Bernstam, E. V. (2006). Accuracy and self correction of information received from an internet breast cancer list: Content analysis. *BMJ (Clinical Research Ed.)*, *332*(7547), 939–942. doi:10.1136/bmj.38753.524201.7C PMID:16513686

European Commission. (2012). eHealth Action Plan 2012-2020 - Innovative healthcare for the 21st century. Report. Brussels: Author.

European Commission. (n.d.). *Personalised Medicine | Health - Research & Innovation - European Commission*. Retrieved January 27, 2017, from http://ec.europa.eu/research/health/index.cfm?pg=policy&policyname=personalised

Evans-Lacko, S., Henderson, C., & Thornicroft, G. (2013). Public knowledge, attitudes and behaviour regarding people with mental illness in England 20092012. *The British Journal of Psychiatry*, *202*(s55), 51–57. doi:10.1192/bjp.bp.112.112979

Eysenbach, G. (2001). What is e-health? *Journal of Medical Internet Research*, *3*(2), e20. doi:10.2196/jmir.3.2.e20 PMID:11720962

Eysenbach, G., Powell, J., Englesakis, M., Rizo, C., & Stern, A. (2004). Health related virtual communities and electronic support groups: Systematic review of the effects of online peer to peer interactions. *BMJ (Clinical Research Ed.)*, 328. PMID:15142921

Facebook Newsroom. (n.d.). *Facebook Company Info.* Retrieved January 27, 2017, from http://newsroom.fb.com/company-info/

Fashler, S. R., Cooper, L. K., Oosenbrug, E. D., Burns, L. C., Razavi, S., Goldberg, L., & Katz, J. (2016). Systematic review of multidisciplinary chronic pain treatment facilities. *Pain Research & Management, 2016*, 1–19. doi:10.1155/2016/5960987 PMID:27445618

Feng, Z., Liu, C., Guan, X., & Mor, V. (2012). Chinas Rapidly Aging Population Creates Policy Challenges In Shaping A Viable Long-Term Care System. *Health Affairs (Project Hope)*, *31*(12), 2764–2773. doi:10.1377/hlthaff.2012.0535 PMID:23213161

Festinger, L. (1954). A theory of social comparison processed. *Human Relations*, *7*(2), 117–140. doi:10.1177/001872675400700202

Fishbein, M. (1967). *Readings in attitude theory and measurement.* New York: John Wiley & Sons, Inc.

Fitch, M. I. (2000). Supportive care for cancer patients. *Hospital Quarterly*, *3*(4), 39–46. PMID:11482268

Fixsen, D. L., Naoom, S. F., Blase, K. A., Friedman, R. M., & Wallace, F. (2005). Implementation Research: A Synthesis of the Literature. Tampa, FL: University of South Florida, Louis de la Parte Florida Mental Health Institute, The National Implementation Research Network (FMHI Publication #231).

Flanagin, A. J., & Metzger, M. J. (2008). Digital media and youth: Unparalleled opportunity and unprecedented responsibilty. The John D. and Catherine T. MacArthur Foundation Series on Digial Media and Learning. Cambridge, MA: MIT Press.

Fletcher, G. J. O., & Fitness, J. (1990). Occurrent social cognition in close relationship interaction: The role of proximal and distal variables. *Journal of Personality and Social Psychology*, *59*(3), 464–474. doi:10.1037/0022-3514.59.3.464

Fogel, J., Ribisl, K. M., Morgan, P. D., Humphreys, K., & Lyons, E. J. (2008). Underrepresentation of African Americans in online cancer support groups. *Journal of the National Medical Association*, *100*(6), 705–712. doi:10.1016/S0027-9684(15)31346-8 PMID:18595573

Fox, S. (2011). Peer-to-peer Health Care. *Pew Research Center.* Retrieved from http://www.pewinternet.org/2011/02/28/peer-to-peer-health-care-2/

Franca, R. D., & Milbourn, B. (2015). A meta-analysis of mindfulness based interventions (MBIs) show that MBIs are effective in reducing acute symptoms of depression but not anxiety. *Australian Occupational Therapy Journal*, *62*(2), 147–148. doi:10.1111/1440-1630.12198 PMID:25865879

Frances, A. (2013). *Saving normal: An insider's revolt against out-of-control psychiatric diagnosis, DSM-5, big pharma and the medicalization of ordinary life.* Retrieved November 15, 2015, from http://search.informit.com.au/documentSummary;dn=464019439257830;res=IELHEA>

Frank, A. (1995). *The wounded storyteller: Body, illness and ethics*. Chicago: The University of Chicago Press. doi:10.7208/chicago/9780226260037.001.0001

Füller, J., Bartl, M., Ernst, H., & Mühlbacher, H. (2006). Community based innovation: How to integrate members of virtual communities into new product development. *Electronic Commerce Research*, *6*(1), 57–73. doi:10.1007/s10660-006-5988-7

Gagliardi, A., & Jadad, A. R. (2002). Examination of instruments used to rate quality of health information on the Internet: Chronicle of a vouage with unclear destination. *British Medical Journal*, *324*(7337), 569–573. doi:10.1136/bmj.324.7337.569 PMID:11884320

Gass, J. S., Weitzen, S., Clark, M., & Dizon, D. S. (2007). Defining social support systems for women with breast cancer. *American Journal of Surgery*, *194*(4), 501–503. doi:10.1016/j.amjsurg.2007.07.005 PMID:17826065

Gatchel, R. J., & Okifuji, A. (2006). Evidence-based scientific data documenting the treatment and cost-effectiveness of comprehensive pain programs for chronic nonmalignant pain. *The Journal of Pain*, *7*(11), 779–793. doi:10.1016/j.jpain.2006.08.005 PMID:17074616

Giddens, A. (1984). *The Constitution of Society*. Cambridge, UK: Polity.

Gigler, K. L., Blomeke, K., Shatil, E., Weintraub, S., & Reber, P. J. (2013). Preliminary evidence for the feasibility of at-home online cognitive training with older adults. *Gerontotechnology*, *12*(1), 26–35. doi:10.4017/gt.2013.12.1.007.00 PMID:26778939

Global, regional, and national incidence, prevalence, and years lived with disability for 310 diseases and injuries, 1990-2015: A systematic analysis for the Global Burden of Disease Study 2015. (2016). *Lancet, 388*(10053), 1545-1602. doi:10.1016/s0140-6736(16)31678-6

Glück, T. M., & Maercker, A. (2011). A randomized controlled pilot study of a brief web-based mindfulness training. *BMC Psychiatry*, *11*(1), 175. doi:10.1186/1471-244X-11-175 PMID:22067058

Goffman, E. (1963). *Stigma: notes on the management of spoiled identity*. New York: Simon and Schuster Inc.

Goldberg, D. S., & McGee, S. J. (2011). Pain as a global public health priority. *BMC Public Health*, *11*(1), 770. doi:10.1186/1471-2458-11-770 PMID:21978149

Goldsmith, D. J. (2004). *Communicating social support*. New York, NY: Cambridge University Press. doi:10.1017/CBO9780511606984

Goldsmith, D. J., & Albrecht, T. L. (2003). Social support, social networks, and health: A guiding framework. In T. L. Thompson, R. Parrot, & J. F. Nusbaum (Eds.), *Handbook of health communication* (pp. 335–348). Mahwah, NJ: Routledge.

Gooden, R. J., Winefield, H. R., Gooden, R. J., & Winefield, H. R. (2007). Breast and prostate cancer online discussion boards: A thematic analysis of gender differences and similarities. *Journal of Health Psychology*, *12*(1), 103–114. doi:10.1177/1359105307071744 PMID:17158844

Government of Canada. (2016). *FedDev Ontario Invests in Health Innovations to Support Canadians Living with Chronic Disease*. Retrieved from http://news.gc.ca/web/article-en.do?nid=1102399

Grande, G. E., Myers, L. B., & Sutton, S. R. (2006). How do patients who participate in cancer support groups differ from those who do not? *Psycho-Oncology*, *15*(4), 321–334. doi:10.1002/pon.956 PMID:16106472

Greenwood, S., Perrin, A., & Duggan, M. (2016). Social Media Update 2016. *Pew Research Centre*. Retrieved from http://www.pewinternet.org/2016/11/11/social-media-update-2016/#fn-17239-1

Griffiths, K. M., Calear, A. L., & Banfield, M. (2009). Systematic review on Internet Support Groups (ISGs) and depression (1): Do ISGs reduce depressive symptoms? *Journal of Medical Internet Research*, *11*(3), e40. doi:10.2196/jmir.1270 PMID:19793719

Grover, S. L., Teo, S. T. T., Pick, D., & Roche, M. (2016). Mindfulness as a personal resource to reduce work stress in the job demands-resources model. *Stress and Health*. doi: 10.1002/smi.2726

Guitton, M. J. (2014). The importance of studying the dark side of social networks. *Computers in Human Behavior*, *31*, 355. doi:10.1016/j.chb.2013.10.055

Guitton, M. J. (2015a). Swimming with mermaids: Communication and social density in the Second Life merfolk community. *Computers in Human Behavior*, *48*, 226–235. doi:10.1016/j.chb.2015.02.004

Guitton, M. J. (2015b). Ethical challenges in online health games. In D. Novak, B. Tulu, & H. Brendryen (Eds.), *Holistic Perspectives in Gamification for Clinical Practice* (pp. 1–9). IGI Global; doi:10.4018/978-1-4666-9522-1.ch001

Guo, T.-C., & Cheng, Z.-C. (2016). Sense of belonging based on novel posting: Individuals processes of social and psychological integration into virtual groups. *Online Information Review*, *40*(2), 204–217. doi:10.1108/OIR-06-2015-0198

Guo, X., Han, X., Zhang, X., Dang, Y., & Chen, C. (2015). Investigating m-health acceptance from a protection motivation theory perspective: Gender and age differences. *Telemedicine Journal and e-Health*, *21*(8), 661–669. doi:10.1089/tmj.2014.0166 PMID:25919800

Gustafson, D. H., Hawkins, R. P., Boberg, E. W., McTavish, F., Owens, B., Wise, M., . . . Pingree, S. (2001). *CHESS: 10 years of research and development in consumer health informatics for broad populations, including the underserved.* Paper presented at the 10th World Congress on Medical Informatics (Medinfo 2001).

Gustafson, D. H., McTavish, F. M., Stengle, W., Ballard, D., Hawkins, R., Shaw, B. R., & Landucci, G. et al. (2005). Use and Impact of eHealth System by Low-income Women With Breast Cancer. *Journal of Health Communication*, *10*(sup1), 195–218. doi:10.1080/10810730500263257 PMID:16377608

Hale, T. M., Pathipati, A. S., Zan, S., & Jethwani, K. (2014). Representation of health conditions on Facebook: Content analysis and evaluation of user engagement. *Journal of Medical Internet Research*, *16*(8), e182. doi:10.2196/jmir.3275 PMID:25092386

Hansson, E., Tuck, A., Lurie, S., & McKenzie, K. (2010). Improving mental health services for immigrant, refugee, ethno-cultural and racialized groups: Issues and options for service improvement. Report for the Task Group of the Services Systems Advisory Committee, Mental Health Commission of Canada.

Hausmann, L. R. M., Parks, A., Youk, A. O., & Kwoh, C. K. (2014). Reduction of bodily pain in response to an online positive activities intervention. *The Journal of Pain*, *15*(5), 560–567. doi:10.1016/j.jpain.2014.02.004 PMID:24568751

Hawkley, L. C., & Cacioppo, J. T. (2010). Loneliness matters: A theoretical and empirical review of consequences and mechanisms. *Annals of Behavioral Medicine*, *40*(2), 218–227. doi:10.1007/s12160-010-9210-8 PMID:20652462

Hayes, S. C., Strosahl, K. D., & Wilson, K. G. (2011). Acceptance and Commitment Therapy: The process and practice of mindful change. Guilford Press. New York, NY: Guilford Press. Retrieved from https://contextualscience.org/ACT_Randomized_Controlled_Trials

Hayes, C., Browne, S., Lantry, G., & Burstal, R. (2002). Neuropathic pain in the acute pain service: A prospective survey. *Acute Pain*, *4*(2), 45–48. doi:10.1016/S1366-0071(02)00026-8

Hayes, M., van Stolk-Cooke, K., & Muench, F. (2015). Understanding Facebook use and the psychological affects of use across generations. *Computers in Human Behavior*, *49*, 507–511. doi:10.1016/j.chb.2015.03.040

He, W., Goodkind, D., & Kowal, P. (2016). An Aging World: 2015: International Population Report. Retrieved from http://cdn.cnsnews.com/attachments/census_bureau-an_aging_world-2015.pdf

Health IT. (2016). *Public Stakeholder consultation on EU-US cooperation in eHealth/Health IT*. Author.

Hefner, J., & Eisenberg, D. (2009). Social support and mental health among college students. *The American Journal of Orthopsychiatry*, *79*(4), 491–499. doi:10.1037/a0016918 PMID:20099940

Heidelberger, C. A., El-Gayar, O., & Sarnikar, S. (2011, January). *Online health social networks and patient health decision behavior: A research agenda.* Paper presented at the Forty-fourth Hawaii International Conference on System Sciences. doi:10.1109/HICSS.2011.328

Helgeson, V. S., & Gottlieb, B. (2000). Support Groups. In S. Cohen, L. Underwood, & B. Gottlieb (Eds.), *Social support measurement and intervention.* Oxford University Press. doi:10.1093/med:psych/9780195126709.003.0007

Herring, S. C. (Ed.). (1996). *Computer-mediated communication: Linguistic, social and cross-cultural perspectives.* Philadelphia, PA: John Benjamins. doi:10.1075/pbns.39

Herring, S., Job-Sluder, K., Scheckler, R., & Barab, S. (2011). Searching for Safety Online: Managing "Trolling" in a Feminist Forum. *The Information Society>. International Journal (Toronto, Ont.), 18*(5), 371–384.

Heyes, K. (2017). *Using virtual ethnography to research vulnerable participants online: A case study of mental health online community support forums.* SAGE Research Methods Online; doi:10.4135/9781526403605

High, A. C., & Solomon, D. H. (2011). Locating computer-mediated social support within online communication environments. In K. B. Wright & L. M. Webb (Eds.), *Computer-mediated communication in personal relationships.* New York: Peter Lang.

Hilgart, M., Thorndike, F. P., Pardo, J., & Ritterband, L. M. (2012). 12 Ethical Issues of Web-Based Interventions and Online Therapy. The Oxford handbook of international psychological ethics, 161.

Hine, C. (2004). Social research methods and the internet: A thematic review. *Sociological Research Online, 9*(2). doi:10.5153/sro.924

Hine, C. (2008). Virtual Ethnography: Modes, Varieties and Affordances. In N. G. Fielding, R. M. Lee, & G. Blank (Eds.), *The SAGE handbook of online research methods.* London: SAGE. doi:10.4135/9780857020055.n14

Hogan, M.-E., Taddio, A., Katz, J., Shah, V., & Krahn, M. (2016a). Health utilities in people with chronic pain using a population-level survey and linked healthcare administrative data. *Pain.* doi:10.1097/j.pain.0000000000000776

Hogan, M.-E., Taddio, A., Katz, J., Shah, V., & Krahn, M. (2016b). Incremental healthcare costs for chronic pain in Ontario, Canada – a population-based matched cohort study of adolescents and adults using administrative data. *Pain, 157,* 1. doi:10.1097/j.pain.0000000000000561 PMID:26447708

Holt-Lunstad, J., Smith, T. B., Baker, M., Harris, T., & Stephenson, D. (2015). Loneliness and social isolation as risk factors for mortality: A Meta-Analytic review. *Perspectives on Psychological Science, 10*(2), 227–237. doi:10.1177/1745691614568352 PMID:25910392

Hong, Y., Peña-Purcell, N. C., & Ory, M. G. (2012). Outcomes of online support and resources for cancer survivors: A systematic literature review. *Patient Education and Counseling*, *86*(3), 288–296. doi:10.1016/j.pec.2011.06.014 PMID:21798685

Hornsey, M. J., & Jetten, J. (2004). The individual within the group: Balancing the need to belong with the need to be different. *Personality and Social Psychology Review*, *8*(3), 248–264. doi:10.1207/s15327957pspr0803_2 PMID:15454348

Hoybye, M. T., Dalton, S. O., Deltour, I., Bidstrup, P. E., Frederiksen, K., & Johansen, C. (n.d.). Effect of Internet peer-support groups on psychosocial adjustment to cancer: A randomised study. *Br J Cancer, 102*(9), 1348–1354.

Hoybye, M. T., Johansen, C., Tjornhoj-Thomsen, T., Hoybye, M. T., Johansen, C., & Tjornhoj-Thomsen, T. (2005). Online interaction. Effects of storytelling in an internet breast cancer support group. *Psycho-Oncology*, *14*(3), 211–220. doi:10.1002/pon.837 PMID:15386774

Hunot, V., Churchill, R., Teixeira, V., & Silva de Lima, M. (2007). Psychological therapies for generalised anxiety disorder. *Cochrane Database of Systematic Reviews*, (1): CD001848. PMID:17253466

Im, E. O., Chee, W., Im, E.-O., & Chee, W. (2008). The use of Internet cancer support groups by ethnic minorities. *Journal of Transcultural Nursing*, *19*(1), 74–82. doi:10.1177/1043659607309140 PMID:18217235

Im, E. O., Chee, W., Tsai, H. M., Lin, L. C., Cheng, C. Y., Im, E.-O., & Cheng, C.-Y. et al. (2005). Internet cancer support groups: A feminist analysis. *Cancer Nursing*, *28*(1), 1–7. doi:10.1097/00002820-200501000-00001 PMID:15681976

Institute of Aging-University of British Columbia. (2007). *The Future is AGING: Institute of Aging Strategic Plan 2007 – 2012*. Retrieved from http://www.cihr-irsc.gc.ca/e/documents/ia_strategic_plan_07-12_e.pdf

Integrating the Healthcare Enterprise. (2017). *Profiles*. Retrieved February 28, 2017, from http://ihe.net/profiles/

Internal Agnecy for Researh on Cancer (IARC). (2014). *GLOBOCAN 2012: Estimated Cancer Incidence, Mortality and Prevalence Worldwide in 2012*. Retrieved from http://globocan.iarc.fr/Pages/fact_sheets_cancer.aspx

InternetLiveStats. (2014). *Internet usage & social media statistics*. Retrieved on January 11, 2017, from http://www.internetlivestats.com

Irvine, I. B., Gelatt, V. A., Seeley, J. R., Macfarlane, P., & Gau, J. M. (2013). Web-based Intervention to Promote Physical Activity by Sedentary Older Adults: Randomized Controlled Trial. *Journal of Medical Internet Research*, *15*(2), e19. doi:10.2196/jmir.2158 PMID:23470322

Jadad, A. R., Enkin, M. W., Glouberman, S., Groff, P., & Stern, A. (2006). Are virtual communities good for our health? *British Medical Journal*, *332*(7547), 925–926. doi:10.1136/bmj.332.7547.925 PMID:16627491

Jadad, A. R., & Gagliardi, A. (1998). Rating health information on the Internet: Navigating to knowledge or to Babel? *Journal of the American Medical Association*, *279*(8), 611–614. doi:10.1001/jama.279.8.611 PMID:9486757

Jamison, R. N., Raymond, S. A., Levine, J. G., Slawsby, E. A., Nedeljkovic, S. S., & Katz, N. P. (2001). Electronic diaries for monitoring chronic pain: 1-year validation study. *Pain*, *91*(3), 277–285. doi:10.1016/S0304-3959(00)00450-4 PMID:11275385

Jefford, M. H. N., & Tattersall, M. H. N. (2002). Informing and involving cancer patients in their own care. *The Lancet Oncology*, *3*(10), 629–637. doi:10.1016/S1470-2045(02)00877-X PMID:12372725

Jensen, T. S., Baron, R., Haanpää, M., Kalso, E., Loeser, J. D., Rice, A. S. C., & Treede, R.-D. (2011). A new definition of neuropathic pain. *Pain*, *152*(10), 2204–2205. doi:10.1016/j.pain.2011.06.017 PMID:21764514

Jha, A. K., Doolan, D., Grandt, D., Scott, T., & Bates, D. W. (2008, December). The Use of Health Information Technology in Seven Nations. *International Journal of Medical Informatics*, *77*(12), 848–854. doi:10.1016/j.ijmedinf.2008.06.007 PMID:18657471

Johnston, A. C., Worrell, J. L., Di Gangi, P. M., & Wasko, M. (2013). Online health communities: An assessment of the influence of participation on patient empowerment outcomes. *Information Technology & People*, *26*(2), 213–235. doi:10.1108/ITP-02-2013-0040

Kabat-Zinn, J. (2003). Mindfulness-based interventions in context: Past, present, and future. *Clinical Psychology: Science and Practice*, *10*(2), 144–156. doi:10.1093/clipsy.bpg016

Kairam, S., Wang, D. J., & Leskovec, J. (2012). The life and death of online groups: predicting growth and longevity. *Proceedings of the Web Search and Data Mining (WSDM) Conference*. doi:10.1145/2124295.2124374

Kann, L., McManu, T., Harris, W. A., Shanklin, S. L., Flin, K. H., Hawkins, J., . . . Zaza, S. (2016). Youth Risk Behavior Surveillance - United States, 2015. *Surveillance Summaries*. Retrieved from http://stateofobesity.org/high-school-obesity/

Kapczinski, F., dos Santos Souza, J. J. S. S., Batista Miralha da Cunha, A. A. B. C., & Schmitt, R. R. S. (2003). Antidepressants for generalized anxiety disorder. *Cochrane Database of Systematic Reviews*, (3): CD003592. PMID:12804478

Kash, K. M., Mago, R., Kunkel, E. J., Kash, K. M., Mago, R., & Kunkel, E. J. S. (2005). Psychosocial oncology: Supportive care for the cancer patient. *Seminars in Oncology*, *32*(2), 211–218. doi:10.1053/j.seminoncol.2004.11.011 PMID:15815967

Katz, J., Weinrib, A., Fashler, S. R., Katznelzon, R., Shah, B. R., Ladak, S. S., ... Clarke, H. (2015). The Toronto General Hospital Transitional Pain Service: Development and implementation of a multidisciplinary program to prevent chronic postsurgical pain. Journal of Pain Research, 8, 695–702. doi:10.2147/JPR.S91924

Katz, J., Pagé, M. G., Fashler, S., Rosenbloom, B. N., & Asmundson, G. J. G. (2014). Chronic pain and the anxiety disorders: Epidemiology, mechanisms and models of comorbidity, and treatment. In *Mental Health and Pain* (pp. 119–155). Springer. doi:10.1007/978-2-8178-0414-9_8

Katz, J., Rosenbloom, B. N., & Fashler, S. (2015). Chronic pain, psychopathology, and DSM-5 somatic symptom disorder. *Canadian Journal of Psychiatry*, *60*(4), 160–167. doi:10.1177/070674371506000402 PMID:26174215

Katz, J., & Seltzer, Z. (2009). Transition from acute to chronic postsurgical pain: Risk factors and protective factors. *Expert Review of Neurotherapeutics*, *9*(5), 723–744. doi:10.1586/ern.09.20 PMID:19402781

Kawachi, I., & Berkman, L. F. (2001). Social Ties and Mental Health. *Journal of Urban Health: Bulletin of the New York Academy of Medicine*, *78*(3), 458–466. doi:10.1093/jurban/78.3.458 PMID:11564849

Kehlet, H., Jensen, T. S., & Woolf, C. J. (2006). Persistent postsurgical pain: Risk factors and prevention. *Lancet*, *367*(9522), 1618–1625. doi:10.1016/S0140-6736(06)68700-X PMID:16698416

Kelly, Y., Sacker, A., Del Bono, E., Francesconi, M., & Marmot, M. (2011). What role for the home learning environment and parenting in reducing the socioeconomic gradient in child development? Findings from the Millennium Cohort Study. *Archives of Disease in Childhood*, *96*(9), 832–837. doi:10.1136/adc.2010.195917 PMID:21666278

Kendall, L. (2002). *Hanging Out in the Virtual Pub: Masculinities and Relationships*. Berkeley, CA: University of California Press. doi:10.1525/california/9780520230361.001.0001

King, S. A., & Moreggi, D. (1998). Internet therapy and self-help groups - the pros and cons. In J. Gackenbach (Ed.), *Psychology and the Internet: Intrapersonal, interpersonal, and transpersonal implications* (pp. 77–109). San Diego, CA: Academic Press.

Klasnja, P., & Pratt, W. (2012). Healthcare in the pocket: Mapping the space of mobile-phone health interventions. *Journal of Biomedical Informatics*, *45*(1), 184–198. doi:10.1016/j.jbi.2011.08.017 PMID:21925288

Klemm, P. (2012). Effects of Online Support Group Format (Moderated vs Peer-Led) on Depressive Symptoms and Extent of Participation in Women With Breast Cancer. *CIN: Computers, Informatics, Nursing*, *30*(1), 9–18.

Klemm, P., Bunnell, D., Cullen, M., Soneji, R., Gibbons, P., & Holecek, A. (2003). Online cancer support groups: a review of the research literature. *CIN: Computers, Informatics, Nursing, 21*(3), 136–142.

Klemm, P., Hurst, M., Dearholt, S. L., & Trone, S. R. (1999). Gender differences on Internet cancer support groups. *Computers in Nursing, 17*(2), 65–72. PMID:10194883

Klemm, P., Reppert, K., & Visich, L. (1998). A nontraditional cancer support group. The Internet. *Computers in Nursing, 16*(1), 31–36. PMID:9454992

Koszycki, D., Thake, J., Mavounza, C., Daoust, J. P., Taljaard, M., & Bradwejn, J. (2016). Preliminary investigation of a mindfulness-based intervention for social anxiety disorder that integrates compassion meditation and mindful exposure. *Journal of Alternative and Complementary Medicine (New York, N.Y.), 22*(5), 363–374. doi:10.1089/acm.2015.0108 PMID:27070853

Kozinets, R. (2015). *Netnography: Redefined.* London: SAGE. doi:10.1002/9781118767771.wbiedcs067

Krusche, A., Cyhlarova, E., & Williams, J. M. G. (2013). Mindfulness online: An evaluation of the feasibility of a web-based mindfulness course for stress, anxiety and depression. *BMJ Open, 3*(11), e003498. doi:10.1136/bmjopen-2013-003498 PMID:24293203

Kwan, J., Croke, J., Panzarella, T., Ubhi, K., Lui, F., Fyles, A., … Bender, J. (2017). *Well breast cancer surivivors perceptions of alternate follow-up care options: A cross-sectional survey.* In Preparation.

Lappalainen, P., Langrial, S., Oinas-Kukkonen, H., Tolvanen, A., & Lappalainen, R. (2015). Web-based acceptance and commitment therapy for depressive symptoms with minimal support: A randomized controlled trial. *Behavior Modification, 39*(6), 805–834. doi:10.1177/0145445515598142 PMID:26253644

Lawrence, G., Lawrence, C. (Producers), & Robinson, P. (Director). (1989). *Field of Dreams.* [Motion Picture]. Universal Pictures.

Lazarus, S., & Folkman, R. (1984). *Stress, appriasial and coping.* New York: Springer.

Learmonth, D., Trosh, J., Rai, S., Sewell, J., & Cavanagh, K. (2008). The role of computer-aided psychotherapy within an NHS CBT specialist service. *Counselling & Psychotherapy Research, 8*(2), 117–123. doi:10.1080/14733140801976290

Lee, F. S., Vogel, D., & Limayem, M. (2003). Virtual community informatics: A review and research agenda. *Journal of Information Technology Theory and Application, 5*(1), 47–61.

Levin, M. E., Hayes, S. C., Pistorello, J., & Seeley, J. R. (2016). Web-based self-help for preventing mental health problems in universities: Comparing acceptance and commitment training to mental health education. *Journal of Clinical Psychology, 72*(3), 207–225. doi:10.1002/jclp.22254 PMID:26784010

Leviss, J., Gugerty, B., & Kaplan, B. (2010). *HIT or Miss: Lessons Learned from Health Information Technology Implementations* (2nd ed.). Chicago: AHIMA Press.

Levula, A., Wilson, A., & Harre, M. (2016). The association between social network factors and mental health at different life stages. *Quality of Life Research: An International Journal of Quality of Life Aspects of Treatment, Care and Rehabilitation, 25*(7), 1725–1733. doi:10.1007/s11136-015-1200-7 PMID:26669317

Lieberman, M. A., Goldstein, B. A., Lieberman, M. A., & Goldstein, B. A. (2006). Not all negative emotions are equal: The role of emotional expression in online support groups for women with breast cancer. *Psycho-Oncology, 15*(2), 160–168. doi:10.1002/pon.932 PMID:15880627

Lin, H. F. (2006). Understanding behavioral intention to participate in virtual communities. *Cyberpsychology & Behavior, 9*(5), 540–547. doi:10.1089/cpb.2006.9.540 PMID:17034320

Link, B. G., Phelan, J. C., Bresnahan, M., Stueve, A., & Pescosolido, B. A. (1999). Public Conceptions of Mental Illness: Labels, Causes, Dangerousness, and Social Distance. *American Journal of Public Health, 89*(9), 1328–1333. doi:10.2105/AJPH.89.9.1328 PMID:10474548

Link, B. G., Struening, E. L., Rahav, M., Phelan, J., & Nuttbrock, L. (1997). On Stigma and Its Consequences: Evidence from a Longitudinal Study of Men with Dual Diagnoses of Mental Illness and Substance Abuse. *Journal of Health and Social Behavior, 38*(2), 177–190. doi:10.2307/2955424 PMID:9212538

Loane, S. S., & DAlessandro, S. (2013). Communication that changes lives: Social support within an online health community for ALS. *Communication Quarterly, 61*(2), 236–251. doi:10.1080/01463373.2012.752397

Lomanowska, A. M., & Guitton, M. J. (2014). My avatar is pregnant! Representation of pregnancy, birth, and maternity in a virtual world. *Computers in Human Behavior, 31*, 322–331. doi:10.1016/j.chb.2013.10.058

Lund, C., Breen, A., Flisher, A. J., Kakuma, R., Corrigall, J., Joska, J. A., & Patel, V. et al. (2010). Poverty and common mental disorders in low and middle income countries: A systematic review. *Social Science & Medicine, 71*(3), 517–528. doi:10.1016/j.socscimed.2010.04.027 PMID:20621748

Ly, K. H., Trüschel, A., Jarl, L., Magnusson, S., Windahl, T., Johansson, R., & Andersson, G. et al. (2014). Behavioural activation versus mindfulness-based guided self-help treatment administered through a smartphone application: A randomised controlled trial. *BMJ Open, 4*(1), e003440. doi:10.1136/bmjopen-2013-003440 PMID:24413342

Maclure, M. (1998). Refutation in epidemiology: why else not? In K. J. Rothman (Ed.), *Causal Inference*. Chestnut Hill, PA: Epidemiology Resources.

Makai, P., Perry, M., Robben, S. H., Schers, H. J., Heinen, M. M., Rikkert, M. G. O., & Melis, R. F. (2014). Evaluation of an eHealth intervention in chronic care for frail older people: Why adherence is the first target. *Journal of Medical Internet Research, 16*(6), e156. doi:10.2196/jmir.3057 PMID:24966146

Maloney-Krichmar, D., & Preece, J. (2005). A multilevel analysis of sociability, usability, and community dynamics in an online health community. *ACM Transactions on Computer-Human Interaction, 12*(2), 201–232. doi:10.1145/1067860.1067864

ManagingLife. (2012). *Cindy's coming to terms with chronic pain.* Retrieved from https://www.managinglife.com/cindy

ManagingLife. (2016). *Manage My Pain (Version 2.63)* [Mobile Application Software]. Retrieved from https://play.google.com/store/apps/details?id=com.lcs.mmp.full&hl=en#details-reviews

Marchand, W. R. (2012). Mindfulness-based stress reduction, mindfulness-based cognitive therapy, and Zen meditation for depression, anxiety, pain, and psychological distress. *Journal of Psychiatric Practice, 18*(4), 233–252. doi:10.1097/01.pra.0000416014.53215.86 PMID:22805898

Marco Leimeister, J., Schweizer, K., Leimeister, S., & Krcmar, H. (2008). Do virtual communities matter for the social support of patients? Antecedents and effects of virtual relationships in online communities. *Information Technology & People, 21*(4), 350–374. doi:10.1108/09593840810919671

Maret, P., Vercouter, L., & El Morr, C. (2011). Special Issue on Web Intelligence and Virtual Communities. *International Journal of Networking and Virtual Organisations, 9*(3), 211–213.

Markham, A. (2004). Internet as research context. In C. Searle, G. Gobo, J. Gubrium, & D. Silverman (Eds.), *Qualitative Research Practice*. London: Sage. doi:10.4135/9781848608191.d28

Marks, J. S. (2008). *Targeting Arthritis: Improving Quality of Life for More Than 46 Million Americans*. Academic Press.

Massimi, M., Bender, J. L., Witteman, H. O., & Ahmed, O. H. (2014). Life transitions and online health communities. In *Proceedings of the 17th ACM conference on Computer supported cooperative work & social computing - CSCW '14* (pp. 1491–1501). New York: ACM Press.

Matura, L. A., McDonough, A., Aglietti, L. M., Herzog, J. L., & Gallant, K. A. (2013). A virtual community: Concerns of patients with pulmonary hypertension. *Clinical Nursing Research, 22*(2), 155–171. doi:10.1177/1054773812462867 PMID:23093554

McKenna, K. Y. A. (2008). MySpace or your place: Relationship initiation and development in the wired and wireless world. In S. Sprechter, A. Wenzel, & J. Harvey (Eds.), *Handbook of Relationship Initiation* (pp. 235–248). New York: Psychology Press.

McKinsey. (2015) *The Internet of Things: Mapping the value beyond the hype*. Author.

McMillan, D. W., & Chavis, D. M. (1986). Sense of community: A definition and theory. *Journal of Community Psychology*, *14*(1), 6–23. doi:10.1002/1520-6629(198601)14:1<6::AID-JCOP2290140103>3.0.CO;2-I

Mead, N., Varnam, R., Rogers, A., & Roland, M. (2003). What predicts patients interest in the Internet as a health resource in primary care in England? *Journal of Health Services Research & Policy*, *8*(1), 33–39. doi:10.1177/135581960300800108 PMID:12683432

Meier, A., Lyons, E. J., Frydman, G., Forlenza, M., Rimer, B. K., Meier, A., & Rimer, B. K. et al. (2007). How cancer survivors provide support on cancer-related Internet mailing lists. *Journal of Medical Internet Research*, *9*(2), e12. doi:10.2196/jmir.9.2.e12 PMID:17513283

Melzer, D., Fryers, T., & Jenkins, R. (2004). *Social inequities and the distribution of common mental disorders*. Hove: Psychology Press.

Meyerowitz, J. (1985). *No sense of place: The impact of electronic media on social behavior*. New York: Oxford University Press.

Mind. (n.d.). *Peer support: Helping each other*. Retrieved September 9, 2014 from http://www.mind.org.uk/information-support/guides-to-support-and-services/peer-support/about-peer-support/?o=10153

Mojtabai, R., & Olfson, M. (2006). Treatment seeking for depression in Canada and the United States. *Psychiatric Services (Washington, D.C.)*, *57*(5), 631–639. doi:10.1176/ps.2006.57.5.631 PMID:16675755

Moore, J. L., & Craig, E. A. (2009). Relationship development and maintenance in a wired world. In J. Park & E. Abels (Eds.), *Interpersonal relations and social patterns in communication technologies: Discourse norms, language structures and cultural variables*. Hershey, PA: IGI Global.

Morledge, T. J., Allexandre, D., Fox, E., Fu, A. Z., Higashi, M. K., Kruzikas, D. T., & Reese, P. R. et al. (2013). Feasibility of an online mindfulness program for stress management - A randomized, controlled trial. *Annals of Behavioral Medicine*, *46*(2), 137–148. doi:10.1007/s12160-013-9490-x PMID:23632913

Morris, J. (2012). *One town for my body, another for my mind*. York, UK: JRF.

Moulin, D. E., Clark, A. J., Speechley, M., & Morley-Forster, P. K. (2002). Chronic pain in Canada-prevalence, treatment, impact and the role of opioid analgesia. *Pain Research & Management*, *7*(4), 179–184. doi:10.1155/2002/323085 PMID:12518174

Mouton, A., & Cloes, M. (2015). Efficacy of a web-based, center-based or combined physical activity intervention among older adults. *Health Education Research*, *30*(3), 422–435. doi:10.1093/her/cyv012 PMID:25772974

Nahm, E. S., Resnick, B., DeGrezia, M., & Brotemarkle, R. (2009). Use of discussion boards in a theory-based health web site for older adults. *Nursing Research*, *58*(6), 419–426. doi:10.1097/NNR.0b013e3181bee6c4 PMID:19918152

Nambisan, S. (2002). Designing virtual customer environments for new product development: Toward a theory. *Academy of Management Review*, *27*(3), 392–413.

Narayan, K. M., Boyle, J. P., Thompson, T. J., Sorensen, S. W., & Williamson, D. F. (2003). Lifetime risk for diabetes mellitus in the United States. *Journal of the American Medical Association*, *290*(14), 1884–1890. doi:10.1001/jama.290.14.1884

Neal, L., Oakley, K., Lindgaard, G., Kaufman, D., Leimeister, J.M., & Selker, T. (2007) Online Health Communities. *Extended Abstracts on Human Factors in Computing Systems,* 2129-2132.

Newton, B. J., Southall, J. L., Raphael, J. H., Ashford, R. L., & LeMarchand, K. (2013). A narrative review of the impact of disbelief in chronic pain. *Pain Management Nursing*, *14*(3), 161–171. doi:10.1016/j.pmn.2010.09.001 PMID:23972867

Noelle-Neumann, E. (1974). The Spiral of Silence: A Theory of Public Opinion. *Journal of Communication*, *24*(2), 43–51. doi:10.1111/j.1460-2466.1974.tb00367.x

Nonnecke, B., & Preece, J. (2000). Lurker demographics: counting the silent. *Proceedings of the SIGCHI conference on Human Factors in Computing Systems*. Retrieved from http://dl.acm.org/citation.cfm?doid=332040.332409

Nonnecke, B., Andrews, D., & Preece, J. (2006). Non-public and public online community participation: Needs, attitudes and behavior. *Electronic Commerce Research*, *6*(1), 7–20. doi:10.1007/s10660-006-5985-x

Norman, C. D., & Skinner, H. A. (2006). eHealth Literacy: Essential Skills for Consumer Health in a Networked World. *Journal of Medical Internet Research*, *8*(2), e9. doi:10.2196/jmir.8.2.e9 PMID:16867972

O Leary, K., & Dockray, S. (2015). The effects of two novel gratitude and mindfulness interventions on well-being. *Journal of Alternative and Complementary Medicine (New York, N.Y.)*, *21*(4), 243–245. doi:10.1089/acm.2014.0119 PMID:25826108

O'Grady, L., Bender, J., Urowitz, S., Wiljer, D., & Jadad, A. R. (2010). Promoting and participating in online health forums : A guide to facilitation and evaluation for health professionals. *Journal of Communication*, *3*(3), 246–258.

O'Reilly, T. (n.d.). *What Is Web 2.0? 7. Rich User Experiences*. Retrieved January 29, 2017, from http://www.oreilly.com/pub/a/web2/archive/what-is-web-20.html?page=5

Ogden, C. L., Carroll, M. D., & Fryar, C. D. (2015). *Prevalence of Obesity Among Adults and Youth: United States, 2011–2014*. Retrieved from https://www.cdc.gov/nchs/data/databriefs/db219.pdf

OGrady, L. A., Bender, J. L., Uroowitz, S., Wiljer, D., & Jadad, A. R. (2010). Promoting and participating in online health forums: A guide to facilitation and evaluation for health professionals. *Journal of Community Health*, *3*(4), 246–257. doi:10.1179/175380710X12870623776478

Orgad, S. (2006). The cultural dimensions of online communities: A study of breast cancer internet spaces. *New Media & Society*, *8*(6), 877–899. doi:10.1177/1461444806069643

Organization, W. H. (2000). World Health Organization disabilty assessment schedule: WHODAS II. Phase 2 field trials. *Health Services Research.*

Ortman, J. M., Velkoff, V. A., & Hogan, H. (2014). An Aging Nation: The Older Population in the United States. Retrieved from https://www.census.gov/prod/2014pubs/p25-1140.pdf

Ostrum, L., Wilhelmsen, C., & Kaplan, B. (1993). Assessing Safety Culture. *Nuclear Safety*, *34*(2), 163–172.

O'Sullivan, P. B. (2000). What you don't know won't hurt me: Impression management functions of communication channels in relationships. *Human Communication Research*, *26*, 403–431.

OToole, L. J. (2000). Research on policy implementation: Assessment and prospects. *Journal of Public Administration: Research and Theory*, *10*(2), 263–288. doi:10.1093/oxfordjournals.jpart.a024270

OToole, L. J. (2004). The Theory-Practice Issue in Policy Implementation Research. *Public Administration*, *82*(2), 309–329. doi:10.1111/j.0033-3298.2004.00396.x

Pagliari, C., Sloan, D., Gregor, P., Sullivan, F., Detmer, D., Kahan, J. P., & MacGillivray, S. et al. (2005). What is e-Health. A Scoping Exercise to Map the Field. *Journal of Medical Internet Research*, *7*(1), e9. doi:10.2196/jmir.7.1.e9 PMID:15829481

Pan-Canadian Clinical Interoperability Steering Committee. (2015). *Clinical Interoperability Action Plan & Notes May 2015*. Retrieved February 28, 2017, from https://ic.infoway-inforoute.ca/en/resources/docs/cistratdocs/254-clinical-interoperability-action-plan-notes-may-2015/file

Pearson, C., Janz, T., & Ali, J. (2013). *Mental and substance use disorders in Canada: health at a glance.* Statistics Canada catalogue no. 82-624-X.

Pecchioni, L. L., Wright, K. B., & Nussbaum, J. F. (2005). *Life-span communication.* Mahwah, NJ: Lawrence Erlbaum Associates.

Pennebaker, J. W. (1999). Psychological factors influencing the reporting of physical symptoms. In A. Stone, J. Turkkan, C. Bachrach, J. Jobe, H. Kurtzman, & V. Cain (Eds.), *The science of self-report: Implications for research and practice* (pp. 299–316). Mahwah, NJ: Erlbaum.

Pennebaker, J. W., & Chung, C. K. (2010). Expressive writing, emotional upheavals, and health. In J. F. Evans (Ed.), *Wellness and writing connections: Writing for better physical, mental, and spiritual health.* Enumclaw, WA: Idyll Arbor, Inc.

Pennebaker, J. W., Kiecolt-Glaser, J. K., & Glaser, R. (1988). Disclosure of traumas and Narrative & Satisfaction, 16 immune function: Health implications for psychotherapy. *Journal of Consulting and Clinical Psychology, 56*, 239–245. doi:10.1037/0022-006X.56.2.239 PMID:3372832

Pennebaker, J. W., & Seagal, J. D. (1999). Forming a story: The health benefits of narrative. *Journal of Clinical Psychology, 55*(10), 1243–1254. doi:10.1002/(SICI)1097-4679(199910)55:10<1243::AID-JCLP6>3.0.CO;2-N PMID:11045774

Pescosolido, B., Martin, J., Long, J., Medina, T., Phelan, J., & Link, B. (2010). A disease like any other? A decade of change in public reactions to schizophrenia, depression, and alcohol dependence. *The American Journal of Psychiatry, 167*(11), 1321–1330. doi:10.1176/appi.ajp.2010.09121743 PMID:20843872

Pewdwell, T. (2016). CRTC declares broadband internet a basic service. *The Toronto Star.*

Pfeil, U., Zaphiris, P., & Wilson, S. (2010). The role of message-sequences in the sustainability of an online support community for older people. *Journal of Computer-Mediated Communication, 15*(2), 336–363. doi:10.1111/j.1083-6101.2010.01523.x

Phillips, W. (2015). *This Is Why We Can't Have Nice Things: Mapping the Relationship Between Online Trolling and Mainstream Culture*. Cambridge, MA: MIT Press.

Pinfold, V., Sweet, D., Porter, I., Quinn, C., Byng, R., Griffiths, C., ... Huxley, P. (2015). Improving community health networks for people with severe mental illness: a case study investigation. *Health Serv Deliv Res, 3*(5).

Pingree, S., Hawkins, R., Baker, T., duBenske, L., Roberts, L. J., & Gustafson, D. H. (2010). The value of theory for enhancing and understanding e-health interventions. *American Journal of Preventive Medicine, 38*(1), 103–109. doi:10.1016/j.amepre.2009.09.035 PMID:20117565

Pitts, V. (2004). Illness and internet empowerment: Writing and reading breast cancer in cyberspace. *Health, 8*(1), 33–59. doi:10.1177/1363459304038794 PMID:15018717

Polk, K., Schoendorff, B., Webster, M., & Olaz, F. (2016). *The Essential Guide to the ACT Matrix: A Step-by-Step Approach to Using the ACT Matrix Model in Clinical Practice*. Oakland, CA: New Harbinger Publications, Inc.

Porter, C. (2004). A typology of virtual communities: A multi-disciplinary foundation for future research. *Journal of Computer-Mediated Communication, 10*(1).

Porter, C. E. (2004). A Typology of Virtual Communities: A Multi-Disciplinary Foundation for Future Research. *Journal of Computer-Mediated Communication.*

Preece, J. (2000). *Online Communities. Designing Usability, Supporting Sociability*. Chichester, UK: Wiley.

Preece, J. (2000). *Online Communities: Designing Usability supporting Sociability*. John Wiley & Sons Ltd.

Preece, J. (2000). *Online communities: Designing usability supporting sociability*. New York: John Wiley & Sons Ltd.

Preece, J. (2001). Sociability and usability in online communities: Determining and measurign success. *Behaviour & Information Technology*, *20*(5), 347–356. doi:10.1080/01449290110084683

Putnam, R. D. (2000). *Bowling alone: The collapse and revival of American community*. New York: Simon & Schuster. doi:10.1145/358916.361990

Rafaeli, S., Ravid, G., & Soroka, V. (2004). *De-lurking in virtual communities: A social communication network approach to measuring the effects of social and cultural capital*. Paper presented at the 37th annual Hawaii international conference on system sciences. doi:10.1109/HICSS.2004.1265478

Rafferty, R. (2011). *Motivations Behind Cyber Bulling and Online Aggression: Cyber Sanctions, Dominance, and Trolling Online*. Retrieved on May 15, 2017, from https://etd.ohiolink.edu/

Rahman, Q. A., Pirbaglou, M., Janmohamed, T., Ritvo, P., Heffernan, D., Clarke, H., & Katz, J. (2017). *Data mining to determine patterns of user engagement with Manage My Pain, an mHealth App for Chronic Pain*. Manuscript submitted.

Ranmuthugala, Plumb, Cunningham, Georgiou, Westbrook, & Braithwaite. (2011). How and why are communities of practice established in the healthcare sector? A systematic review of the literature. *BMC Health Services Research, 11*(273).

Redelmeier, D. A., Katz, J., & Kahneman, D. (2003). Memories of colonoscopy: A randomized trial. *Pain, 104*(1), 187–194. doi:10.1016/S0304-3959(03)00003-4 PMID:12855328

Reed, M., Larwood, D., Lindop, C., Macerola, B., & Picton, P. (2016). *Cross Enterprise Remote Reading Clinical Requirements*. Retrieved February 28, 2017, from https://ic.infoway-inforoute.ca/en/resources/docs/imagingdocs/736-cross-enterprise-remote-reading-clinical-requirements-26aug15

Ren, Y., Harper, F. M., Drenner, S., Terveen, L., Kiesler, S., Riedl, J., & Kraut, R. E. (2012). Building member attachment in online communities: Applying theories of group identity and interpersonal bonds. *Management Information Systems Quarterly, 36*(3), 841–864.

Rheingold, H. (1994). *The virtual community: Finding connection in a computerized world*. London: Secker & Warburg.

Rheingold, H. (2000). *The Virtual Community: Homesteading on the Electronic Frontier*. Cambridge, MA: MIT Press.

Richardson, L-J. (2015). Micro-blogging and Online Community. *Internet Archaeology,* 39.

Richardson, C. R., Buis, L. R., Janney, A. W., Goodrich, D. E., Sen, A., Hess, M. L., & Strecher, V. J. et al. (2010). An online community improves adherence in an internet-mediated walking program. Part 1: Results of a randomized controlled trial. *Journal of Medical Internet Research*, *12*(4), e71. doi:10.2196/jmir.1338 PMID:21169160

Ridings, C. M., & Gefen, D. (2004). Virtual community attraction: Why people hang out online. *Journal of Computer-Mediated Communication*, *10*(1). Retrieved from http://jcmc.indiana.edu/vol10/issue1/ridings_gefen.html

Rodham, K., McCabe, C., & Blake, D. (2009). Seeking support: An interpretative phenomenological analysis of an Internet message board for people with Complex Regional Pain Syndrome. *Psychology & Health*, *24*(6), 619–634. doi:10.1080/08870440802563245 PMID:20205016

Röll, M. (2004). Distributed KM – improving knowledge worker's productivity and organizational knowledge sharing with weblog-based personal publishing. *BlogTalk 2.0 – The European Conference on Weblogs*. Retrieved from http://www.roell.net/publikationen/distributedkm.pdf

Rubin, J., & Chisnell, D. (2008). *Handbook of usability testing: how to plan, design and conduct effective tests*. Hoboken, NJ: John Wiley & Sons.

Russek, L. G., & Schwartz, G. E. (1997). Feelings of parental caring predict health status in midlife: A 35-year follow-up of the Harvard Mastery Study of Stress. *Journal of Behavioral Medicine*, *30*(1), 1–13. doi:10.1023/A:1025525428213 PMID:9058175

Ryff, C. D., & Singer, B. H. (2008). Know thyself and become what you are: An eudemonic approach to psychological wellbieng. *Journal of Happiness Studies*, *9*(1), 13–39. doi:10.1007/s10902-006-9019-0

Rysman, M. (2009). The economics of two-sided markets. *The Journal of Economic Perspectives*, *23*(3), 125–144. doi:10.1257/jep.23.3.125

Salzer, M. S., Palmer, S. C., Kaplan, K., Brusilovskiy, E., Ten Have, T., Hampshire, M., & Coyne, J. C. et al. (2010). A randomized, controlled study of Internet peer-to-peer interactions among women newly diagnosed with breast cancer. *Psycho-Oncology*, *19*(4), 441–446. doi:10.1002/pon.1586 PMID:19484712

Sandaunet, A. G., & Sandaunet, A.-G. (2008). The challenge of fitting in: Non-participation and withdrawal from an online self-help group for breast cancer patients. *Sociology of Health & Illness*, *30*(1), 131–144. doi:10.1111/j.1467-9566.2007.01041.x PMID:18254837

Sandaunet, A.-G. (2008). A space for suffering? Communicating breast cancer in an online self-help context. *Qualitative Health Research*, *18*(12), 1631–1641. doi:10.1177/1049732308327076 PMID:18955462

Scascighini, L., Toma, V., & Sprott, H. (2008). *Multidisciplinary treatment for chronic pain: A systematic review of interventions and outcomes*. 10.1093/rheumatology/ken021

Schiel, T. (2005). Modernity, Ambivalence and the Gardening State. *Thesis Eleven, 83*, 78 -89

Schmalensee, R., & Evans, D. S. (2007). The industrial organization of two-sided platforms. *Competition Policy Int.*, *3*(1), 151–179.

Schneider, A., von Krogh, G., & Jager, P. (2013). Whats coming next? Epistemic curiosity and lurking behaviour in online communities. *Computers in Human Behavior*, *29*(1), 293–303. doi:10.1016/j.chb.2012.09.008

Schneiderman, B. (2003). *Leonardo's laptop: Human needs and the new computing technologies*. Cambridge, MA: The MIT Press.

Schomerus, G., Angemeyer, M. C., Baumeister, S. E., Stolzenberg, S., Link, B. G., & Phelan, J. C. (2016). An online intervention using information on the mental health-mental illness continuum to reduce stigma. *European Psychiatry*, *32*, 21–27. doi:10.1016/j.eurpsy.2015.11.006 PMID:26802980

Schopflocher, D., Taenzer, P., & Jovey, R. (2011). The prevalence of chronic pain in Canada. *Pain Research & Management: The Journal of the Canadian Pain Society = Journal de La Société Canadienne Pour Le Traitement de La Douleur, 16*(6), 445–50. Retrieved from http://www.pubmedcentral.nih.gov/articlerender.fcgi?artid=3298051&tool=pmcentrez&rendertype=abstract

Schork, N. J. (2015). Personalized medicine: Time for one-person trials. *Nature*, *520*(7549), 609–611. doi:10.1038/520609a PMID:25925459

Schubert, P., & Hampe, J. F. (2005). *Business Models for Mobile Communities*. Paper presented at the 38th Annual Hawaii International Conference on System Sciences(HICSS '05). doi:10.1109/HICSS.2005.132

Seale, C., Anderson, E., & Kinnersley, P. (2006). Treatment advice in primary care: A comparative study of nurse practitioners and general practitioners. *Journal of Advanced Nursing*, *54*(5), 534–541. doi:10.1111/j.1365-2648.2006.03865.x PMID:16722950

Segrin, C. (1998). Disrupted interpersonal relationships and mental health problems. In B. H. Spitzberg & W. R. Cupach (Eds.), *The dark side of close relationships* (pp. 327–365). Mahwah, NJ: Erlbaum.

Sharf, B. F. (1997). Communicating breast cancer on-line: Support and empowerment on the Internet. *Women & Health*, *26*(1), 65–84. doi:10.1300/J013v26n01_05 PMID:9311100

Siddall, P. J., & Cousins, M. (2004). *Persistent pain as a disease entity: Implications for clinical management*. 10.1213/01.ANE.0000133383.17666.3A

Simco, R., McCusker, J., & Sewitch, M. (2014). Adherence to self-care interventions for depression or anxiety: A systematic review. *Health Education Journal*, *73*(6), 714–730. doi:10.1177/0017896913514738

Singh, M., & Waddell, D. (2004). *E-business Innovation and Change Management*. IRM Press. doi:10.4018/978-1-59140-138-4

Slatcher, R. B., & Pennebaker, J. W. (2007). Emotional expression and health. In S. Ayers, A. Baum, C. McManus, S. Newman, K. Wallston, J. Weinman, & R. West (Eds.), *Cambridge Handbook of Psychology, Health & Medicine* (2nd ed.; pp. 84–86). Cambridge, UK: Cambridge University Press. doi:10.1017/CBO9780511543579.019

Slevin, J. (2000). The Internet and Society. Cornwall, UK: Polity Press.

Smit, W., van Uden-Kraan, C. F., Drossaert, C. H. C., Seydel, E. R., Taal, E., & Van der Laar, M. (2007). Patients with breast cancer feel empowered by their participation in online support groups. In *Proceedings of the American Society for Clinical Oncology (ASCO) Conference*. Chicago: ASCO Press.

SNOMED International. (2017). *What is SNOMED CT?*. Retrieved February 28, 2017, from http://www.snomed.org/snomed-ct/what-is-snomed-ct

Snyder, D. K., Gordon, K., & Baucom, D. H. (2004). Treating affair couples. Extending the written disclosure paradigm to relationship trauma. *Clinical Psychology: Science and Practice*, *11*(2), 155–159. doi:10.1093/clipsy.bph066

Spiegel, D., & Classen, C. (2000). *Group therapy for cancer patients*. New York: Basic Books.

Star, S. (1955, November). *The public's ideas about mental illness*. Paper presented at the Annual Meeting of the National Association for Mental Health, Indianapolis, IN.

Statistics Canada. (2012). *Canadian Internet Use Survey, 2012*. Author.

Statistics Canada. (2015). *Canada's population estimates: Age and sex, July 1, 2015*. Retrieved from http://www.statcan.gc.ca/daily-quotidien/150929/dq150929b-eng.htm

Steffens, N. K., Haslam, S. A., Schuh, S. C., Jetten, J., & van Dick, R. (2016). A Meta-Analytic review of social identification and health in organizational contexts. *Personality and Social Psychology Review*. https://doi.org/10.1177/1088868316656701

Stellefson, M., Chaney, B., Barry, A. E., Chavarria, E., Tennant, B., Walsh-Childers, K., & Zagora, J. et al. (2013). Web 2.0 chronic disease self-management for older adults: A systematic review. *Journal of Medical Internet Research*, *15*(2), e35. doi:10.2196/jmir.2439 PMID:23410671

Steptoe, A., Shankar, A., Demakakos, P., & Wardle, J. (2013). Social isolation, loneliness, and all-cause mortality in older men and women. *Proceedings of the National Academy of Sciences of the United States of America*, *110*(15), 5797–5801. doi:10.1073/pnas.1219686110 PMID:23530191

Subercaze, J., El Morr, C., Maret, P., Joly, A., Koivisto, M., Antoniadis, P., & Ihara, M. (2009). Towards Successful Virtual Communities. In J. Filipe & J. Cordeiro (Eds.), *Enterprise Information Systems: 11th International Conference, ICEIS 2009* (*Vol. 24*, pp. 677-688). Milan, Italy: Springer Berlin Heidelberg.

Suler, J. (2004). The online disinhibition effect. *Cyberpsychology & Behavior*, *7*(3), 321–326. doi:10.1089/1094931041291295 PMID:15257832

Sullivan, C. F. (2003). Gendered cybersupport: A thematic analysis of two online cancer support groups. *Journal of Health Psychology*, *8*(1), 83–103. doi:10.1177/1359105303008001446 PMID:22113903

Sum, S., Mathews, R. M., Pourghasem, M., & Hughes, I. (2009). Internet use as a predictor of sense of community in older people. *Cyberpsychology & Behavior*, *12*(2), 235–239. doi:10.1089/cpb.2008.0150 PMID:19250013

Szasz, T. S. (1961). The uses of naming and the origin of the myth of mental illness. *The American Psychologist*, *16*(2), 59–65. doi:10.1037/h0040842

Tajfel, H., & Turner, J. C. (1979). An integrative theory of intergroup conflict. In W. G. Austin & S. Worchel (Eds.), *The Social Psychology of Intergroup Relations* (pp. 33–47). Monterey, CA: Brooks/Cole.

Tanis, M. (2008). Health-related on-line forums: Whats the big attraction? *Journal of Health Communication*, *13*(7), 698–714. doi:10.1080/10810730802415316 PMID:18958781

Tate, D. F., & Zabinski, M. F. (2004). Computer and Internet applications for psychological treatment: Update for clinicians. *Journal of Clinical Psychology*, *60*(2), 209–220. doi:10.1002/jclp.10247 PMID:14724928

Taylor, S. E. (1983). Adjustment to threatening events: A theory of cognitive adaptation. *The American Psychologist*, *38*(11), 1161–1173. doi:10.1037/0003-066X.38.11.1161

Taylor, S. E., & Lobel, M. (1989). Social comparison activity under threat: Downward evaluation and upward contacts. *Psychological Review*, *96*(4), 569–575. doi:10.1037/0033-295X.96.4.569 PMID:2678204

Taylor, S., & Todd, P. A. (1995). Assessing IT usage: A test of competing models. *Information Systems Research*, *6*, 144–176. doi:10.1287/isre.6.2.144

Temesgen, Z., Knappe-Langworthy, J. E., St Marie, M. M., Smith, B. A., & Dierkhising, R. A. (2006). Comprehensive Health Enhancement Support System (CHESS) for people with HIV infection. *AIDS and Behavior*, *10*(1), 35–40. doi:10.1007/s10461-005-9026-x PMID:16400508

The National Academies Press. (2011). *Relieving Pain in America: A Blueprint for Transforming Prevention, Care, Education, and Research*. Washington, DC: The National Academies Press.

Third, A., Forrest-Lawrence, P., & Collier, A. (2014). *Addressing the cyber-safety challenge*. Retrieved September 7, 2015, from https://www.telstra.com.au/content/dam/tcom/about-us/community-environment/pdf/cyber-safety-challenge-risk-resillience.pdf

Tracey, I., & Bushnell, M. C. (2009). How neuroimaging studies have challenged us to rethink: Is chronic pain a disease? *The Journal of Pain*, *10*(11), 1113–1120. doi:10.1016/j.jpain.2009.09.001 PMID:19878862

Treede, R., Rief, W., Barke, A., Aziz, Q., Bennett, M. I., Benoliel, R., ... Wang, S. (2015). *A classification of chronic pain for ICD-11*. Academic Press.

Turk, D. C., Dworkin, R. H., Allen, R. R., Bellamy, N., Brandenburg, N., Carr, D. B., & Galer, B. S. et al. (2003). Core outcome domains for chronic pain clinical trials: IMMPACT recommendations. *Pain*, *106*(3), 337–345. doi:10.1016/j.pain.2003.08.001 PMID:14659516

Uchino, B. N. (2004). *Social support and physical health: Understanding the health consequences of relationships*. New Haven, CT: Yale University Press. doi:10.12987/yale/9780300102185.001.0001

Uchino, B. N. (2006). Social support and health: A review of physiological processes potentially underlying links to disease outcomes. *Journal of Behavioral Medicine*, *29*(4), 377–387. doi:10.1007/s10865-006-9056-5 PMID:16758315

Uchino, B. N., Cacioppo, J. T., & Kiercolt-Glaser, J. K. (1996). The relationship between social support and physiological processes: A review with emphasis on underlying mechanisms and implications for health. *Psychological Bulletin*, *119*(3), 488–531. doi:10.1037/0033-2909.119.3.488 PMID:8668748

Usability of consumer products and products for public use - Part 2: Summative test method. (1998). Retrieved from https://www.iso.org/obp/ui/#iso:std:iso:ts:20282:-2:ed-2:v1:en

Ussher, J., Kirsten, L., Butow, P., & Sandoval, M. (2006). What do cancer support groups provide which other supportive relationships do not? The experience of peer support groups for people with cancer. *Social Science & Medicine*, *62*(10), 2565–2576. doi:10.1016/j.socscimed.2005.10.034 PMID:16303220

van der Eijk, M., Faber, M. J., Aarts, J. W., Kremer, J. A., Munneke, M., & Bloem, B. R. (2013). Using online health communities to deliver patient-centered care to people with chronic conditions. *Journal of Medical Internet Research*, *15*(6), e115. doi:10.2196/jmir.2476 PMID:23803284

van Uden-Kraan, C. F., Drossaert, C. H. C., Taal, E., Seydel, E. R., & van de Laar, M. A. F. (2010). Patient-intitated online support groups: Motives for initation, extent of success and success factors. *Journal of Telemedicine and Telecare*, *16*(1), 30–34. doi:10.1258/jtt.2009.001009 PMID:20086265 van Uden-Kraan, C. F., Drossaert, C. H. C., Taal, E., Smit, W. M., Moens, H. J. B., Siesling, S., & van de Laar, M. A. F. J. et al. (2009). Health-related Internet use by patients with somatic diseases: Frequency of use and characteristics of users. *Informatics for Health & Social Care, 34*(1), 18–29. doi:10.1080/17538150902773272 PMID:19306196

van Uden-Kraan, C. F., Drossaert, C. H., Taal, E., Seydel, E. R., van de Laar, M. A., van Uden-Kraan, C. F., & van de Laar, M. A. F. J. et al. (2008). Self-reported differences in empowerment between lurkers and posters in online patient support groups. *Journal of Medical Internet Research, 10*(2), e18. doi:10.2196/jmir.992 PMID:18653442

van Uden-Kraan, C. F., Drossaert, C. H., Taal, E., Shaw, B. R., Seydel, E. R., van de Laar, M. A., & van de Laar, M. A. F. J. (2008). Empowering processes and outcomes of participation in online support groups for patients with breast cancer, arthritis, or fibromyalgia. *Qualitative Health Research, 18*(3), 405–417. doi:10.1177/1049732307313429 PMID:18235163

Vasconcellos-Silva, P. R., Carvalho, D., & Lucena, C. (2013). Word frequency and content analysis approach to identify demand patterns in a virtual community of carriers of Hepatitis C. *Interactive Journal of Medical Research, 2*(2), e12. doi:10.2196/ijmr.2384 PMID:23827772

Veldel, I., Akhlaghpour, S., Vaghefi, I., Bergman, H., & Lapointe, L. (2013). Health information technologies in geriatrics and gerontology: A mixed systematic review. *Journal of the American Medical Informatics Association, 20*(6), 1109–1119. doi:10.1136/amiajnl-2013-001705 PMID:23666776

Veroff, J., Kulka, R. A., & Douvan, E. (1981). *Mental health in America: Patterns of help-seeking from 1957-1976*. New York: Basic Books.

Vilhauer, R. P., & Vilhauer, R. P. (2009). Perceived benefits of online support groups for women with metastatic breast cancer. *Women & Health, 49*(5), 381–404. doi:10.1080/03630240903238719 PMID:19851944

Vimarlund, V. (Ed.). (2016). E-Health Two-sided markets. Academic Press.

Vimarlund, V., & Keller, C. (2014). The many faces of implementation. Vinnova Report 2014:06.

Vimarlund, V., Timpka, T., & Patel, V. (1999). Information Technology and Knowledge Exchange in Health-Care Organizations. *Proceedings of AMIA*, 632-636.

Vimarlund. (2011). *Att fånga nyttan av IT-investeringar inom vård och omsorg.En analysmodell förplanering och uppföljning av IT-investeringar- ehälsonätverk*. Forskningsrapport. (in Swedish)

Vimarlund, V., Davoody, N., & Koch, S. (2013). Steps to consider for effective decision making when selecting and prioritizing eHealth services. *Studies in Health Technology and Informatics, 192*, 239–243. PMID:23920552

Vimarlund, V., & Koch, S. (2012). *Identifying where the values come from IT-innovations in health and social care*. Intelligent Information Management.

Vivar, C. G., & McQueen, A. (2005). Informational and emotional needs of long-term survivors of breast cancer. *Journal of Advanced Nursing*, *51*(5), 520–528. doi:10.1111/j.1365-2648.2005.03524.x PMID:16098169

Vowles, K. E., Fink, B. C., & Cohen, L. L. (2014). Acceptance and Commitment Therapy for chronic pain: A diary study of treatment process in relation to reliable change in disability. *Journal of Contextual Behavioral Science*, *3*(2), 74–80. doi:10.1016/j.jcbs.2014.04.003 PMID:27818931

Wagner, C., & Bolloju, N. (2005). Supporting knowledge management in organizations with conversational technologies: Discussion forums, weblogs, and wikis. *Journal of Database Management*, *16*(2), 1–8.

Wall, P. D., & Jones, M. (1991). Defeating pain: The war against a silent epidemic. New York: Plenum Press.

Walther, J. B., Pingree, S., Hawkins, R. P., Buller, D. B., Walther, J. B., Pingree, S., & Buller, D. B. et al. (2005). Attributes of interactive online health information systems. *Journal of Medical Internet Research*, *7*(3), e33. doi:10.2196/jmir.7.3.e33 PMID:15998624

Webb, T. L., Joseph, J., Yardley, L., Michie, S., Webb, T. L., Joseph, J., … Michie, S. (n.d.). Using the internet to promote health behavior change: A systematic review and meta-analysis of the impact of theoretical basis, use of behavior change techniques, and mode of delivery on efficacy. *Journal of Medical Internet Research, 12*(1), e4.

Weinrib, A. (2016). *Manage My Pain*. Retrieved from https://www.managinglife.com/faq?id=9

Weinrib, A. Z., Azam, M. A., Birnie, K., Burns, L. C., Clarke, H., & Katz, J. (2017). (in press). The psychology of persisting post-surgical pain: New frontiers in risk factor identification, prevention, and management. *British Journal of Pain*.

Weissman, D. (2000). *A social ontology*. Yale University Press.

Weiss, R. (1974). The provisions of social relationships. In *Doing unto others*. Prentice Hall.

Welbourne, J. L., Blanchard, A. L., & Wadsworth, M. B. (2013). Motivation in virtual health communities and their relationship to community, connectedness and stress. *Computers in Human Behavior*, *29*(1), 129–139. doi:10.1016/j.chb.2012.07.024

White, K. M., Starfelt, L. C., Young, R. M., Hawkes, A. L., Cleary, C., Leske, S., & Wihardjo, K. (2015). A randomised controlled trial of an online theory-based intervention to improve adult Australians sun-protective behaviours. *Preventive Medicine*, *72*, 19–22. doi:10.1016/j.ypmed.2014.12.025 PMID:25572618

WHO European Region. (2016). *From innovation to implementation – eHealth in the WHO European Region*. Author.

WHO. (2005). *Promoting mental health.* Retrieved August 8, 2016, from http://www.who.int/mental_health/evidence/MH_Promotion_Book.pdf

WHO. (2015). *Global health workforce, finances remain low for mental health.* World Health Organization. Retrieved January 11, 2017, from http://www.who.int/mediacentre/news/notes/2015/finances-mental-health/en/

Whybrow, P., & Heyes, K. (2016). *Caring for Carers.* Research report. Retrieved from Cost of Living Official URL: http://www.cost-ofliving.net/caring-for-carers/

Williams, J. M. G., Teasdale, J. D., Segal, Z. V., & Kabat-Zinn, J. (2007). *The mindful way through depression: Freeing yourself from chronic unhappiness.* New York: The Guilford Press.

Winzelberg, A. J., Classen, C., Alpers, G. W., Roberts, H., Koopman, C., Adams, R. E., & Taylor, C. B. et al. (2003). Evaluation of an internet support group for women with primary breast cancer. *Cancer, 97*(5), 1164–1173. doi:10.1002/cncr.11174 PMID:12599221

Wittel, A. (2001). Toward a network sociality. *Theory, Culture & Society, 18*(6), 51–76. doi:10.1177/02632760122052048

Wolever, R. Q., Bobinet, K. J., McCabe, K., Mackenzie, E. R., Fekete, E., Kusnick, C., & Baime, M. (2012). Effective and viable mind-body stress reductin in the workplace: A randomized controlled trial. *Journal of Occupational Health Psychology, 17*(2), 246–258. doi:10.1037/a0027278 PMID:22352291

Wood, J. T. (2000). *Relational communication: Continuity and change in personal relationships.* Belmont, CA: Wadsworth.

Wood, J. V. (1989). Theory and research concerning social comparisons of personal attributes. *Psychological Bulletin, 106*(2), 231–248. doi:10.1037/0033-2909.106.2.231

Woong Yun, G., & Park, S.-Y. (2011). Selective posting: Willingness to post a message online. *Journal of Computer-Mediated Communication, 16*(2), 201–227. doi:10.1111/j.1083-6101.2010.01533.x

World Health Organization and the Calouste Gulbenkian Foundation. (2014). *Social determinants of mental health.* Geneva: World Health Organization.

World Health Organization. (2005). *Preventing Chronic Disease: A Vital Investment.* Geneva, Switzerland: WHO.

World Health Organization. (2015). *WHO | Cancer Fact Sheet Number 297.* WHO.

World Health Organization. (2017). *Depression and other common mental disorders: Global health estimates.* Geneva: World Health Organization.

World Wide Web Consortium. (2000). *A Little History of the World Wide Web.* Retrieved from https://www.w3.org/History.html

Wright, K. (2002). Social support within an online cancer community: An assessment of emotional support, perceptions of advantages and disadvantage, and motives for using the community from a communication perspective. *Journal of Applied Communication Research*, *30*(3), 195–209. doi:10.1080/00909880216586

Wright, K. B. (2004). On-line relational maintenance strategies and perceptions of partners within exclusively internet-based and primarily internet-based relationships. *Communication Studies*, *55*(2), 239–253. doi:10.1080/10510970409388617

Wright, K. B., Bell, S. B., Wright, K. B., & Bell, S. B. (2003). Health-related Support Groups on the Internet: Linking Empirical Findings to Social Support and Computer-mediated Communication Theory. *Journal of Health Psychology*, *8*(1), 39–54. doi:10.1177/1359105303008001429 PMID:22113899

Wright, K. B., & Miller, C. H. (2010). A measure of weak-tie / strong-tie support network preference. *Communication Monographs*, *77*(4), 502–520. doi:10.1080/03637751.2010.502538

Wright, K. B., & Muhtaseb, A. (2011). Personal relationships and computer mediated support groups. In K. B. Wright & L. M. Webb (Eds.), *Computer-mediated communication in personal relationships*. New York: Peter Lang.

Würtzen, H., Dalton, S. O., Christensen, J., Andersen, K. K., Elsass, P., Flyger, H. L., & Johansen, C. et al. (2015). Effect of mindfulness-based stress reduction on somatic symptoms, distress, mindfulness and spiritual wellbeing in women with breast cancer: Results of a randomized controlled trial. *Acta Oncologica*, *54*(5), 712–719. doi:10.3109/0284186X.2014.997371 PMID:25752972

Xu, Y., & Burleson, B. R. (2001). Effects of sex, culture, and support type on perceptions of spousal social support: An assessment of the support gap hypothesis in early marriage. *Human Communication Research*, *24*(4), 535–566. doi:10.1111/j.1468-2958.2001.tb00792.x

Yach, D., Leeder, S. R., Bell, J., & Kistnasamy, B. (2005). Global Chronic Diseases. *Science*, *307*(5708), 317. doi:10.1126/science.307.5708.317 PMID:15661976

Yalom, I. (1995). *Theory and practice of group pscyhotherapy*. New York: Basic Books.

Yalom, I., & Leszcz, M. (2005). *Theory and Practice of Group Psychotherapy* (5th ed.). New York: Basic Books.

Yamasaki, J. (2016). Communicating health and connection in supportive communities. In J. Yamasaki, P. Geist-Martin, & B. F. Sharf (Eds.), *Storied health and illness: Communicating personal, cultural, and political complexities*. Long Grove, IL: Waveland Press.

Yeo, A., Legard, R., Keegan, J., Ward, K., McNaughton Nicholls, C., & Lewis, J. (2014). In-Depth Interviews. In J. Ritchie, J. Lewis, C. McNaughton Nicholls, & R. Ormston (Eds.), *A Guide for Social Science Students and Researchers*. London: SAGE.

Young, C. (2013). Community management that works: How to build and sustain a thriving online health community. *Journal of Medical Internet Research*, *15*(6), e119. doi:10.2196/jmir.2501 PMID:23759312

Yuill, C., Crinson, I., & Duncan, E. (2010). *Key concepts in health studies*. London: SAGE Publications Ltd. doi:10.4135/9781446251676

Zabora, J., BrintzenhofeSzoc, K., Curbow, B., Hooker, C., & Piantadosi, S. (2001). The prevalence of psychological distress by cancer site. *Psycho-Oncology*, *10*(1), 19–28. doi:10.1002/1099-1611(200101/02)10:1<19::AID-PON501>3.0.CO;2-6 PMID:11180574

Zhang, X., Guo, X., Lai, K. H., Guo, F., & Li, C. (2014). Understanding gender differences in m-health adoption: A modified theory of reasoned action model. *Telemedicine Journal and e-Health*, *20*(1), 39–46. doi:10.1089/tmj.2013.0092 PMID:24161004

Zhou, T., Li, X., Pei, Y., Gao, J., & Kong, J. (2016). Internet-based cognitive behavioural therapy for subthreshold depression: A systematic review and meta-analysis. *BMC Psychiatry*, *16*(1), 356. doi:10.1186/s12888-016-1061-9 PMID:27769266

About the Contributors

Christo El Morr is a Health Informatics researcher at the school of Health Policy and Management at York University. His cross-disciplinary research covers health informatics and health services. His research interests focus on Health Virtual Communities, e-Collaboration, particularly in the domain of Chronic Disease Management and health promotion: Peripheral Arterial Disease, Kidney Diseases and Mental Health. He also has research interests in Global eHealth and equity, Hospital Patient Services and Patient Quality of Care (e.g. readmission patterns). He has published books, chapters, and articles in these areas. He received funds from the Ontario Center of Excellence (OCE) and the Canadian Institute for Health Research (CIHR) and is a Research Scientist at North York General Hospital. In 2016, he received a recognition as York University Research Leader.

* * *

Farah Ahmad is a health services researcher with a focus on psychosocial health, vulnerable communities, primary care and eHealth innovations. She has training in medicine (Punjab University) and a master's (Harvard University) and doctorate (University of Toronto) in public health sciences. She applies health promotion and equity perspective in her research to understand and improve health and health care systems.

Muhammad Abid Azam is a doctoral candidate in the Clinical Psychology program at York University. He specializes in health psychology and mindfulness and acceptance-based interventions for chronic pain. He is currently working at the Toronto General Hospital Transitional Pain Service developing interventions based on Acceptance & Commitment Therapy and mindfulness meditation to prevent and manage chronic pain and opioid misuse after surgery.

Elisabeth Beaunoyer is a PhD candidate at Laval University, interested in how new technologies and virtual spaces can be used to answer the needs of aged people. Her research interest also includes health literacy and mental health literacy – the subject of her master thesis. In addition to her research work, she is very active in her community and received the Quebec provincial government award "Hommage bénévolat Québec - Claude Masson" for her volunteer implication with community seniors.

Jackie Bender is a social and behavioral health scientist. She holds the position of Scientist at the ELLICSR Health, Wellness and Cancer Survivorship Centre, Princess Margaret Cancer Centre at the University Health Network, and Assistant Professor in the Dalla Lana School of Public Health at the University of Toronto. Her research focuses on designing and evaluating ways to improve the health and health care experience of people affected by cancer through the use of social support and information and communication technologies. Dr. Bender has presented and published extensively on the topic of virtual communities and social media for health.

Hance Clarke is the Director of Pain Services and the Medical Director of the Pain Research Unit at the Toronto General Hospital. After his medical doctor (MD) and anesthesia subspecialty training in Toronto he received his PhD from the Institute of Medical Sciences at the University of Toronto and is a member of the Royal College Clinician Scientist Program. His research interests identifying novel acute pain treatments following major surgery, identifying the factors involved in the transition of acute postsurgical pain to chronic pain and identifying risk factors associated with continued opioid use and poor health related quality of life after major surgery. He has further subspecialty training in Hyperbaric Medicine and Interventional Chronic Pain Management. Dr. Clarke was recently awarded the 2016 Early Career Award from the Canadian Pain Society and recognized nationally and internationally for his research productivity and improvements to patient care such as the development of his novel Transitional Pain Program.

Gina DeBenedetti holds a public health designation, tenure in the pharmaceutical industry, leadership of international communications firm and independent consulting practice respectively. She has contributed to and developed virtual education and engagement platforms in many areas of healthcare.

Matthieu J. Guitton, PhD, is Associate Professor and Secretary of the Faculty of Medicine at Laval University (Quebec City, QC, Canada), and Senior Researcher/ Group Leader in the Department of Integrative Neuroscience and Experimental Therapeutics at the ''Institut Universitaire en Santé Mentale de Québec''. A former

Koshland Scholar-Postdoctoral Fellow of Excellence at the Weizmann Institute of Science (Rehovot, Israel), he obtained his PhD from the Faculty of Medicine at the University of Montpellier (France), and is a graduate of the Université Pierre et Marie Curie - Paris VI (France) and the University of Rouen (France). He is a Fellow of the Royal Anthropological Institute of Great Britain, and is member of several Editorial Boards of peer-reviewed journals. He is since January 2017 the Editor-in-Chief of "Computers in Human Behavior". His research interests are on cyberbehavior, ranging from virtual communities to eHealth.

Kim Heyes is a Lecturer and PhD candidate at Manchester Metropolitan University. She has been teaching Abuse Studies at MMU since 2012, and has worked extensively with people with mental health problems. Kim is an advocate for ensuring that mental health is treated as seriously as physical health.

Tahir Janmohamed is passionate about expanding the role of mHealth in chronic disease management. Tahir founded ManagingLife to use technology and analytics to reduce the human and financial cost of pain.

Joel Katz is a Distinguished Research Professor of Psychology and Tier 1 Canada Research Chair in Health Psychology at York University in Toronto. He is the Research Director of the Pain Research Unit, in the Department of Anesthesia and Pain Management at the Toronto General Hospital and a Professor in the Department of Anesthesia at the University of Toronto. He is the inaugural Editor-in-Chief of the Canadian Journal of Pain, the official journal of the Canadian Pain society. Dr. Katz's has published more than 250 articles and book chapters and has been invited to present his work at professional and scientific meetings in North America, Europe, the Middle East, and Asia. Dr. Katz's research program is aimed at understanding the psychological, emotional, and biomedical factors involved in acute and chronic pain. He and his students and colleagues are exploring factors involved in the transition of acute, time-limited pain to chronic, pathological pain after surgery, accidents, and spinal cord injury. They are also evaluating interventions designed to prevent acute post-operative pain and the transition to chronicity.

Kelly Kuru has worked in digital health strategy development, vendor liaison through Infoway's national certification service, and most recently, in strategic communications and stakeholder engagement within the organization's clinical interoperability and standards program. Kelly thrives on communicating organizational vision, priorities and successes with meaning for stakeholders and influencers.

Vered Valeria Latman holds a B.Sc. in Psychology from University of Toronto, and M.A & M.Ed. in Counseling Psychology from Columbia University. During her graduate studies, she completed an extensive internship at the Lehman College Counseling Center in New York, and a practicum at the Dean Hope Center at Columbia University, where she developed a strong interest in health psychology. While working with underserved populations and volunteering with survivors with PTSD, she became aware of the growing need for affordable and accessible treatments for chronic conditions. This led her to continue her education at York University in order to research potential solutions at the graduate level. Currently, her research interests focus on studying the effects of mobile and internet based interventions in individuals with chronic pain and illness. To accomplish these goals, she uses her experience as a co-founder of two technological startups and knowledge of user experience.

Linda Monico is a business analyst on Canada Health Infoway's Clinical Systems Integration team, with over 10 years of experience in data management, reporting, analytics and research. As an administrator of Infoway's InfoCentral platform, she has authored many of the online guides and collaboration resources currently serving as detailed reference tools for communities of interest.

Jessica Moore is Chair of the Department of Human Communication and Organizational Leadership in the College of Communication at Butler University. Dr. Moore's research explores communication processes in interpersonal relationships and how communication impacts health and wellbeing. Dr. Moore teaches courses in interpersonal communication, relational communication, health communication, and research methods, among others, and she is an active member of the International Association of Relationship Researchers and the National Communication Association.

Peter Picton is a biomedical engineer and healthcare system specialist. He has worked in areas ranging from physiological research, digital health research and development, interoperability standards and health technology evaluation.

Vivian Vimarlund has since 1989 conducted research within the area of Informatics with special focus on issues such as: a) Methods and models to evaluate the impact of the implementation and use of IT-based innovations in healthcare. b) Business models for Public Information Systems and Electronic Markets c) E-health governance and innovation. Professor Vimarlund has a wide experience on management and leadership. Academic leadership is practiced as, Director of the Research Center (CENIT/IS), as a Member of the American Medical Informatics

(AMIA) Mentorship Programme, and as the scientific leader of a series of research projects. Vimarlund is also the coordinator of the national eHealth network, scientific secretary at SFMI and the Swedish project leader for the project eHealth Research Network, supported by the Nordic Council of Ministers. Vimarlund has been opponent and member of the evaluation committee of a number of PhD and licentiate theses in Scandinavian. She has also been evaluator of numerous lecturer positions and professorships in Sweden, Canada, Europe, South Arabia, and the Nordic countries. Vimarlund is also reviewer for numerous journals and conferences as well as SPC member in the fields of health and medical informatics. Evaluator for a number of national grants offices (VR, Vinnova, SIDA, Forte) and international research councils (EU, Norway Research Council and MITACS-Canada).

Tasha Shaw-Verbic is part of Canada Health Infoway's Clinical Systems Integration team and serves as the primary contact for InfoCentral operations. Tasha has led the onboarding, training and technical support for all of InfoCentral's communities and working groups. Routinely engaging directly with community members, she shares many operational best practices during group onboarding and training. Additionally, she supporting the efforts of the team to raise awareness of the accomplishments and activities through timely promotion.

Jamie Wang is an experienced clinical research associate specialized in the fields of e-health initiatives and mental health. Graduated in 2014 from York University with an Hon. Bachelor's Degree of Health Science - Specialized in Health Informatics, she is a Summa Cum Laude recipient and was listed on the Dean's Honor Roll. She has been involved in multiple health policy and service based research projects and has participated in various research-related activities such as protocol handling, literature search and review, data management and analysis, manuscript writing, academic conference presentation (poster). She, as the second author, has assisted the publication of a peer-reviewed journal article regarding the association between re-evaluation of nursing home residing seniors' goals of care and the outcomes of care. She holds First Professional Degree in Medicine and had been working in the healthcare setting for a number of years.

Aliza Weinrib (Ph.D., C.Pscyh) is a registered clinical psychologist and pain specialist. She serves as the clinical lead for the pain psychology program at Toronto General Hospital and Toronto Western Hospital.

Index

L

M

N

O

P

R

S

T

U

V

W

www.ingramcontent.com/pod-product-compliance
Lightning Source LLC
LaVergne TN
LVHW081325300926
849161LV00008B/1879